# Dermatopathology

*Editor*

THOMAS BRENN

# SURGICAL PATHOLOGY CLINICS

www.surgpath.theclinics.com

*Consulting Editor*

JASON L. HORNICK

June 2017 • Volume 10 • Number 2

**ELSEVIER**

1600 John F. Kennedy Boulevard • Suite 1800 • Philadelphia, Pennsylvania, 19103-2899

http://www.theclinics.com

**SURGICAL PATHOLOGY CLINICS Volume 10, Number 2**
**June 2017 ISSN 1875-9181, ISBN-13: 978-0-323-53035-4**

Editor: Stacy Eastman
Developmental Editor: Donald Mumford

*Surgical Pathology Clinics* (ISSN 1875-9181) is published quarterly by Elsevier Inc., 360 Park Avenue South, New York, NY 10010. Months of issue are March, June, September, and December. Business and Editorial Office: Elsevier Inc., 1600 John F. Kennedy Blvd., Ste. 1800, Philadelphia, PA 19103-2899. Accounting and Circulation Offices: Elsevier Inc., 3251 Riverport Lane, Maryland Heights, MO 63043. Periodicals postage paid at New York, NY and at additional mailing offices. Subscription prices are $206.00 per year (US individuals), $274.00 per year (US institutions), $100.00 per year (US students/residents), $258.00 per year (Canadian individuals), $312.00 per year (Canadian Institutions), $258.00 per year (foreign individuals), $312.00 per year (foreign institutions), and $120.00 per year (international & Canadian students/residents). Foreign air speed delivery is included in all *Clinics'* subscription prices. All prices are subject to change without notice. **POSTMASTER:** Send address changes to *Surgical Pathology Clinics*, Elsevier, 3251 Riverport Lane, Maryland Heights, MO 63043. **Customer Service: 1-800-654-2452 (US). From outside the United States, call 1-314-447-8871. Fax: 1-314-447-8029. E-mail: JournalsCustomerServiceusa@elsevier.com (for print support)** and **JournalsOnlineSupport-usa@elsevier.com (for online support)**.

*Reprints.* For copies of 100 or more, of articles in this publication, please contact the Commercial Reprints Department, Elsevier Inc., 360 Park Avenue South, New York, NY 10010-1710. Tel. 212-633-3874; Fax: 212-633-3820; E-mail: reprints@elsevier.com.

*Surgical Pathology Clinics of North America* is covered in *MEDLINE/PubMed (Index Medicus)*.

# Contributors

## CONSULTING EDITOR

**JASON L. HORNICK, MD, PhD**
Director of Surgical Pathology, Director,
Immunohistochemistry Laboratory, Brigham
and Women's Hospital, Associate Professor of
Pathology, Harvard Medical School, Boston,
Massachusetts

## EDITOR

**THOMAS BRENN, MD, PhD, FRCPath**
Head, Dermatopathology Service, NHS
Lothian University Hospitals Trust, Honorary
Senior Lecturer, Department of Pathology,
Western General Hospital, University of
Edinburgh, Edinburgh, Scotland

## AUTHORS

**STEVEN D. BILLINGS, MD**
Professor of Pathology, Lerner College of
Medicine, Department of Pathology, Cleveland
Clinic, Cleveland, Ohio

**THOMAS BRENN, MD, PhD, FRCPath**
Head, Dermatopathology Service, NHS
Lothian University Hospitals Trust, Honorary
Senior Lecturer, Department of Pathology,
Western General Hospital, University of
Edinburgh, Edinburgh, Scotland

**EDUARDO CALONJE, MD, DipRCPath**
Dermatopathology Laboratory, St John's
Institute of Dermatology, St Thomas' Hospital,
London, United Kingdom

**LEIGH A. COMPTON, MD, PhD**
Department of Pathology, Brigham and
Women's Hospital, Harvard Medical School,
Boston, Massachusetts

**GILLES F. DIERCKS, MD, PhD**
Department of Dermatology, Center for
Blistering Diseases, University Medical Center
Groningen, University of Groningen,
Groningen, The Netherlands

**LEONA A. DOYLE, MD**
Department of Pathology, Brigham and
Women's Hospital, Harvard Medical School,
Boston, Massachusetts

**GIOVANNI FALCONIERI, MD**
Department of Pathology, University of Trieste
School of Medicine, Trieste, Italy

**KATHARINA FLUX, MD**
Labor für Dermatohistologie und
Oralpathologie, Munich; Department of
Dermatology, University of Heidelberg,
Heidelberg, Germany

**ADRIANA GARCÍA-HERRERA, MD, PhD**
Department of Pathology, Hospital Clínic de
Barcelona, Barcelona, Spain

**JOHN R. GOODLAD, MBChB, MD**
Haematological Malignancy Diagnostic
Services (HMDS), St James's University
Hospital, Leeds, United Kingdom

**SCOTT R. GRANTER, MD**
Associate Professor, Department of Pathology, Brigham and Women's Hospital, Harvard Medical School, Boston, Massachusetts

**MARCEL F. JONKMAN, MD, PhD**
Department of Dermatology, Center for Blistering Diseases, University Medical Center Groningen, University of Groningen, Groningen, The Netherlands

**WERNER KEMPF, MD**
Kempf & Pfaltz, Histologische Diagnostik; Department of Dermatology, University Hospital Zurich, Zurich, Switzerland

**ALVARO C. LAGA, MD, MMSc**
Assistant Professor, Department of Pathology, Brigham and Women's Hospital, Harvard Medical School, Boston, Massachusetts

**ALLISON LARSON, MD**
Assistant Dean of Academic Affairs, Assistant Professor of Dermatology, Boston University School of Medicine, Boston, Massachusetts

**BOŠTJAN LUZAR, MD, PhD**
Professor, Institute of Pathology, Medical Faculty, University of Ljubljana, Ljubljana, Slovenia

**ZLATKO MARUŠIĆ, MD, PhD**
Department of Pathology, University Hospital Center Zagreb, Zagreb, Croatia

**F.D. MENEZES, MD**
Senior Resident, Department of Pathology, Instituto Portugues de Oncologia do Porto FG, Porto, Portugal

**THOMAS MENTZEL, MD**
Dermatopathology, Bodensee, Friedrichshafen, Germany

**CHRISTINA MITTELDORF, MD**
Department of Dermatology, HELIOS Klinikum Hildesheim, Hildesheim, Germany

**W.J. MOOI, MD, PhD**
Professor, Department of Pathology, VU University Medical Center, Amsterdam, The Netherlands

**HENDRI H. PAS, PhD**
Department of Dermatology, Center for Blistering Diseases, University Medical Center Groningen, University of Groningen, Groningen, The Netherlands

**MELISSA PULITZER, MD**
Associate Attending Pathologist, Department of Pathology, Memorial Sloan Kettering Cancer Center, New York, New York

**LUIS REQUENA, MD**
Department of Dermatology, Fundacion Jimenez Diaz, Madrid, Spain

**MICHIEL P.J. VAN DER HORST, MD**
Department of Pathology, Groene Hart Ziekenhuis, Gouda, The Netherlands

# Contents

Spitz tumors are melanocytic neoplasms hallmarked by large cell size, lack of high-grade atypia, and a regular architecture. Most are nonpigmented or poorly pigmented. Malignant potential ranges from absent (Spitz nevus), to fully present (spitzoid melanoma), with a further, ill-defined group of Spitz tumors with limited metastatic potential. Microscopic evaluation may prove inconclusive in some instances, resulting in a verdict of Spitz tumor of uncertain malignant potential (STUMP). STUMP is, therefore, not an entity, and should not be equated with Spitz tumors with limited metastatic potential. Novel diagnostic techniques are yielding promising results, and further evaluation is ongoing.

Cutaneous mesenchymal neoplasms often pose significant diagnostic challenges; many such entities are rare or show clinical and histologic overlap with both other mesenchymal and nonmesenchymal lesions. Recent advances in the genetic classification of many cutaneous mesenchymal neoplasms have not only helped define unique pathologic entities and increase our understanding of their biology, but have also provided new diagnostic markers. This review details these recent discoveries, with a focus on their implications for tumor classification and diagnosis.

Atypical fibroxanthoma (AFX) represents a rare mesenchymal neoplasm arising predominantly in the head and neck area of elderly patients. Clinically, the neoplasm is characterized by a rapid and exophytic growth with frequent ulceration of the epidermis. Histopathologically, AFX represents a well-circumscribed, dermal-based neoplasm composed of a variable admixture of large histiocytoid cells, enlarged spindled and epithelioid tumor cells, and multinucleated tumor giant cells with bizarre and pleomorphic nuclei. If strict diagnostic criteria are applied, the clinical behavior of AFX is benign in most cases, and complete excision represents the treatment of choice.

Cutaneous malignant peripheral nerve sheath tumors (MPNSTs) are rare sarcomas of neuroectodermal origin arising in the dermis and/or subcutis. In contrast with their deep soft tissue and visceral counterparts, cutaneous MPNST are rarely associated with neurofibromatosis type 1. Two main subtypes of cutaneous MPNST can be distinguished histologically: conventional (ie, spindle cell) and epithelioid MPNST. The 2 subtypes also differ in predilection for deep versus superficial locations, association with preexistent benign peripheral nerve sheath tumors and S100 immunohistochemistry. Herein, we review current knowledge of cutaneous MPNST and discuss its differential diagnosis.

Vascular tumors with a spindled morphology represent a diagnostic challenge in soft tissue pathology. It may be difficult to distinguish certain benign entities in this category from spindled vascular tumors of intermediate malignancy or even spindled variants of angiosarcoma. This article focuses on vascular tumors characterized by a predominantly spindled morphology, including spindle cell hemangioma, acquired tufted angioma (angioblastoma of Nakagawa), kaposiform hemangioendothelioma, Kaposi sarcoma, and spindle cell variants of angiosarcoma.

Sebaceous skin tumors are classified into sebaceous adenoma, sebaceoma, and sebaceous carcinoma. An additional group of cystic sebaceous tumors indicate the Muir-Torre syndrome (MTS). Cystic sebaceous tumors are considered as morphologic variants of the 3 main categories. Multilineage adnexal tumors with partly sebaceous differentiation may pose a challenge to categorize. Sebaceous hyperplasia and nevus sebaceus are not considered as true sebaceous tumor entities. Recently, attention has been drawn to morphologic clues of sebaceous differentiation. Immunohistochemistry using the mismatch repair proteins and/or genetic microsatellite instability testing should be performed on sebaceous neoplasms to diagnose MTS as early as possible.

Malignant sweat gland tumors are rare cutaneous neoplasms, traditionally separated according to their behavior into low- and high-grade malignant. There is significant morphologic overlap, and outright malignant tumors may show relatively bland histologic features. They may, therefore, be mistaken easily for benign neoplasms. Recognition of these tumors and accurate diagnosis is important for early treatment to prevent aggressive behavior and adverse outcome. This article provides an overview of 4 important entities with emphasis on diagnostic pitfalls, differential diagnosis and recent developments. Microcystic adnexal carcinoma, squamoid eccrine ductal carcinoma, aggressive digital papillary adenocarcinoma, and spiradenocarcinoma are discussed in detail.

Merkel cell carcinoma (MCC) encompasses neuroendocrine carcinomas primary to skin and occurs most commonly in association with clonally integrated Merkel cell polyomavirus with related retinoblastoma protein sequestration or in association with UV radiation–induced alterations involving the TP53 gene and mutations, heterozygous deletion, and hypermethylation of the *Retinoblastoma* gene. Molecular genetic signatures may provide therapeutic guidance. Morphologic features, although patterned, are associated with predictable diagnostic pitfalls, usually resolvable by immunohistochemistry. Therapeutic options for MCC, traditionally limited to surgical intervention and later chemotherapy and radiation, are growing, given promising early results of immunotherapeutic regimens.

## Cutaneous Lymphomas with Cytotoxic Phenotype

Adriana García-Herrera and Eduardo Calonje

Primary cutaneous cytotoxic lymphomas are T-cell or natural killer–cell lymphomas that express 1 or more cytotoxic markers. These neoplasms constitute a spectrum of diseases. In this review, an overview of clinical, morphologic, and phenotypical features of each subtype is provided. Differential diagnosis is discussed with attention to scenarios in which diagnostic difficulties are most frequently encountered.

## Epstein-Barr Virus–associated Lymphoproliferative Disorders in the Skin

John R. Goodlad

Epstein-Barr virus (EBV)–associated lymphoproliferations involving the skin are a rare but important group of diseases with a broad spectrum of behavior, ranging from self-limiting spontaneously resolving disorders to highly aggressive malignancies. They may be of B, T, or natural killer (NK) cell type and include EBV-positive mucocutaneous ulcer, lymphomatoid granulomatosis, EBV-positive diffuse large B-cell lymphoma, hydroa vacciniforme–like lymphoproliferative disorder, and extranodal NK/T-cell lymphoma of nasal type. Recognition and distinction of these entities is important in view of their differing prognoses and treatments. An association with EBV may be the first indication that a patient is immunosuppressed.

## Cutaneous Pseudolymphoma

Christina Mitteldorf and Werner Kempf

The term, *cutaneous pseudolymphoma (PSL)*, refers to a group of lymphocyte-rich infiltrates, which either clinically and/or histologically simulate cutaneous lymphomas. Clinicopathologic correlation is essential to achieve the final diagnosis in cutaneous PSL and to differentiate it from cutaneous lymphomas. A wide range of causative agents (eg, *Borrelia*, injections, tattoo, and arthropod bite) has been described. Based on clinical and/or histologic presentation, 4 main groups of cutaneous PSL can be distinguished: (1) nodular PSL, (2) pseudo–mycosis fungoides, (3) other PSLs (representing distinct clinical entities), and (4) intravascular PSL. The article gives an overview of the clinical and histologic characteristics of cutaneous PSLs.

## Histopathologic Spectrum of Connective Tissue Diseases Commonly Affecting the Skin

Alvaro C. Laga, Allison Larson, and Scott R. Granter

Connective tissue disorders (CTDs), also known as collagen vascular diseases, are a heterogeneous group of diseases with a common pathogenic mechanism: autoimmunity. Precise classification of CTDs requires clinical, serologic, and pathologic correlation and may be difficult because of overlapping clinical and histologic features. The main contribution of histopathology in the diagnosis of these disorders is to confirm, rule out, or alert clinicians to the possibility of CTD as a disease category, rather than producing definitive diagnoses of specific entities. This article discusses the histopathologic spectrum of 3 common rheumatologic skin disorders: lupus erythematosus, dermatomyositis, and morphea (localized scleroderma).

Gilles F. Diercks, Hendri H. Pas, and Marcel F. Jonkman

Autoimmmune bullous diseases of skin and mucosa are uncommon, disabling, and potentially lethal diseases. For a quick and reliable diagnosis immunofluorescence is essential. This article describes two variants of immunofluorescence. The direct method uses a skin or mucosal biopsy of the patient to detect in vivo bound antibodies. Indirect immunofluorescence uses a patient's serum and a substrate to visualize circulating autoantibodies. These two methods supplemented with advanced techniques allow reliable classification of autoimmune bullous diseases; not only the main entities pemphigus and pemphigoid, but also subclasses within these groups. This is important because prognosis and therapy vary among different variants of autoimmune bullous diseases.

# SURGICAL PATHOLOGY CLINICS

---

### RELATED INTEREST

*Dermatologic Clinics,* October 2015 (Volume 33, Issue 4)
**Cutaneous Lymphoma**
Elise A. Olsen, *Editor*

---

**THE CLINICS ARE AVAILABLE ONLINE!**
Access your subscription at:
www.theclinics.com

# SURGICAL PATHOLOGY CLINICS

## FORTHCOMING ISSUES

**September 2017**
**Bone Tumor Pathology**
Judith V.M.G. Bovée, Editor

**December 2017**
**Gastrointestinal Pathology: Common**
**Questions and Diagnostic Dilemmas**
Rhonda K. Yantiss, Editor

**March 2018**
**Breast Pathology**
Laura C. Collins, Editor

## RECENT ISSUES

**March 2017**
**Head and Neck Pathology**
Raja R. Seethala, Editor

**December 2016**
**Pancreatic Pathology**
Laura Wood and Lodewijk Brosens, Editors

**September 2016**
**Molecular Pathology: Predictive, Prognostic,**
**and Diagnostic Markers in Tumors**
Lynette M. Sholl, Editor

### ISSUE OF RELATED INTEREST

*Dermatologic Clinics* (October 2015, Volume 33, Issue 4)
**Cutaneous Lymphoma**
Elise A. Olsen, Editor

# Preface
# Diagnostic Challenges in Dermatopathology

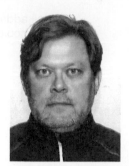

Thomas Brenn, MD, PhD, FRCPath
*Editor*

One of the main challenges in the practice of dermatopathology is being confronted with a broad spectrum of diseases, both inflammatory and neoplastic, many of which are unique to the skin or show specific features when affecting the skin. Since the last dedicated review issue to dermatopathology in the *Surgical Pathology Clinics* in 2009, our understanding of the molecular genetics of cutaneous disorders has evolved significantly, and many novel forms of treatment have been developed and introduced into clinical practice. Pathologists are frequently faced with the challenge of rendering more definitive diagnoses on even smaller tissue samples. The judicious use and adequate interpretation of immunohistochemistry and molecular testing have become an invaluable adjunct in the routine diagnostic setting.

The current review issue provides an update on selected and difficult topics across the clinical spectrum of dermatopathology, in the hope of providing the reader with an understanding of recent advances in the field and the diagnostic tools to tackle these challenges. The diagnosis of melanocytic tumors continues to represent one of the most challenging areas in surgical pathology, and Spitzoid tumors in particular remain a problematic and contentious topic. Significant progress has been made over the past years in our understanding of the underlying genetics and the behavior of these distinctive melanocytic tumors, which is discussed here in detail. Molecular advances have also had a particular impact on mesenchymal tumor pathology. The current body of knowledge as it relates to cutaneous mesenchymal tumors is reviewed with an emphasis on the development of novel markers. This is complemented by additional overviews on atypical fibroxanthoma, cutaneous malignant nerve sheath tumor, and vascular tumors with spindle cell morphology. Updates on skin adnexal tumor pathology include a review of the morphological spectrum of sebaceous neoplasms, a discussion of diagnostically challenging malignant sweat gland tumors, and Merkel cell carcinoma. The topic of cutaneous lymphoproliferative disorders is focused on the spectrum of tumors with a cytotoxic phenotype and Epstein-Barr virus–associated disorders. This is contrasted with an overview of reactive and inflammatory conditions mimicking lymphoproliferative disease, the so-called pseudolymphomas. Two articles dealing with inflammatory skin disorders conclude this review: an overview

Surgical Pathology 10 (2017) xi–xii
http://dx.doi.org/10.1016/j.path.2017.03.001
1875-9181/17/© 2017 Published by Elsevier Inc.

of the histologic spectrum of connective tissue disease in the skin and an outline of the significance of immunofluorescence in autoimmunone bullous disorders.

I wish to express my sincere thanks to all the contributing authors for sharing their vast knowledge and for making this a fantastic educational resource. Editing this text has been an absolute pleasure and an important educational experience.

Thomas Brenn, MD, PhD, FRCPath
Department of Pathology
Western General Hospital
Alexander Donald Building, 1st Floor
Crewe Road
Edinburgh EH4 2XU, Scotland

E-mail address:
t_brenn@yahoo.com

# Spitz Tumors of the Skin

F.D. Menezes, MD[a], W.J. Mooi, MD, PhD[b],*

## KEYWORDS

- Spitz nevus • Spitzoid melanoma • STUMP • Childhood melanoma • Melanoma diagnosis

## Key points

- Spitz tumors are a group of cutaneous (and, more rarely, mucosal) melanocytic neoplasms, hallmarked by large cell size, lack of high-grade atypia, and a regular architecture.

- Malignant potential ranges from absent (Spitz nevus), to fully present (spitzoid melanoma). A further, as yet incompletely defined, group of Spitz tumors shows potential for regional spread but not for distant metastasis.

- Diagnosis hinges on microscopic evaluation, which commonly (but not always) yields an unequivocal diagnosis of case of Spitz nevus or spitzoid melanoma, but cannot reliably identify the cases with potential for regional spread only.

- When microscopic evaluation fails to yield diagnostic certainty, a verdict of Spitz tumor of uncertain malignant potential (STUMP) is appropriate. Such uncertainty may have many causes, including avoidable ones, such as suboptimal biopsy quality. STUMP is, therefore, not an entity, and should not be equated with Spitz tumors with potential for regional spread but not for distant metastasis.

- Novel diagnostic techniques are yielding promising results, and further evaluation is ongoing. They require substantial technical and interpretative expertise and are not yet generally available.

## ABSTRACT

Spitz tumors are melanocytic neoplasms hallmarked by large cell size, lack of high-grade atypia, and a regular architecture. Most are nonpigmented or poorly pigmented. Malignant potential ranges from absent (Spitz nevus), to fully present (spitzoid melanoma), with a further, ill-defined group of Spitz tumors with limited metastatic potential. Microscopic evaluation may prove inconclusive in some instances, resulting in a verdict of Spitz tumor of uncertain malignant potential (STUMP). STUMP is, therefore, not an entity, and should not be equated with Spitz tumors with limited metastatic potential. Novel diagnostic techniques are yielding promising results, and further evaluation is ongoing.

## OVERVIEW

Spitz nevus is a benign tumor of melanocytes, distinguished histologically by the large size of the neoplastic melanocytes, as well as several architectural features that to some degree resemble those of melanoma. As a result of these similarities, the histologic differential diagnosis between Spitz nevus and melanoma is a common source of diagnostic uncertainty and error. These diagnostic problems are compounded by the occurrence of a small group of melanomas (referred to colloquially as spitzoid melanomas) that display a striking resemblance to Spitz nevus. In addition, there is a group of Spitz tumors that commonly spread to a regional lymph node, but very rarely metastasize to distant sites; this apparent propensity for regional spread but lack

Disclosure: The authors have nothing to disclose.

[a] Department of Pathology, Instituto Portugues de Oncologia do Porto FG, Rua Dr Antonio Bernardino de Almeida, Porto 4200-072, Portugal; [b] Department of Pathology, VU University Medical Center, PO Box 7057, Amsterdam 1007 MB, The Netherlands

* Corresponding author.

*E-mail address:* wj.mooi@vumc.nl

Surgical Pathology 10 (2017) 281–298

http://dx.doi.org/10.1016/j.path.2017.01.004

of hematogenous metastatic potential challenges the traditional dichotomy of melanocytic tumors into fully benign and fully malignant groups, and constitutes another level of complexity in the differential diagnosis within the group of Spitz tumors.

The practical and conceptual difficulties associated with the differential diagnosis within this group of lesions have resulted in an extensive literature, with controversies resulting from discrepant data as well as from divergence of interpretation of data. Novel diagnostic modalities, focusing on abnormalities within the lesions' genomes, are now raising the prospect of improved prediction of biological behavior. These modalities are highly interesting, but the necessary techniques are not yet generally available, are sometimes costly, and involve technical and interpretative pitfalls. Thus, pathologists dealing with a difficult Spitz tumor face a variety of unsolved problems, and are challenged by ongoing scientific and technical developments.

This article provides guidance to pathologists working in a standard, routine diagnostic setting, and therefore focuses primarily on histology and immunohistochemistry, as well as on clinical-pathologic correlation. It outlines the distinguishing features of the various groups of Spitz tumors, with emphasis on the various histologic pitfalls, the differential diagnosis, as well as any uncertainties associated with histologic diagnosis, and how to deal with them.

## SPITZ NEVUS: CLINICAL FEATURES

Spitz nevus, being a nevus, is benign by definition. If there is doubt about the biological potential, a lesion should not be labeled Spitz nevus.

Spitz nevus occurs mainly in white people. As is the case with most benign skin lesions, reliable incidence figures are impossible to obtain, because many do not come to clinical attention. Most are diagnosed in children and adolescents, but a few are encountered beyond middle age. Age is a factor to take into account diagnostically: a Spitz tumor in an infant or young child is usually a Spitz nevus; in a teenager, this is no longer the case, because spitzoid melanomas are not rare in this age group. In middle-aged and elderly patients, spitzoid lesions should be scrutinized with an increased level of concern, because with advancing age the a priori chance of melanoma steadily increases, whereas that of Spitz nevus declines.

In infants and children, most Spitz nevi present on the face and ear, whereas later in life the extremities (especially the thighs and upper legs)

and, to a lesser extent, the trunk, are favored sites.[1,2] No site precludes the diagnosis of Spitz nevus, and an occasional example presents in a juxtacutaneous mucous membrane (upper digestive tract, genitalia). Some occur as part of a congenital nevus, or a speckled lentiginous nevus.[3] Spitz nevi may occur multiply, either agminated[4] or disseminated, sometimes after excision of a solitary lesion, and rare cases of eruptive Spitz nevi are on record.[5]

As a group, Spitz nevi are more commonly non-pigmented or poorly pigmented than other nevi. Most are at least lightly pigmented on diascopy, and pigment is evenly distributed and homogeneously colored. Associated vasodilatation and vascular proliferation result in erythema, especially in infants and children. Shapes vary from polypoid to dome shaped to almost flat, and most are less than 1 cm across, with a regular, symmetric shape. Consistency varies from soft (especially at an early age) to firm (common in adults). There may be an initial rapid growth phase, but after the nevus reaches stability there is little, if any, further change. The affected skin is usually intact, but trauma may result in erosion or ulceration, especially in soft and polypoid examples.

Spitz nevi are commonly mistaken clinically for other benign skin lesions, such as hemangioma, dermatofibroma, or melanocytic nevus of another type.[1,2,6,7] Most are regarded as unsuspicious, except some darkly pigmented examples, usually of the pigmented spindle cell nevus subtype,[8] which clinically resemble a small and heavily pigmented nodular melanoma. Agminated[4] or disseminated Spitz nevi may raise concern of melanoma with multiple cutaneous metastases.

Dermatoscopically, starburst, globular, and mixed patterns are most common. Most are interpreted as benign or probably benign, but sometimes an irregular distribution of different patterns, or the presence of a blue-white veil, raises suspicion.[9]

## SPITZ NEVUS: HISTOLOGIC FEATURES

Spitz nevi are junctional, compound, or intradermal proliferations of large melanocytes with increased cytoplasm and enlarged, regular nuclei (Figs. 1 and 2). Shapes vary from epithelioid (rounded or polygonal) to oval and spindle shaped. Epithelioid cells tend to predominate in infancy and early childhood (Fig. 3), whereas spindle cells are most common in adolescence and adulthood (Fig. 4). However, there are many exceptions, and most Spitz nevi contain a mixture of spindle-shaped and epithelioid cells. Cells are largest in the central and superficial part; they gradually

Fig. 1. Spitz nevus, removed from the leg of a 21-year-old woman. Note the regular overall architecture, with numerous junctional nests with a preferentially vertical orientation associated with epidermal hyperplasia and hyperkeratosis. There is a minor dermal component that does not form compact nodules or a pushing border with the underlying preexistent dermis (H&E, original magnification, ×5).

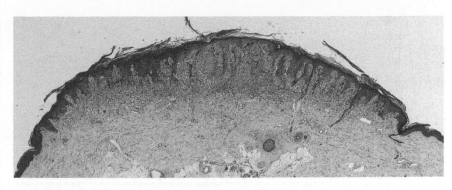

diminish in size toward the dermal deep border and, to a lesser extent, toward the dermal lateral periphery. Any pigment present is generally granular, and pigmentation (and associated HMB-45-postivity) tends to be restricted to the superficial part of the nevus. There is generally some shrinkage of the cytoplasm, which is especially conspicuous in junctional nests (see **Fig.** 1). This shrinkage is diagnostically relevant: when cytoplasm-rich junctional cells do not show any shrinkage, and especially when they contain dust-like rather than granular melanin, the lesion is more likely to be a melanoma.

Nuclei tend to have a regular, rounded, or oval shape, with peripheral margination of chromatin and a central rounded nucleolus. Scattered hyperchromatic nuclei are often present and carry little or no diagnostic significance. Nuclear enlargement, anisochromasia, and polymorphism can be marked in lesions presenting in infancy, especially when the epithelioid cell type predominates.

At the junction and in the upper dermis, the nevi usually aggregate into nests. Nests are often oval and vertically oriented, but horizontal orientation is seen as well, as is confluence of adjacent nests resulting in irregular cell masses. However, large,

Fig. 2. Spitz nevus, same case as **Fig.** 1. At higher power, the predominantly oval to fusiform nevus cells cluster in nests and show some shrinkage of the cytoplasm, resulting in formation of small cleftlike spaces (H&E, original magnification, ×5).

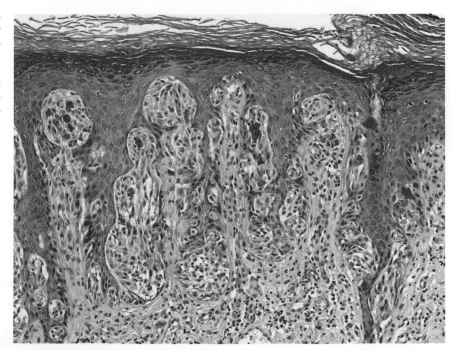

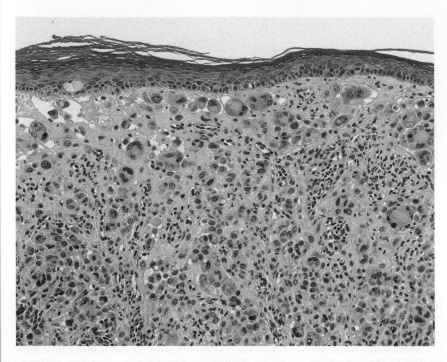

*Fig. 3.* The cells of this Spitz nevus, removed from the lower arm of a 3-year-old girl, show an almost exclusively epithelioid cell type (H&E, original magnification, ×10).

rounded, cannonball-like nests are not a feature of Spitz nevus. Junctional or compound Spitz nevi generally show epidermal hyperplasia, with some hypergranulosis and hyperkeratosis, as well as some degree of keratinocyte hypertrophy. Epidermal flattening and thinning (epidermal consumption), especially when associated with a subepidermal confluent mass of spitzoid melanocytes pushing against it, usually indicates melanoma. Transepidermal elimination of junctional nests is common in Spitz nevi, and may be striking. In addition, some ascent of solitary nevus cells is often detectable. Ascending cells and their nuclei tend to become progressively smaller toward the

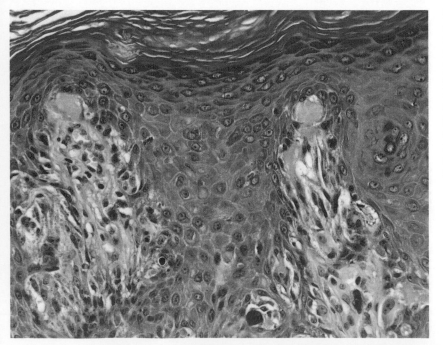

*Fig. 4.* Spitz nevus, same case as **Fig. 1**. Note the oval to spindled cell type. At the tips of 2 papillae, small amorphic eosinophilic Kamino bodies are seen. These aggregates of basement membrane matrix are common in Spitz nevi and much rarer in melanomas (H&E, original magnification, ×10).

upper epidermal cell layers, and they are most common where the junctional component is most cellular, which is usually the center of the lesion. At the junction, Kamino bodies,[10] which are small eosinophilic aggregates of matrix containing basement membrane proteins, may be detected (see **Fig. 4**). They have some diagnostic relevance, because they are more common in Spitz nevus than in melanoma.

The dermal periphery of Spitz nevi is characteristically less densely cellular, with solitary cells and small cell groups insinuating themselves between the preexistent connective tissue. A compact, pushing architecture at the deep border is characteristically absent. Its presence, especially when associated with deep mitotic activity, is an important indicator of malignancy, because mitotic figures are generally absent from the deep invasion front of a Spitz nevus. Immune stains are of help: Ki-67/MIB1 immunostaining is largely restricted to upper parts of the lesion. This finding contrasts with melanoma, in which it is generally higher and expressed at all levels, including the deep border.[11,12]

At low power, Spitz nevus shows a regular and symmetric architecture, which is most apparent in S-100 and melan-A immune stains. This regularity and symmetry holds for the cellular features, the architecture, distribution of pigment, as well as reactive epidermal and dermal changes. The presence of abrupt transitions in histologic features from area to area is a suspicious finding, far more so than variation between individual cells throughout the lesion. However, some spitzoid melanomas show a deceptively regular architecture as well.

Note that reliable diagnosis of Spitz nevus requires an excisional biopsy. A punch biopsy does not contain the lateral periphery of the lesion, and a shave biopsy often lacks the deepest part. In both situations, potentially essential diagnostic information is unavailable. A completion excisional biopsy is required when incisional biopsy evaluation has not yielded a conclusive diagnosis. Histologic evaluation of such a subsequent excisional biopsy specimen is complicated by the tissue damage and reactive changes induced by it so an unequivocal diagnosis may again be impossible. Therefore, clinicians who consider the possibility of a Spitz nevus are well advised to opt for an excisional biopsy as the initial procedure.

## SPITZ NEVUS VARIANTS

Through the years, many Spitz nevus variants have been recognized. The common denominator of all of these variants is the key feature of Spitz nevus:

increased nevus cell size, with at least some of the architectural features of Spitz nevus outlined earlier.

Desmoplastic Spitz nevus[13] is a lesion of late adolescence and of adulthood, and presents as an ill-defined, firm, skin-colored, or light-brown papule, most commonly on the extremities, especially the upper leg. On histology, it is an intradermal or almost exclusively intradermal proliferation of spitzoid melanocytes, usually spindle shaped, and associated with increased amounts of collagen. In the superficial central upper part, nesting is usually evident, whereas the periphery shows the cells in a more dispersed arrangement. Cells in the periphery, especially those at the deep border, are smaller than the nested central-superficial cells (**Fig. 5**). No deep mitotic activity is seen, but some mitotic figures may be encountered more superficially. Deep nodules are absent.

Pigmented spindle cell nevus (Reed nevus)[8] is hallmarked by a compact and densely cellular architecture (**Fig. 6**), and a spindle-shaped cell type that is usually smaller and more slender than the spindle cells of most Spitz nevi (**Fig. 7**). Most Reed nevi produce substantial amounts of melanin, transferred to epidermal keratinocytes and accumulating in dermal melanophages. The junctional component usually consists of confluent nests, associated with epidermal hyperplasia, and there is often melanocyte ascent, which may be marked in some patients. A dermal component is often present and is restricted to the superficial dermis, with a more densely cellular, less infiltrative deep border than that of most other Spitz nevi. Mitotic activity is usually present. There is no basal bandlike inflammatory infiltrate. As a whole, the lesion, although densely cellular, has a regular architecture. Large rounded melanocytes, expansile deep nodules, or substantial variations in cell type or lesional architecture are absent.

Combined Spitz nevus shows a component of Spitz nevus and a component of another nevus subtype, such as common acquired nevus or, rarely, blue nevus. Each component shows the classic features of its type; the difference between the two components may inappropriately suggest intralesional malignant transformation.

Recurrent Spitz nevus[14] is a diagnostic problem, clinically as well as histologically. Because the diagnosis of Spitz nevus is already difficult, recurrent lesions are viewed with suspicion, especially if such a recurrence is multifocal (agminate recurrent Spitz nevus), a rare phenomenon most common in patients in the first years of life. In essence, the histologic criteria are the same as in the undisturbed lesion, but with superimposed posttraumatic scarring and some irregularity of architecture within

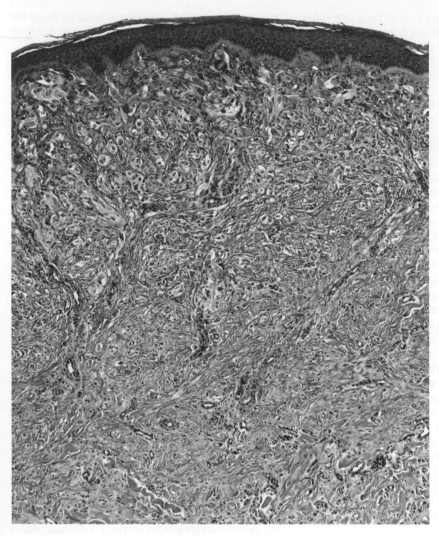

*Fig.    5.* Desmoplastic Spitz nevus, removed from the upper leg of a 42-year-old    woman. Note the gradual transition from a large cell type to a small cell type from top to bottom, and the presence of small compact strands and nests in superficial parts, but a more dissociative architecture in the deep part. The formation of new collagen is evident from the small diameter and the orientation of collagen fibers between the melanocytes. Like most desmoplastic nevi, there is no junctional component in this example (H&E, original magnification, ×5).

and adjacent to the scar tissue. Reevaluation of the initial excisional specimen, and comparison of its histology with the recurrent lesion, is very helpful.

Halo Spitz nevus[15] is a Spitz nevus diffusely infiltrated by a dense lymphocytic inflammatory infiltrate. The inflammatory response is often noted clinically as recent change (growth, erythema, itch) of a previously stable nevus. Usually, no halo of depigmentation is evident clinically, because most examples are nonpigmented or poorly pigmented, and the lesions are generally removed before any such halo becomes apparent clinically.

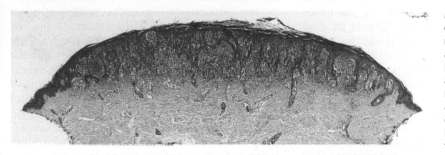

*Fig. 6.* Pigmented spindle cell nevus (Reed nevus) removed from the upper arm of a 31-year-old man. Note the dense cellularity and compactness of this nevus. Junctional nests are preferentially vertically oriented and often become confluent to form larger and irregular masses (H&E, original magnification, ×5).

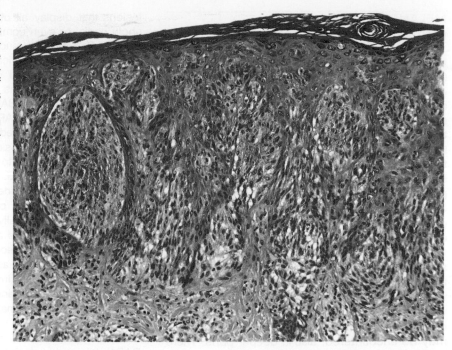

*Fig. 7.* At higher power it is apparent that the cells of this pigmented spindle cell nevus are more slender, and more pigmented, than those of many other Spitz nevus variants. Note the presence of some ascending melanocytes (H&E, original magnification, ×5).

Pagetoid Spitz nevus[16,17] shows unusually prominent intraepidermal pagetoid spread of nevus cells. Most are entirely or predominantly epidermal. In the authors' opinion, the differential diagnosis with melanoma in situ can be problematic, so it is usually wise to insist on histologically verified free margins.

Tubular Spitz nevus[18] is a rare Spitz nevus variant with formation of intradermal small, rounded, epithelioid nevus cells nests, arranged around an optically empty center. There is commonly a dense stromal inflammatory infiltrate. The epithelioid cell type and the infiltrate may raise the possibility of melanocytic BRCA-associated protein 1 (BAP1)–associated intradermal tumor (MBAIT; discussed later); however, the one case the authors have stained for BAP1 showed nuclear BAP1 positivity.

The cells of balloon cell Spitz nevus[19] have copious and finely vacuolated cytoplasm. This ballooning also occurs in some common acquired nevi and blue nevi, especially cellular blue nevi. As a focal change in small numbers of cells, it is common, but a nevus with large numbers of such balloon cells is a rarity. Because ballooning makes the affected cells stand out, it may inappropriately be regarded as an indication of intralesional malignant transformation, and ascending nevus cells showing this feature may stand out in the upper epidermis, and may thus be inappropriately be regarded as ascending melanoma cells.

Myxoid or hyalinizing changes in intralesional matrix deposition can result in myxoid Spitz nevus[20] or hyalinizing Spitz nevus,[21] respectively.

Spitzoid proliferations showing a prominent fascicular dermal growth have been designated plexiform Spitz nevus.[22] The compact dermal architecture of these lesions deviates from that of Spitz nevus, including its many variants, and this may force pathologists to refrain from an unequivocal diagnosis of Spitz nevus and place these lesions in the STUMP category (discussed later).

Angiomatoid Spitz nevus[23] is a Spitz nevus with markedly increased numbers of blood vessels, associated with endothelial hyperplasia and prominence. Because these vascular reactive changes are common in Spitz nevus in general, the authors regard these findings as insufficient reason to label such lesions as a separate Spitz nevus subtype. Similarly, polypoid Spitz nevus[24] and verrucous Spitz nevus, which have a conspicuous polypoid or papillated, exophytic architecture, can be regarded as examples of the exophytic architecture of many Spitz nevi, especially in childhood. We do not regard these as sufficiently distinctive Spitz nevus variants.

In addition, MBAIT[25] has been put forward as yet another Spitz nevus subtype. Because of its divergent features and the broader potential implications on the diagnosis, it is discussed separately in the next section.

## MELANOCYTIC BRCA-ASSOCIATED INTRADERMAL TUMOR

Melanocytic brca-associated intradermal tumor (MBAIT) is regarded by many clinicians as an epithelioid Spitz nevus subtype. This lesion deviates in several respects from other Spitz nevus subtypes; the authors think that its inclusion into the group of Spitz nevi has been rightly challenged.[26] Nonetheless, a brief discussion is justified here. MBAIT generally presents as a small, shining, smooth-surfaced, reddish or brownish papule, and consists of an entirely or largely intradermal population of large, round or polygonal, generally nonpigmented melanocytes (**Figs. 8 and 9**). These melanocytes are dispersed, with or without formation of admixed compact nests, and are often (but not always) associated with a lymphocytic infiltrate. Maturation is often absent, which is in stark contrast with other Spitz nevus variants, in which it is a diagnostically important indicator of benignity. One or a few mitotic figures may be encountered, also in deeper parts. There is often a banal intradermal or compound nevus component at the periphery.

MBAIT often harbors a *BRAF* mutation, which again sets these lesions apart from other Spitz nevus types. *HRAS* mutations are lacking. There is often loss of nuclear BAP1 immunoreactivity, which contrasts with the normal positivity that is found in preexistent cells such as epidermal cells, as well as in the nevus-NOS component, if present (**Fig. 10**). BAP1 is a deubiquitinating enzyme that acts in diverse cellular processes, including cell cycle control and DNA damage responses. In the authors' experience some lesions that display all other features of MBAIT show partial or even complete BAP1 immunopositivity. Possibly, in such lesions there is a defect functionally identical to loss of BAP1 protein but not associated with loss of the BAP1 epitope. BAP1 mutations are occasionally unassociated with loss of BAP1 immunoreactivity.[27] In contrast, loss of BAP1 immunoreactivity is occasionally encountered in melanocytic neoplasms lacking the classic morphologic features of MBAIT.[26] It remains to be seen how such lesions are best classified.

Some MBAITs are index lesions of a familial cancer risk syndrome caused by a germline BAP1 mutation, especially when there are multiple lesions or if there is a history of (cutaneous or uveal) melanoma. Recent evidence indicates that other malignancies associate with the BAP1 loss familial cancer syndrome: these include malignant mesothelioma, renal cancer, and possibly some other visceral malignancies.[28] A recent study suggests that MBAIT positive for BRAFV600E immunostaining but negative for BAP1 staining is especially linked to the cancer syndrome.[26]

Available evidence indicates that MBAIT is usually benign, but the authors think that additional experience needs to accumulate before there is sufficient evidence to conclude that there are no pitfalls. This hesitation to accept all of these lesions as benign is fueled by the fact that germline BAP1 mutations are associated with increased risk of cutaneous melanoma, and that there is as yet no detailed information on the histopathologic features of such BAP1-associated melanomas.

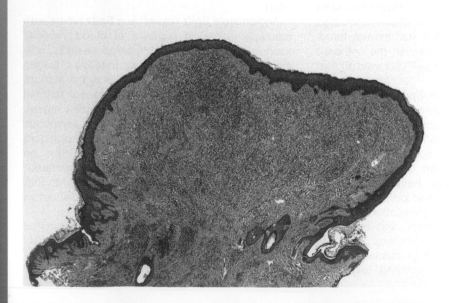

*Fig. 8.* MBAIT, removed from the scalp of a 20-year-old woman. A dermal population of nonpigmented melanocytes associated with an inflammatory infiltrate is covered by a flattened epidermis, resulting in a smooth-surfaced papule. The melanocytes do not form a solid mass that pushes against the epidermis (H&E, original magnification, ×5).

*Fig. 9.* MBAIT, same case as **Fig. 8**. At higher power, the large melanocytes rich in cytoplasm and with variable and often conspicuous nuclear enlargement are loosely scattered in a background of numerous lymphocytes (H&E, original magnification, ×10).

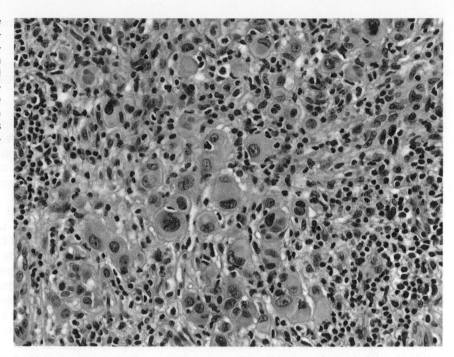

## SPITZOID MELANOMA: CLINICAL AND HISTOLOGIC FEATURES

Some melanomas show a striking resemblance to Spitz nevi.[2,29,30] Because the degree of resemblance is difficult, if not impossible, to specify reliably, the term spitzoid melanoma does not reflect

a well-defined subset of melanomas. Nonetheless, some general remarks can be made, in order to provide some diagnostic guidance to identify them as melanomas.

Implicitly, many of the features of these spitzoid melanomas have been dealt with earlier, because the features indicating malignancy are the

*Fig. 10.* MBAIT, same case as **Fig. 8**. A BAP1 immune stain shows the absence of nuclear staining in the large melanocytes, contrasting with positive staining in lymphocytes (as well as many other preexistent cells types, not visible in this picture) (H&E, original magnification, ×10).

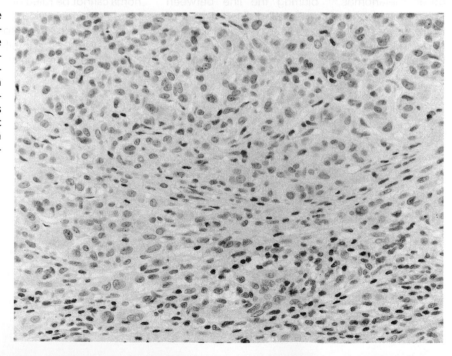

opposite to the features of benignity of Spitz nevi. In short, spitzoid melanoma is a lesion that at first sight shows a resemblance to Spitz nevus, but at close inspection shows unequivocal features of malignancy. These features of malignancy include various combinations of the following: irregular architecture and variations in cell type, resulting in substantial asymmetry (however, some are remarkably regular in architecture; **Fig. 11**); presence of mitotic activity at the deepest dermal border (**Fig. 12**); presence of atypical mitotic figures; ascent of large melanocytes rich in cytoplasm, also where the junctional component is paucicellular; a central area of epidermal flattening and thinning (so-called epidermal consumption) above a mass of junctional/dermal melanocytes, which may culminate in ulceration; presence of dermal compact and round cellular nodules; irregular distribution of dermal inflammatory infiltrate and fibrosis; presence of a dermal bandlike inflammatory infiltrate below the deep invasion front; presence of plasmocellular inflammatory infiltrates; abrupt variations in architecture and/or cytologic details between different areas, indicating outgrowth of different lesional subclones; high-grade nuclear atypia; and presence of copious, nonshrinking cytoplasm that may contain dustlike pigment. A more comprehensive listing of the various distinguishing features is given in **Table 1**; key pitfalls are tabulated in **Table 2**.

There is some indirect evidence that, as a group, spitzoid melanomas have a lower chance of tumor recurrence and progression than do other melanomas,[31] blurring the line between spitzoid melanoma and the ill-defined group of Spitz tumors that may spread to a regional lymph node basin but not beyond (discussed later). However, some spitzoid melanomas clearly progress to visceral metastasis and the death of the patient.

## SPITZ TUMORS OF UNCERTAIN MALIGNANT POTENTIAL

The diagnosis of (spitzoid) melanoma is not difficult when many of the features discussed earlier are present, but diagnostic problems emerge when atypical features are few and present in conjunction with other features that seem to indicate a benign lesion.

A different source of diagnostic uncertainty drives from suboptimal biopsy quality and lack of clinical information. If the specimen is traumatized, or very incomplete, the histologic evaluation is to some degree compromised. The question of whether a complete and optimal biopsy specimen would have yielded diagnostically relevant information that is unavailable in the submitted biopsy cannot be answered. If the histologic findings do not point unequivocally to Spitz nevus or spitzoid melanoma, or when the biopsy shows a Spitz lesion but is very incomplete or otherwise suboptimal, a diagnostic verdict of Spitz tumor of uncertain malignant potential (STUMP) is appropriate.

However, STUMP should not be regarded as a diagnostic entity. Any Spitz nevus can receive a verdict of STUMP when the specimen is traumatized to the degree that it can still be recognized as a spitzoid melanocytic proliferation but melanoma cannot be ruled out. Similarly, a very incomplete incisional biopsy of a Spitz nevus is insufficient to rule out spitzoid melanoma. Thus, in these and similar situations, the verdict of STUMP does not point to an entity but to a

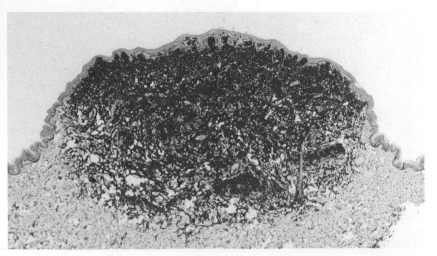

*Fig. 11.* Spitzoid melanoma, removed from the upper arm of a 30-year-old man. There is a deceptively regular and infiltrative architecture that is striking in this Melan-A immune stain. It is important to bear in mind that such a regular architecture does not rule out spitzoid melanoma (H&E, original magnification, ×5).

*Fig. 12.* Spitzoid melanoma, same case as Fig. 11. At higher power, this deepest part of the lesion shows a large cell type with large nuclei and mitotic activity (mitotic figures were numerous at this deep invasion front). Note the cell with dustlike melanin pigment. In this example, the cellular details and deep mitotic activity rather than the overall architecture led to the correct diagnosis (H&E, original magnification, ×40).

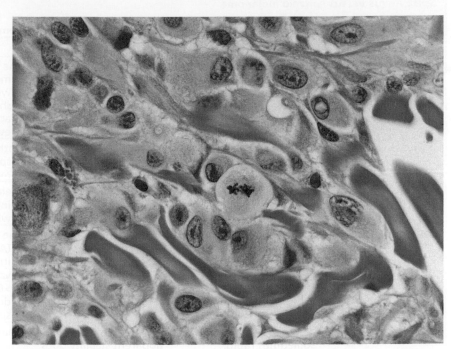

situation: the situation is that the pathologist, after having completed the diagnostic evaluation, is unable to either diagnose or rule out melanoma.

When the lesion is less than 1 mm in thickness and lacks ulceration or dermal mitotic activity, so that the differential diagnosis is between T1a melanoma and (Spitz) nevus, the authors prefer not to issue a verdict of STUMP, but of spitzoid superficial atypical melanocytic proliferation of uncertain significance (spitzoid SAMPUS).[32–34] This term avoids the T of tumor and M of malignancy, and therefore does more justice to the fact that, after complete removal of such a small and thin lesion, the chance of future trouble is vanishingly small.

Some pathologists prefer not to use terms such as STUMP, melanocytic tumors of uncertain malignant potential, or SAMPUS, and describe rather than categorize such lesions. As long as the reports unequivocally state that there is diagnostic uncertainty that cannot be eliminated, and provide some guidance to clinicians about how to proceed from this uncertainty, there is no problem. However, such cases should never be called atypical Spitz nevus or some similar designation, because the term nevus indicates that the lesion is benign.

Note that sentinel node biopsy is contraindicated in this group of lesions. A recent meta-analysis of atypical Spitz tumors for which sentinel node biopsy was performed revealed that a positive sentinel node does not predict a poorer outcome.[35]

## SPITZ TUMORS WITH INCOMPLETE METASTATIC POTENTIAL

So far, this article has discussed Spitz nevi, spitzoid melanomas, and lesions for which, either because of intrinsic difficulties in interpretation or because of suboptimal biopsy quality, a diagnosis of nevus or melanoma is impossible, and that are therefore categorized as STUMP or spitzoid SAMPUS.

It is self-evident that, in aggregate, STUMPs, which must be a group of undiagnosable spitzoid tumors that is likely to consist of a mixture of Spitz nevi and melanomas, have a better prognosis than a group of unequivocal melanomas, and a worse one than a group of unequivocal Spitz nevi. However, in the case of Spitz tumors, the situation is more complex than that. In the past decades, it has become apparent that there is a group of spitzoid tumors that commonly spreads to a regional lymph node, but only rarely metastasizes to distant sites. Such behavior cannot be explained by the assumption that this group of lesions is just a mixture of benign nevi and fully malignant melanomas. This point is self-evident: it would be expected that, within the group of STUMP, the subgroup of fully malignant spitzoid melanoma

*Table 1*
Spitz nevus versus spitzoid melanoma

| Feature | Spitz Nevus | Spitzoid Melanoma | Remarks |
|---|---|---|---|
| **Clinical Findings** | | | |
| Age | Mostly in first 2 decades, but may occur at all ages | Mostly adolescents and adults | The a priori chance of melanoma increases with age, and this should be taken into account in the evaluation of the lesion |
| Site | Head and neck area in children; extremities and trunk in adults | Wide variety of sites | Both Spitz nevi and spitzoid melanomas may affect any body site |
| Size | Most ≤1 cm | Any size | Melanomas are increasingly diagnosed when they are still small |
| Shape and color | Usually evenly pigmented or erythematous; symmetric | May be irregular, but some are quite regular in shape and color | The ABCDE rule (Asymmetry; Border irregularity; Color variations; Diameter >6 mm; Enlarging) often does not apply in spitzoid melanoma |
| Evolution | Initial phase of growth, sometimes rapid, followed by prolonged period of stability | Continued growth, but apparent stability does not rule out melanoma | Change after a period of apparent stability is a suspicious finding |
| Dermoscopic findings | Various | Various | Dermoscopy is often not discriminatory |
| **Architectural Findings** | | | |
| Overall | Generally regular, resulting in symmetry | Irregular or regular | Irregularity (distribution of cells; aspect of cells; epidermal and dermal reactive changes) is a significant and concerning finding; regularity does not rule out melanoma |
| Epidermal component | Often prominent nesting, with epidermal hyperplasia | Nesting and/or lentiginous arrangement of cells, sometimes epidermal flattening and thinning (epidermal consumption) that may culminate in ulceration | Traumatic ulceration may also occur in Spitz nevus |
| Transepidermal elimination of nests | May be present | May be present | Not a distinguishing feature |
| Ascent of solitary cells and very small cell groups | May be common, especially in childhood and in the presence of a richly cellular junctional component (mostly situated centrally). Ascending cells tend to become progressively smaller | May or may not be common. Absence of ascent does not rule out melanoma. Ascent in a flattened epidermis and in presence of a paucicellular junctional component, and ascent of large cells rich in cytoplasm, are concerning findings | Ascent, or absence of ascent, is a common source of melanoma overdiagnosis and melanoma underdiagnosis |

(*continued on next page*)

**Table 1**
*(continued)*

| Feature | Spitz Nevus | Spitzoid Melanoma | Remarks |
|---|---|---|---|
| Lateral junctional border | Consists most commonly of nests, but may be lentiginous | Consists most commonly of nests, but may be lentiginous | Not a rewarding diagnostic parameter. There are many exceptions to the idea that Spitz nevus is well circumscribed and melanoma is not |
| Dermal architecture | Generally symmetric, with an ill-defined, infiltrative rather than pushing periphery (toward the base but also toward the lateral periphery) | Deep nodules and micronodules (pushing base) are an important indicator of malignancy. They are commonly associated with deep mitotic activity | Superficial Spitz nevi and especially pigmented spindle cell (Reed) nevi may have a more densely cellular, noninfiltrative dermal periphery |
| Maturation | Generally obvious, unless the lesion is very superficial | Some degree of diminution of cell size at the base is common in melanoma, including spitzoid melanoma. Changes in cell size are often more abrupt than in nevi | |
| Distribution of mitotic activity | Mitotic figures, when present, tend to be restricted to superficial parts (but occasionally detected in deeper parts) | Mitotic activity at the deep border is highly suspicious. Atypical mitotic figures are highly suspicious. Their absence carries little diagnostic significance | |
| **Cellular Details** | | | |
| Pigment | Uncommon; regularly distributed granular pigment, gradually disappearing toward base | Variable; deep and irregularly distributed dustlike pigment worrisome for malignancy | |
| Shrinkage artifact | Often present, creating retraction spaces | Usually absent; large or grouped melanocytes, devoid of shrinkage artifact, are worrisome | |
| Kamino bodies | Sometimes present; cluster into larger irregular aggregates | Uncommon; small if present | |
| Inflammatory infiltrate | Perivascular; similar throughout lesion | Irregularly distributed/bandlike at the base | Plasmacytic infiltrate is rare in spitzoid melanoma, but if present strongly favors malignancy |
| **Immunohistochemical Findings** | | | |
| S-100 and Melan-A | Usually positive throughout | Usually positive throughout | |
| MIB-1/Ki-67 | Varying numbers; diminishing numbers toward the base | Varying numbers; numbers may not diminish toward the base | |

*(continued on next page)*

**Table 1**
**(continued)**

| Feature | Spitz Nevus | Spitzoid Melanoma | Remarks |
|---|---|---|---|
| Cyclin D1 | Varying numbers; diminishing numbers toward the base | Varying numbers; numbers may not diminish toward the base | |
| HMB-45 | Positivity usually, but not always, limited to upper parts | Variable positivity often not limited to upper parts | |
| p16 | Often strong positivity | Variable | Complete loss of p16 is a rare but probably a significant indicator of malignancy |
| BAP1 | Normal (positive nuclear staining) except in MBAIT | Usually normal (positive nuclear staining) | |

**Table 2**
**Pitfalls in the diagnosis of Spitz nevus**

| Pitfall/Mistake | Comment |
|---|---|
| Incomplete histologic evaluation | The diagnosis of melanoma may be missed when only a punch biopsy or superficial shave biopsy is available. Sampling error and misinterpretation caused by lack of complete overview may lead to melanoma underdiagnosis |
| Over-reliance on the diagnostic significance of melanocyte ascent, or its absence | Melanocyte ascent may be substantial in Spitz nevi, especially in young children, in acral sites and in the presence of a richly cellular junctional component. In contrast, ascent is absent or almost absent in some spitzoid melanomas |
| Over-reliance on the diagnostic significance of maturation | In many melanomas, cells in the deep part are smaller than superficial ones. Transitions tend to be abrupt and irregular rather than smooth and gradual, as is the case in Spitz nevus. In very superficial Spitz nevi and variants, especially pigmented spindle cell nevus, maturation is not obvious |
| Misinterpretation of reactive/posttraumatic changes | Ulceration caused by trauma (picking), fibrosis caused by compression of raised part, or recurrence in scar tissue after incomplete shave excision may inappropriately suggest melanoma |
| Tunnel vision: focus on a few histologic findings, with disregard for clinical context | A small Spitz tumor in a child is hardly ever a melanoma. An extensive Spitz tumor in an adult is highly suspicious. A high level of clinical suspicion based on the lesion's history and its macroscopic and dermatoscopic appearance should never be lightly dismissed |
| Positive sentinel node of a Spitz tumor indicates melanoma | Atypical Spitz tumors have a high likelihood of sentinel node involvement but rarely metastasize to distant sites. In this group of lesions, a positive sentinel node does not have prognostic significance |
| Erroneous first impression that a skin tumor is a Spitz tumor | Consider nonmelanocytic neoplasms in the differential diagnosis and perform the appropriate immune stains. Immune stains may inappropriately confirm the first impression in cases of PEComa and, especially, cutaneous clear cell sarcoma |

*Abbreviation:* PEComa, perivascular epithelioid cell tumor.

that subsequently betrays itself by metastasizing to a regional lymph node would have the same prognosis as similar unequivocal melanomas with a regional lymph node metastasis. However, this is not the case. An early report of Spitz tumors involving a regional node but not progressing to distant metastasis,[36] and resulting in an awkward designation of 'benign metastasizing Spitz nevus', met with aggressive early criticism[37] but the essential findings of that early report were later reproduced manyfold.[38–42] There is now no doubt that there is a group of Spitz tumors that has a propensity for regional spread but not, or to a very limited extent, for distant metastasis. A large number of Spitz tumors about which the pathologist feels uncertain (ie, STUMP) because of equivocal histologic findings, seem to belong to this group. In a systematic review of published literature, Lallas and colleagues[35] provided a meta-analysis of 541 such cases. Of these, 303 (56%) underwent sentinel node biopsy, of which 119 (39%) were positive. Of the latter, 97 (82%) underwent completion lymph node dissection, yielding additional positive nodes in 18 (19%). Of the entire group, only 6 patients (1%) died of distant metastatic disease. It was concluded from these and further data in this meta-analysis that positive sentinel node in this group is not associated with poorer outcome.

This finding adds to the complexity of the Spitz tumor typing. It seems that pathologists need to distinguish not 2 but 3 groups: Spitz nevi, spitzoid melanomas that can metastasize to distant body sites and kill the patient, and a group of Spitz tumors with incomplete metastatic potential.

At present, it is impossible to make a confident diagnosis of that intermediate group of Spitz tumors at the level of the individual lesion/patient, with the possible exception of Spitz tumors that arise before puberty. In the latter subgroup, Spitz tumors with deep dermal spread, often with deep nodular outgrowth and mitotic activity that would otherwise result in a diagnosis of spitzoid melanoma, regional spread is common, but distant metastasis is distinctly rare.[40] Nonetheless, here, too, exceptions do occur: the authors recently saw a Spitz tumor arising in a congenital nevus of a 3-year-old, which in the next months progressed to regional and then distant metastasis, leading to death within one year.

In sum, if a confident diagnosis of Spitz nevus is deemed impossible, it is impossible to guarantee absence of distant metastatic potential in any individual case, and we therefore prefer to limit ourselves to a statement that prognosis is fair, without guaranteeing that there will be no distant metastasis. It is hoped that the accumulating experience with novel diagnostic modalities will allow a more precise prediction of the behavior of these rare tumors.

## NOVEL DIAGNOSTIC MODALITIES

In recent years, genetic analyses of Spitz tumors have yielded novel data of substantial diagnostic interest.

Conventional melanomas are characterized by high genetic instability and multiple copy number variations when studied by comparative genomic hybridization (CGH). Spitz nevi generally lack chromosomal aberrations besides gains in 11p (15%–20%) or tetraploidy (5%–10%).[43] Increases in 11p are sometimes associated with an activating mutation in the HRAS gene, and show an association with the desmoplastic Spitz nevus subtype.[44,45] Although HRAS mutations have been described in Spitz nevi, they are rare in melanoma,[46–48] which provides some diagnostic applicability. In contrast, BRAF and NRAS mutations, commonly found in conventional melanoma, are rare in Spitz nevi and uncommon in STUMPs but also in spitzoid melanomas,[48–50] detracting from their applicability.

Fluorescence in situ hybridization (FISH) based on a panel with higher sensitivity for spitzoid melanoma carries promise for increased diagnostic accuracy.[51] It studies alterations in 6p25 (RREB1), 8q24 (C-MYC), 9p21 (CDKN2A), and 11q13 (CCND1) and can be used to help determine the clinical risk of STUMPs[52]: low with no alterations, intermediate with 6p25 and 11q13 gains, and high with 9p21 homozygous deletion.

Lesions regarded as STUMP often have chromosomal aberrations lacking in Spitz nevi and, although less numerous than in melanomas and not in its common locations,[53] they may be associated with poorer prognosis, most notably the homozygous deletion of 9p21 (CDKN2A), which leads to loss of p16 expression.[54,55]

Although CGH still seems to offer most information, its applicability is largely limited to research centers. FISH analysis is more affordable and widely available (although less sensitive and specific than CGH), allowing quick evaluation of specific loci. In addition, telomerase reverse transcriptase promoter (TERT-p) mutation has been identified as a predictor of poorer outcome,[56] but requires further validation.

Recently it has been found that approximately half of all spitzoid lesions with no HRAS mutation have kinase fusions, affecting ROS1 (10%), NTRK1 (10%), ALK (10%), BRAF (5%), RET (5%), or MET (1%).[48,57] These oncogenic fusions are rare in other melanocytic lesions and some have been related to specific histologic phenotypes of Spitz tumor. Besides offering potential therapeutic targets, they might constitute an indication that spitzoid lesions are related. However, these kinase fusions apparently do not help in distinguishing benign from malignant Spitz tumors.

## NONMELANOCYTIC SIMULATORS OF SPITZ NEVUS AND SPITZOID MELANOMA

A variety of benign and malignant skin tumors consisting of large pale cells with ample cytoplasm may show some resemblance to Spitz nevus. Because none of these shows the involution toward the base that is an important indicator of benignity in Spitz tumors, failure to recognize the nonmelanocytic nature of the lesion may result in overdiagnosis of malignancy. With a small number of notable exceptions (discussed later), diagnostic problems are quickly solved with immune stains. The danger of misdiagnosis generally results from failure to consider nonmelanocytic lesions. It is good practice to confirm melanocytic lineage whenever a lesion resembling a Spitz tumor is devoid of pigment and lacks an obvious junctional component.

Intraepidermal lesions that, to varying extents, simulate junctional Spitz nevus (and in situ melanoma) include benign and malignant epithelial neoplasms with Borst-Jadassohn phenomenon or pagetoid architecture. Examples include clonal seborrheic keratosis, hidroacanthoma simplex, mammary and extramammary Paget disease, and pagetoid actinic keratosis. Several nonepithelial lesions can be added to this list: mycosis fungoides with extensive epidermotropism (pagetoid reticulosis, Woringer-Kolopp disease), and a variety of soft tissue tumors spreading to a limited extent into the epidermal compartment. Dermal lesions simulating Spitz tumors are more commonly a source of confusion. Lesions that have given rise to confusion include epithelioid histiocytoma, plexiform histiocytoma, spindle cell atypical fibroxanthoma, cellular neurothekeoma, (clear cell) leiomyoma, epithelioid leiomyoma, spindle cell carcinoma, and metastatic cancers of various types.

A special pitfall is provided by a small number of tumors that show morphologic as well as immunohistochemical overlap with Spitz tumors. These tumors include the (almost always benign) cutaneous PEComa (perivascular epithelioid cell tumor), a dermal tumor of pale epithelioid and spindled cells arranged in coalescent sheets round thin-walled blood vessels. The tumor cells are positive for Melan-A, MITF, and HMB-45

(focally). An important clue, in addition to the morphology, which is fairly characteristic, is the S-100 negativity of these tumors. Primary cutaneous clear cell sarcoma is an especially difficult diagnosis: this rare sarcoma, which may arise in the skin, shows the full spectrum of melanocytic differentiation, with melanin production (occasionally), positivity for a range of markers of melanocytic differentiation, and S-100 positivity. A history of slow but relentless growth beyond the sizes seen in most Spitz tumors, and subtle histologic clues such as the formation of islands of pale oval to fusiform cells embedded in paucicellular sclerotic stroma, may raise this diagnostic possibility. Demonstration of the diagnostic t(12;22) and/or an *EWSR1/ATF1* fusion gene transcript clinches the diagnosis. It might even explain the melanocytic differentiation phenotype: *MITF*, a key melanocytic differentiation inducer, is a transcriptional target of the protein encoded by the abnormal fusion gene.

## SUMMARY

The histologic diagnosis of a Spitz tumor is an especially challenging one, and requires an optimal excisional biopsy as well as detailed clinical information. A confident diagnosis of either nevus or melanoma is not always possible, and diagnostic uncertainty should be communicated in precise and unequivocal terms to the clinician. The differential diagnosis is complicated by the existence of a group of Spitz tumors with limited metastatic potential and that commonly affect a regional lymph node but only exceptionally result in distant metastasis. Sentinel node biopsy is contraindicated for this reason, because a positive sentinel node inappropriately raises the possibility of stage III melanoma. Novel diagnostic modalities are currently under intensive study and may yield robust and significant diagnostic information. They require extensive technical and interpretative experience and are not yet generally available. In addition, nonmelanocytic tumors of the skin should be included in the differential diagnosis when the first impression is of a Spitz tumor.

## REFERENCES

1. Requena C, Requena L, Kutzner H, et al. Spitz nevus: a clinicopathological study of 349 cases. Am J Dermatopathol 2009;31(2):107–16.
2. Lott JP, Wititsuwannakul J, Lee JJ, et al. Clinical characteristics associated with Spitz nevi and spitzoid malignant melanomas: the Yale University Spitzoid Neoplasm Repository experience, 1991 to 2008. J Am Acad Dermatol 2014;71(6):1077–82.

3. Torti DC, Brennick JB, Storm CA, et al. Spitz nevi arising in speckled lentiginous nevus: clinical, histologic, and molecular evaluation of two cases. Pediatr Dermatol 2011;28(5):561–7.

4. Zeng MH, Kong QT, Sang H, et al. Agminated Spitz nevi: case report and review of the literature. Pediatr Dermatol 2013;30(5):e104–5.

5. Levy RM, Ming ME, Shapiro M, et al. Eruptive disseminated Spitz nevi. J Am Acad Dermatol 2007;57(3):519–23.

6. Weedon D, Little JH. Spindle and epithelioid cell nevi in children and adults. A review of 211 cases of the Spitz nevus. Cancer 1977;40(1):217–25.

7. Paniago-Pereira C, Maize JC, Ackerman AB. Nevus of large spindle and/or epithelioid cells (Spitz's nevus). Arch Dermatol 1978;114(12):1811–23.

8. Reed RJ, Ichinose H, Clark WH Jr, et al. Common and uncommon melanocytic nevi and borderline melanomas. Semin Oncol 1975;2(2):119–47.

9. Marghoon AA, Malvehy J, Braun RP. Spitz and reed nevi. Atlas of dermoscopy. 2nd edition. London: Informa Healthcare; 2012. p. 189–97.

10. Kamino H, Flotte TJ, Misheloff E, et al. Eosinophilic globules in Spitz's nevi. New findings and a diagnostic sign. Am J Dermatopathol 1979;1(4):319–24.

11. Kapur P, Selim MA, Roy LC, et al. Spitz nevi and atypical Spitz nevi/tumors: a histologic and immunohistochemical analysis. Mod Pathol 2005;18(2):197–204.

12. Garrido-Ruiz MC, Requena L, Ortiz P, et al. The immunohistochemical profile of Spitz nevi and conventional (non-Spitzoid) melanomas: a baseline study. Mod Pathol 2010;23(9):1215–24.

13. Barr RJ, Morales RV, Graham JH. Desmoplastic nevus: a distinct histologic variant of mixed spindle cell and epithelioid cell nevus. Cancer 1980;46(3): 557–64.

14. Gambini C, Rongioletti F. Recurrent Spitz nevus. Case report and review of the literature. Am J Dermatopathol 1994;16(4):409–13.

15. Yasaka N, Furue M, Tamaki K. Histopathological evaluation of halo phenomenon in Spitz nevus. Am J Dermatopathol 1995;17(5):484–6.

16. Busam KJ, Barnhill RL. Pagetoid Spitz nevus. Intraepidermal Spitz tumor with prominent pagetoid spread. Am J Dermatopathol 1995;19(9):1061–7.

17. Fernandez AP, Billings SD, Bergfeld WF, et al. Pagetoid Spitz nevi: clinicopathologic characterization of a series of 12 cases. J Cutan Pathol 2016;43(11): 932–9.

18. Burg G, Kempf W, Hochli M, et al. 'Tubular' epithelioid cell nevus: a new variant of Spitz's nevus. J Cutan Pathol 1998;25(9):475–8.

19. Valdivielso-Ramos M, Burdaspal A, Conde E, et al. Balloon-cell variant of the Spitz nevus. J Eur Acad Dermatol Venereol 2016;30(9):1621–2.

20. Hoang MP. Myxoid Spitz nevus. J Cutan Pathol 2003;30(9):566–8.

21. Suster S. Hyalinizing spindle and epithelioid cell nevus. A study of five cases of a distinctive histologic variant of Spitz's nevus. Am J Dermatopathol 1994;16(6):593–8.

22. Barnhill RL, Mihm MC Jr, Magro CM. Plexiform spindle cell naevus: a distinctive variant of plexiform melanocytic naevus. Histopathology 1991;18(3):243–7.

23. Diaz-Cascajo C, Borghi S, Weyers W. Angiomatoid Spitz nevus: a distinct variant of desmoplastic Spitz nevus with prominent vasculature. Am J Dermatopathol 2000;22(2):135–9.

24. Fabrizi G, Massi G. Polypoid Spitz naevus: the benign counterpart of polypoid malignant melanoma. Br J Dermatol 2000;142(1):128–32.

25. Wiesner T, Murali R, Fried I, et al. A distinct subset of atypical Spitz tumors is characterized by BRAF mutation and loss of BAP1 expression. Am J Surg Pathol 2012;36(6):818–30.

26. Piris A, Mihm MC Jr, Hoang MP. BAP1 and BRAFV600E expression in benign and malignant melanocytic proliferations. Hum Pathol 2015;46(2): 239–45.

27. Klebe S, Driml J, Nasu M, et al. BAP1 hereditary cancer predisposition syndrome: a case report and review of literature. Biomark Res 2015;3:14.

28. Murali R, Wiesner T, Scolyer RA. Tumours associated with BAP1 mutations. Pathology 2013;45(2):116–26.

29. Kamino H. Spitzoid melanoma. Clin Dermatol 2009; 27(6):545–55.

30. Requena C, Botella R, Nagore E, et al. Characteristics of spitzoid melanoma and clues for differential diagnosis with Spitz nevus. Am J Dermatopathol 2012;34(5):478–86.

31. Hung T, Piris A, Lobo A, et al. Sentinel lymph node metastasis is not predictive of poor outcome in patients with problematic spitzoid melanocytic tumors. Hum Pathol 2013;44(1):87–94.

32. Elder DE, Xu X. The approach to the patient with a difficult melanocytic lesion. Pathology 2004;36(5): 428–34.

33. Elder DE, Murphy GF. Management of "uncertain" melanocytic neoplasms: superficial atypical melanocytic proliferations of uncertain significance (SAMPUS) and melanocytic tumors of uncertain malignant potential (MELTUMP). Melanocytic tumors of the skin (AFIP atlas of tumor pathology: series 4). Am Registry Pathol 2010;12:264–8.

34. Pusiol T, Morichetti D, Piscioli F, et al. Theory and practical application of superficial atypical melanocytic proliferations of uncertain significance (SAMPUS) and melanocytic tumours of uncertain malignant potential (MELTUMP) terminology: experience with second opinion consultation. Pathologica 2012;104(2):70–7.

35. Lallas A, Kyrgidis A, Ferrara G, et al. Atypical Spitz tumours and sentinel lymph node biopsy: a systematic review. Lancet Oncol 2014;15(4):e178–83.

36. Smith KJ, Barrett TL, Skelton HG 3rd, et al. Spindle cell and epithelioid cell nevi with atypia and metastasis (malignant Spitz nevus). Am J Surg Pathol 1989;13(11):931–9.

37. Mones JM, Ackerman AB. "Atypical" Spitz's nevus, "malignant" Spitz's nevus, and "metastasizing" Spitz's nevus: a critique in historical perspective of three concepts flawed fatally. Am J Surg Pathol 2004;26(4):310–33.

38. Lohmann CM, Coit DG, Brady MS, et al. Sentinel lymph node biopsy in patients with diagnostically controversial spitzoid melanocytic tumors. Am J Surg Pathol 2002;26(1):47–55.

39. Barnhill RL. The Spitzoid lesion: rethinking Spitz tumors, atypical variants, 'Spitzoid melanoma' and risk assessment. Mod Pathol 2006;19(Suppl 2):S21–33.

40. Mooi WJ, Krausz T. Spitz nevus versus spitzoid melanoma: diagnostic difficulties, conceptual controversies. Adv Anat Pathol 2006;13(4):147–56.

41. Ludgate MW, Fullen DR, Lee J, et al. The atypical Spitz tumor of uncertain biologic potential: a series of 67 patients from a single institution. Cancer 2009;115(3):631–41.

42. McCormack CJ, Conyers RK, Scolyer RA, et al. Atypical Spitzoid neoplasms: a review of potential markers of biological behavior including sentinel node biopsy. Melanoma Res 2014;24(5):437–47.

43. Bastian BC, Wesselmann U, Pinkel D, et al. Molecular cytogenetic analysis of Spitz nevi shows clear differences to melanoma. J Invest Dermatol 1999;113(6):1065–9.

44. Bastian BC, LeBoit PE, Pinkel D. Mutations and copy number increase of HRAS in Spitz nevi with distinctive histopathological features. Am J Pathol 2000;157(3):967–72.

45. van Engen-van Grunsven AC, van Dijk MC, Ruiter DJ, et al. HRAS-mutated Spitz tumors: a subtype of Spitz tumors with distinct features. Am J Surg Pathol 2010;34(10):1436–41.

46. Takata M, Lin J, Takayanagi S, et al. Genetic and epigenetic alterations in the differential diagnosis of malignant melanoma and spitzoid lesion. Br J Dermatol 2007;156(6):1287–94.

47. van Dijk MC, Bernsen MR, Ruiter DJ. Analysis of mutations in B-RAF, N-RAS, and H-RAS genes in the differential diagnosis of Spitz nevus and spitzoid melanoma. Am J Surg Pathol 2005;29(9):1145–51.

48. Wiesner T, Kutzner H, Cerroni L, et al. Genomic aberrations in spitzoid melanocytic tumours and their implications for diagnosis, prognosis and therapy. Pathology 2016;48(2):113–31.

49. Da Forno PD, Pringle JH, Fletcher A, et al. BRAF, NRAS and HRAS mutations in spitzoid tumours and their possible pathogenetic significance. Br J Dermatol 2009;161(2):364–72.

50. Fullen DR, Poynter JN, Lowe L, et al. BRAF and NRAS mutations in spitzoid melanocytic lesions. Mod Pathol 2006;19(10):1324–32.

51. Gerami P, Li G, Pouryazdanparast P, et al. A highly specific and discriminatory FISH assay for distinguishing between benign and malignant melanocytic neoplasms. Am J Surg Pathol 2012;36(6):808–17.

52. Gerami P, Scolyer RA, Xu X, et al. Risk assessment for atypical spitzoid melanocytic neoplasms using FISH to identify chromosomal copy number aberrations. Am J Surg Pathol 2013;37(5):676–84.

53. Raskin L, Ludgate M, Iyer RK, et al. Copy number variations and clinical outcome in atypical Spitz tumors. Am J Surg Pathol 2011;35(2):243–52.

54. Yazdan P, Cooper C, Sholl LM, et al. Comparative analysis of atypical Spitz tumors with heterozygous versus homozygous 9p21 deletions for clinical outcomes, histomorphology, BRAF mutation, and p16 expression. Am J Surg Pathol 2014;38(5):638–45.

55. Mason A, Wititsuwannakul J, Klump VR, et al. Expression of p16 alone does not differentiate between Spitz nevi and Spitzoid melanoma. J Cutan Pathol Dec 2012;39(12):1062–74.

56. Lee S, Barnhill RL, Dummer R, et al. TERT promoter mutations are predictive of aggressive clinical behavior in patients with spitzoid melanocytic neoplasms. Sci Rep 2015;5:11200.

57. Wiesner T, He J, Yelensky R, et al. Kinase fusions are frequent in Spitz tumours and spitzoid melanomas. Nat Commun 2014;5:3116.

# Advances in the Genetic Characterization of Cutaneous Mesenchymal Neoplasms
## Implications for Tumor Classification and Novel Diagnostic Markers

Leigh A. Compton, MD, PhD, Leona A. Doyle, MD*

## KEYWORDS

• Soft tissue tumor • Immunohistochemistry • Sarcoma • Mesenchymal • Neoplasm

## Key Points

- Cutaneous mesenchymal neoplasms often pose significant diagnostic challenges; many such entities are rare or show clinical and histologic overlap with both other mesenchymal and non-mesenchymal lesions.

- Recent advances in the genetic classification of many cutaneous mesenchymal neoplasms have not only helped define unique pathologic entities and increase our understanding of their biology, but have also provided new diagnostic markers.

- Except for very difficult or unusual cases, molecular studies such as fluorescence in situ hybridization or real-time polymerase chain reaction–based methods are not routinely used for the diagnosis of cutaneous mesenchymal neoplasms, but many of the recent molecular discoveries have resulted in the development of new and useful immunohistochemical markers, such as FOSB, CAMTA1, and ALK.

## ABSTRACT

Cutaneous mesenchymal neoplasms often pose significant diagnostic challenges; many such entities are rare or show clinical and histologic overlap with both other mesenchymal and non-mesenchymal lesions. Recent advances in the genetic classification of many cutaneous mesenchymal neoplasms have not only helped define unique pathologic entities and increase our understanding of their biology, but have also provided new diagnostic markers. This review details these recent discoveries, with a focus on their implications for tumor classification and diagnosis.

## OVERVIEW

Cutaneous mesenchymal neoplasms often pose significant diagnostic challenges; many such entities are rare or show clinical and histologic overlap with both other mesenchymal and non-mesenchymal lesions. Recent advances in the

The authors have no conflicts of interest to declare.
Department of Pathology, Brigham and Women's Hospital, Harvard Medical School, 75 Francis Street, Boston, MA 02115, USA
* Corresponding author.
E-mail address: ladoyle@partners.org

Surgical Pathology 10 (2017) 299–317
http://dx.doi.org/10.1016/j.path.2017.01.005

genetic classification of many cutaneous mesenchymal neoplasms have not only helped define unique pathologic entities and increase our understanding of their biology, but have also provided new diagnostic markers. Except for very difficult or unusual cases, molecular studies such as fluorescence in situ hybridization (FISH) or real-time polymerase chain reaction (RT-PCR)-based methods are not routinely used for the diagnosis of cutaneous mesenchymal neoplasms, with the exception of distinguishing clear cell sarcoma from melanoma, but many of the recent molecular discoveries have resulted in the development of new and useful immunohistochemical markers that act as surrogate markers for underlying genetic changes. This review details these recent discoveries, with a focus on their implications for tumor classification and diagnosis.

## PSEUDOMYOGENIC HEMANGIOENDOTHELIOMA

In 1992, Mirra and colleagues[1] described a spindle-cell tumor thought to be a histologic variant of epithelioid sarcoma based on similarities in clinical features (arising on the extremities of young adults) and shared diffuse positivity for cytokeratin. A larger clinicopathologic study of 50 cases later defined this entity as pseudomyogenic hemangioendothelioma (PMHE), a tumor with distinct clinical, histologic, and immunohistochemical features showing endothelial differentiation.[2] Subsequent studies demonstrated the presence of a novel and recurrent chromosomal translocation in PMHE, establishing it as a distinct tumor type. PMHE characteristically presents as either painful or painless nodules on the extremities of young to middle-age adult men. Imaging studies often reveal multiple tumors arising in separate tissue planes within the same anatomic region of the body.[2] PMHE is currently considered to be of intermediate biologic potential, given the high rate of local recurrence of 50%, but only very rare propensity for distant metastases.[3] The current recommended therapy is conservative excision with close clinical follow-up.

PMHE may arise in the dermis, subcutaneous tissue, or deep soft tissues, including skeletal muscle and bone (Fig. 1). Most tumors are smaller than 3 cm in greatest dimension and have a gray-white cut surface with ill-defined borders.[2] Tumors are composed of loose fascicles or sheets of plump spindle cells with vesicular chromatin, variably prominent nucleoli, and abundant

brightly eosinophilic cytoplasm, imparting a myoid appearance (see Fig. 1). Most tumors have a minor population of epithelioid cells and some may show areas of striking rhabdomyoblast-like differentiation. Nuclear atypia is generally mild with just a minority of cases showing focal pleomorphism. Mitoses may be present but are not numerous (average 2 per 10 high-power fields, range of 0–10). Inductive epidermal hyperplasia is observed in some cases, similar to that seen in benign fibrous histiocytoma (dermatofibroma).[2]

Tumor cells show strong diffuse staining for cytokeratin AE1/AE3, FLI1, and ERG, and variable expression of CD31, consistent with endothelial differentiation (see Fig. 1). Some cases show focal positivity for Cam5.2, smooth muscle actin (SMA), EMA, and pancytokeratin. CD34, desmin, and S100 are negative.[2] INI-1 expression, in contrast to epithelioid sarcoma, is intact.[2,4]

The description of PMHE as a distinct endothelial neoplasm was validated by the identification of a novel and recurrent chromosomal translocation, t(7;19) (q22;q13), present in the vast majority of tumors.[5,6] This translocation situates the FOSB gene on chromosome 19 adjacent to the transcriptional regulatory elements upstream of the SERPINE1 locus on chromosome 7. Gene expression studies performed on a small number of tumors suggest this translocation results in overexpression of FOSB[6] and recent studies have validated the utility of nuclear FOSB expression by immunohistochemistry in confirming the diagnosis of PHE, as most other endothelial vascular tumors and epithelioid sarcoma are negative for FOSB.[7,8] The SERPINE-1 locus encodes a serine protease inhibitor, plasminogen activator inhibitor type 1 (PAI-1). It is highly expressed in vascular endothelial cells, among a variety of other normal tissue types and tumors, and plays a role in angiogenesis and cell invasion.[9,10] FOSB encodes a member of the larger family of FOS transcription factors and heterodimerizes with JUN proteins and together form the major components of the activating-protein-1 complex, which regulates a wide range of biologic processes, including cell proliferation, tumor invasion, and angiogenesis.[11,12] Multiple isoforms of the FOSB protein exist and may have opposing effects on transcriptional activity of target genes.[13–15] Interestingly, a subset of epithelioid hemangiomas, particularly cellular and intraosseous variants, have been found to harbor a rearrangement involving the FOSB locus.[16,17]

## EPITHELIOID HEMANGIOENDOTHELIOMA

Epithelioid hemangioendothelioma (EHE) is a malignant tumor showing endothelial differentiation that occurs in the skin, soft tissue, viscera, and bone. Given the broad differential of epithelioid tumors at these various anatomic sites, these tumors can pose a significant diagnostic challenge. Fortunately, the recent identification of translocations associated with EHE have not only provided initial insights into their biology, but have also led to the identification of useful diagnostic immunohistochemical markers.

EHE of the skin or superficial soft tissues typically presents as a solitary, painful nodule in middle-aged adults. The 2013 World Health Organization Classification of Tumors of Soft Tissues and Bone classifies EHE as a malignant neoplasm clinicopathologic studies demonstrate a metastatic rate of approximately 21% and mortality rate of 17% for tumors arising in soft tissues, and metastatic and mortality rates for primary EHE of visceral sites are approximately 40%.[18,19] Treatment approaches are determined by site and disease burden: solitary cutaneous and soft tissue tumors are typically amenable to surgical excision alone, whereas for recurrent, locally extensive, or metastatic disease, radiation and systemic therapies may be used.[20–22]

Cutaneous lesions tend to be small, have well-circumscribed borders, and do not arise in association with a vessel. In contrast, deep soft tissue and visceral lesions are frequently large and infiltrative, and 50% arise in association with medium-sized vessels, usually veins.[20] Microscopically, EHE consists of strands, cords, or nests of epithelioid cells in a myxohyaline stroma

(**Fig. 2**). Vasoformative growth is generally not a feature of EHE but may be found in a small subset of tumors. Tumor cells have moderate amounts of glassy eosinophilic cytoplasm and round nuclei with inconspicuous nucleoli. Intracytoplasmic vacuoles are sometimes present and may contain an erythrocyte. A number of degenerative architectural features can be seen, including cystic degeneration, hemorrhage, sclerosis, and necrosis.[20–22] Features such as tumor size >3 cm, sheetlike growth, nuclear atypia, pleomorphism, necrosis, mitotic activity greater than 3 per 50 high-power fields, and a prominent spindle-cell component have been associated with a more aggressive clinical course.[20,23,24] The tumor cells of EHE express the endothelial markers CD31, CD34, ERG, and FLI-1; however, with the exception of ERG, expression of these markers is variable and often multifocal (see **Fig. 2**).[25,26] Therefore, in practice, evaluation of multiple endothelial markers is often needed. ERG is the most sensitive and specific marker of endothelial differentiation, but expression may be seen in a small subset of epithelioid sarcomas, depending on the specific antibody used. Keratin positivity is found in approximately 25% to 50% of cases, but EMA is usually negative.[20,21,27–29]

EHE harbors a recurrent t(1;3) (p36.3;q25) that results in a novel *WWTR1-CAMTA1* gene fusion. This translocation was identified in EHE across all anatomic sites and in tumors of varying clinical behavior, and appears to be present in at least 90% of EHE.[30–33] *WWTR1*, also known as TAZ, encodes a downstream transcriptional mediator of the Hippo pathway that mediates a number of biologic events in epithelial cells, including proliferation and cell adhesion.[34–37] *CAMTA1* on chromosome 1 belongs to a family of calmodulin-binding transcription factors important in cell-cycle regulation.[38] The biologic significance of this fusion protein is unknown, but its discovery led to the identification of CAMTA1 as a useful immunohistochemical marker for EHE (see **Fig. 2**). At least 90% of EHE shows strong and diffuse nuclear positivity for CAMTA1, including tumors with high-grade features, such as solid growth, marked cytologic atypia, and high mitotic activity. Histologic mimics of EHE, including epithelioid vascular tumors (epithelioid hemangioma, epithelioid angiosarcoma, and PMHE), other epithelioid mesenchymal neoplasms, such as epithelioid sarcoma and myoepithelioma, and many epithelial neoplasms, are negative for CAMTA1.[39] Accordingly, CAMTA1 is a useful and reliable marker of EHE, and reflects the presence of a *WWTR1-CAMTA1* fusion gene.

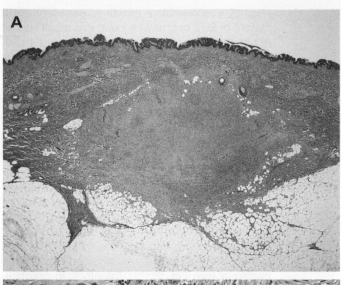

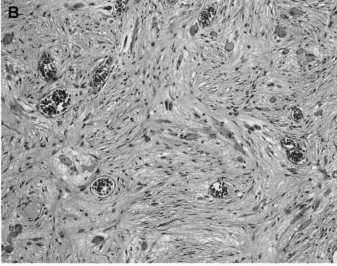

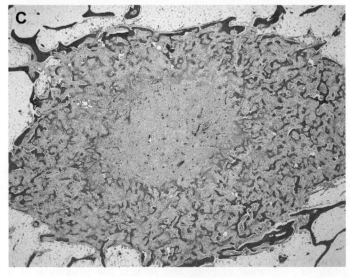

*Fig. 1.* Pseudomyogenic hemangioendothelioma involving dermis, with infiltrative edges (*A*). The tumor cells grow in sheets or fascicles and are spindled with abundant eosinophilic cytoplasm, imparting a myoid appearance (*B*). These tumors are often multifocal within the same anatomic region, involving different tissue planes, as in this case in which bone lesions were also present (*C*).

*Fig. 1.* (*continued*). Tumor cells are positive for cytokeratin AE1/AE3 (*D*) and show nuclear positivity for the endothelial marker ERG (*E*).

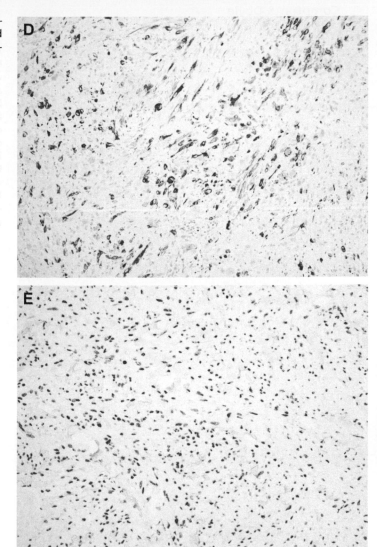

A separate translocation event has been identified in a subset of EHE with distinct morphologic features. Tumors that show at least focal vasoformative activity, solid architecture, and have bright eosinophilic cytoplasm are associated with *YAP1-TFE3* fusion gene.[40] YAP1, similar to WWTR1, is also a downstream transcriptional regulator of the Hippo pathway and there is significant sequence homology between the two proteins.[41] TFE3 is a known oncogenic transcription factor and translocation events involving TFE3 also occur in alveolar soft part sarcoma and a subset of renal cell carcinoma.[42–46] Although strong diffuse nuclear positivity for TFE3 is seen in these tumors, TFE3 is a less-specific surrogate marker for the *YAP1-TFE3* gene fusion of EHE, and some tumors that show expression of TFE3 are not associated with the presence of the fusion gene: in a recent study, only positive cases with a strong diffuse staining pattern correlated with the presence of *YAP1-TFE3*.[33]

## *Key Points*
### Cutaneous Epithelioid Hemangioendothelioma

- Solitary painful nodule; usually not associated with a vessel

- Strands, cords, and nests of epithelioid cells with moderate amounts of pale, glassy cytoplasm (+/− intracytoplasmic vacuoles) in a myxohyaline stroma

- Immunohistochemical expression of CD31, CD34, ERG, and cytokeratin (50%)

- t(1;3) (p36.3;q25) in greater than 95% results in a *WWTR1-CAMTA1* fusion gene and nuclear expression of CAMTA1 protein

- A subset (<5%) with vasoformative features and brightly eosinophilic cytoplasm have *YAP1-TFE3* fusion

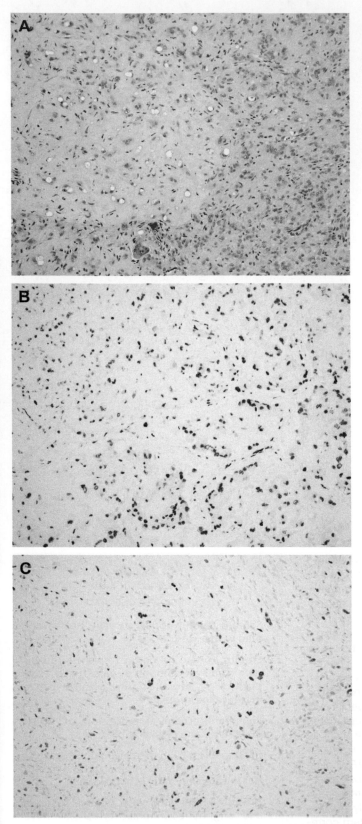

*Fig.* 2. Epithelioid hemangioendothelioma is composed of endothelial cells
with abundant eosinophilic cytoplasm
and round nuclei, intracytoplasmic
lumina (often containing erythrocytes),
and mild cytologic atypia (*A*). Expression
of ERG, a transcription factor present in
cells showing endothelial differentiation,
is present in the vast majority of epithelioid hemangioendotheliomas (*B*). Nuclear expression of CAMTA1 is seen in at
least 95% of cases, and reflects the presence of the *WWTR1-CAMTA1* fusion
gene (*C*).

features of EFH suggested it may be a distinct biologic entity, and this has been further supported by recent studies identifying recurrent *ALK* translocations in EFH.[69–71] Similar to conventional FH, EFH most often arises on the lower extremities of young to middle-age adults, forming papular or polypoid, solitary, skin-colored lesions. EFH is a benign tumor, with only exceptional cases of recurrence or metastasis reported in the literature.[72,73]

Like conventional FH, EFH is dermal-based, but may show focal extension into subcutaneous tissue. It differs, however, from all other varieties of FH in that it frequently has an epidermal collarette and does not show peripheral dermal collagen entrapment (**Fig. 4**). The tumor cells have round to oval nuclei with vesicular chromatin and small eosinophilic nucleoli, and moderate amounts of palely eosinophilic cytoplasm, imparting an epithelioid appearance. By definition, more than 50% of the cells should have an epithelioid appearance, although typically almost all tumor cells within a given lesion are epithelioid. Binucleate forms are frequently seen, whereas multinucleated cells are less common than in conventional FH (see **Fig. 4**). The stroma is loosely collagenous or hyalinized and contains numerous thin-walled and thick-walled small vessels.[68,72,74–76] Approximately 60% of EFH show diffuse membranous positivity for EMA, a finding not seen in conventional FH,[75] and approximately 50% show focal positivity for D2-40. SMA and desmin, which show variable positivity in conventional FH, and are typically negative in EFH, as are S100, AE1/AE3, CD45, CD34 and CD163.[75,77,78]

Two small recent studies demonstrated recurrent *ALK* rearrangements in 2 cases each of "atypical FH with epithelioid features" and EFH; in the latter study *ALK* gene rearrangements resulted in the formation of *VCL-ALK* and *SQSTM1-ALK* gene fusions.[70,71] Subsequently, a large clinicopathologic study of 33 cases of EFH demonstrated consistent diffuse cytoplasmic expression of ALK by immunohistochemistry, which correlated to the presence of *ALK* gene rearrangement by FISH (see **Fig. 4**). Several histologic mimics, including cutaneous syncytial myoepithelioma and atypical fibroxanthoma were negative for ALK.[69] ALK expression by immunohistochemistry is therefore a useful surrogate for genetic testing and is helpful in distinguishing EFH from histologic mimics. Of note, approximately 10% of Spitz nevi harbor *ALK* rearrangements and ALK expression.[79] Melanocytic markers, such as S100 protein and Mart-1, are positive in Spitz nevi, and therefore can distinguish from EFH in difficult cases.

ALK is a receptor tyrosine kinase that transmits extracellular signals via MAPK, PI3K, and NFk-B pathways. Genomic alterations in *ALK* have been implicated in the pathogenesis of a variety of tumor types, including lymphoma, lung adenocarcinoma, inflammatory myofibroblastic tumor, and neuroblastoma.[80–85] Although all these events appear to lead to increased ALK expression and activity, it remains unclear why some *ALK*-rearranged tumors follow a benign course and others show highly aggressive malignant behavior.

**Key Points**
**EPITHELIOID FIBROUS HISTIOCYTOMA**

- Skin-colored papule on the lower extremities of young to middle-aged adults

- Epidermal collarette, epithelioid cells, commonly with binucleate forms

- Fine collagenous stroma with prominent small vessels

- Positive for EMA and ALK

- *ALK* gene rearrangement is common and results in overexpression of ALK

## CUTANEOUS MYOEPITHELIAL TUMORS

Cutaneous myoepithelial tumors include chondroid syringoma, myoepithelioma, and myoepithelial carcinoma. Chondroid syringoma, also known as mixed tumor, is a benign neoplasm analogous to pleomorphic adenoma of the salivary gland. The typical presentation is a solitary, painless nodule on the head and neck area, usually in males. They arise in the dermis or subcutis, have a lobulated architecture and well-circumscribed borders. Epithelial and myoepithelial cells are present in varying proportions in a chondromyxoid or hyalinized stroma. The epithelial cells may be distributed as single cells, cords, nests, or as ductal structures. The myoepithelial cells are frequently spindled and may form a wide array of architectural patterns. Areas of chondroid differentiation may be present. By immunohistochemistry, the epithelial component is positive for keratins and EMA, whereas the myoepithelial component is positive for S100 and less commonly other markers of myoepithelial differentiation including p63, GFAP, and SMA.[86,87] Molecular studies of cutaneous mixed tumor reveal the presence of *PLAG1* rearrangements similar to that seen in pleomorphic adenoma. As a result of this translocation, tumor cells show strong diffuse nuclear positivity for PLAG1 protein by immunohistochemistry.[88–90]

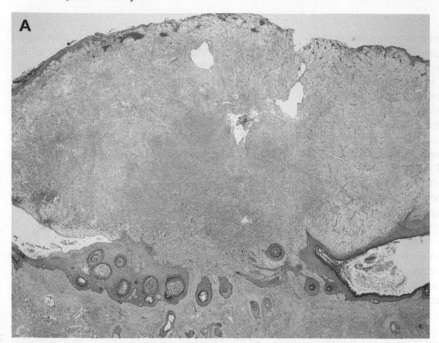

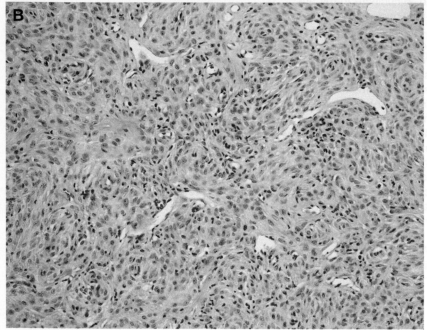

*Fig. 4.* Epithelioid fibrous histiocytoma is usually exophytic and has an epidermal collarette (*A*). The tumor cells show a sheetlike or storiform growth pattern, and prominent small to medium-sized blood vessels are common (*B*).

Cutaneous myoepitheliomas are composed of a pure myoepithelial cell population that lacks the epithelial component found in chondroid syringoma. Cutaneous syncytial myoepithelioma is a variant of cutaneous myoepithelioma with distinct histologic and immunohistochemical characteristics. These dermal tumors show a solid, sheetlike growth of a uniform population of ovoid to spindled cells with pale eosinophilic cytoplasm and ill-defined cell borders that impart a syncytial appearance to the cells (**Fig. 5**). Little intercellular stroma is present. Almost all cases show expression of both EMA and S100 by immunohistochemistry and are negative for cytokeratin (see **Fig. 5**). More than 80% of cutaneous syncytial myoepitheliomas harbor an *EWSR1* arrangement by FISH studies; however, no fusion partners have been identified to date.[91,92] The main differential diagnosis is EFH; immunohistochemistry for EMA, S100, and ALK readily distinguishes the two.

*Fig. 4.* (*continued*). The cells are round to polygonal and have abundant palely eosinophilic cytoplasm and frequent binucleate forms (*C*). Diffuse cytoplasmic expression of ALK is present in the vast majority of cases, reflecting the presence of an *ALK* gene rearrangement (*D*).

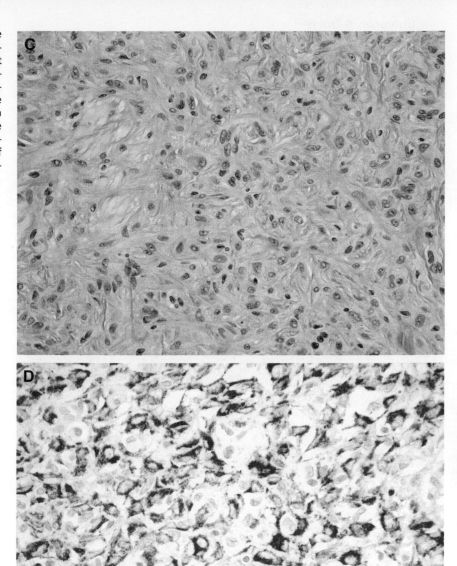

## Key Points
### CUTANEOUS SYNCYTIAL MYOEPITHELIOMA

- Painless nodule on the extremities, dermal-based

- Sheets of epithelioid to spindled cells with pale cytoplasm and minimal stroma

- Tumor cells express EMA and S100

- *EWSR1* rearrangement in greater than 80%

## CLEAR CELL SARCOMA

The main role that molecular diagnostics plays in the evaluation of cutaneous mesenchymal neoplasms is in the diagnosis of clear cell sarcoma (CCS). CCS arises on the extremities (usually ankle or foot) of young to middle-age adults in association with tendons and aponeuroses and often involves superficial subcutis or dermis.[93] Local recurrence is common and as many as 50% of patients will develop metastases, although distant spread tends to occur after many years.[94–97]

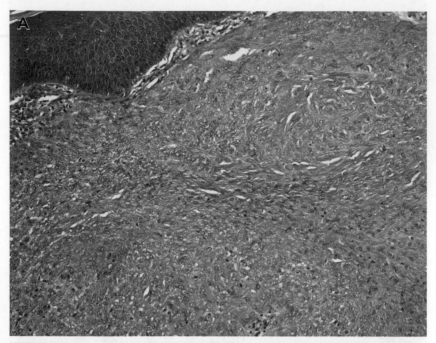

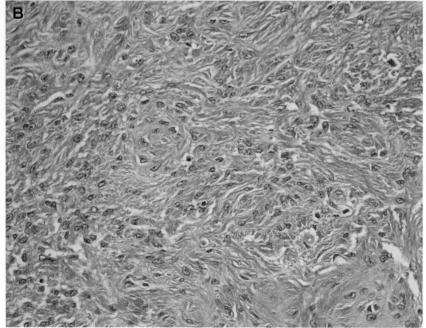

*Fig. 5.* Cutaneous syncytial myoepithelioma is usually well circumscribed and located in the superficial dermis (*A*). Tumor cells are ovoid and relatively monotonous with minimal atypia and pale eosinophilic cytoplasm with indistinct cell borders, which imparts a syncytial appearance (*B*).

Wide surgical excision and adjuvant radiotherapy is the standard of care.

Most tumors are smaller than 5 cm at the time of diagnosis and have well-circumscribed borders and a yellow to white-gray cut surface. Histologically, CCS is composed of nests and fascicles of epithelioid to spindled cells within a delicate fibrocollagenous stroma (**Fig. 6**). The cells have indistinct cell borders, palely eosinophilic to amphophilic cytoplasm, round nucleoli, and prominent macronucleoli. Cells with clear cytoplasm are uncommon. Multinucleate, Touton-like cells are commonly present (see **Fig. 6**). Mitotic activity is typically low and necrosis is rare. Scattered cells may contain melanin pigment.[94,95,98,99]

*Fig. 5. (continued).* The characteristic immuno-profile of cutaneous syncytial myoepithelioma is that of coexpression of S100 protein (*C*) and EMA (*D*).

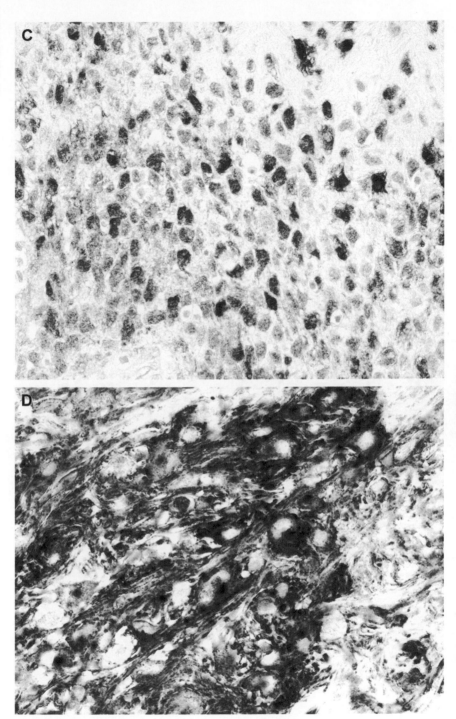

The tumor cells of CCS express at least one marker of melanocytic differentiation. Nearly all tumors are positive for S100 and most express HMB45, Mart-1, and/or Mitf (see **Fig. 6**).[99,100] Most CCS harbor a recurrent t(12;22) (q13;q12) that creates a fusion protein composed of the N-terminal portion of EWSR1, whose gene is located on chromosome 22, and the basic leucine zipper of ATF1, a transcriptional activator located on chromosome 12.[99,101–103] The fusion results in cAMP-independent gene activation, including activation of *MITF*, a master regulator of melanocytic differentiation. An alternate translocation t(2;22) (q34;q12) involving *EWSR1* and *CREB1* occurs in a smaller number of cases.[99,104]

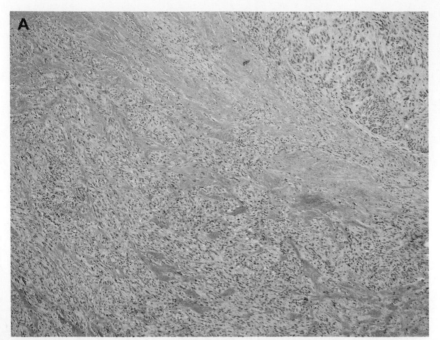

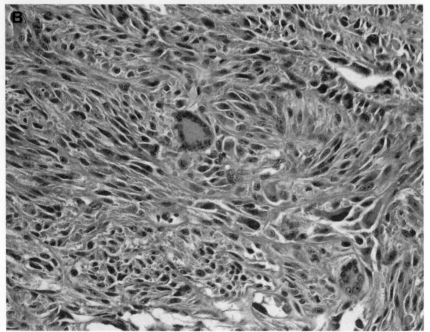

*Fig. 6.* CCS characteristically has a nested architecture (*A*), and is composed of spindle cells with variable amounts of palely eosinophilic cytoplasm, prominent nucleoli, and minimal mitotic activity; Touton-type giant cells are commonly present (*B*).

The main differential diagnosis of CCS is malignant melanoma. Distinguishing melanoma from CCS can be extremely difficult, particularly in core biopsy samples, due to overlapping histologic and immunohistochemical features. The tumor cells of CCS characteristically show more intense or diffuse staining for HMB-45 compared with S100, a finding that is uncommon in melanoma. However, this feature alone is generally not reliable enough in a given case to distinguish these two tumor types, and distinction relies on a combination of clinicopathologic and molecular features. Histologic features that favor a diagnosis of CCS include lack of a superficial epidermal component, infiltration of tendinous tissue by tumor in a nested pattern, multinucleate tumor cells, and the presence of only mild atypia and pleomorphism. However, in many cases, the histologic and

*Fig. 6. (continued).* Tumor cells show expression of S100 protein (*C*) and HMB-45 (*D*), as well as other melanocytic markers.

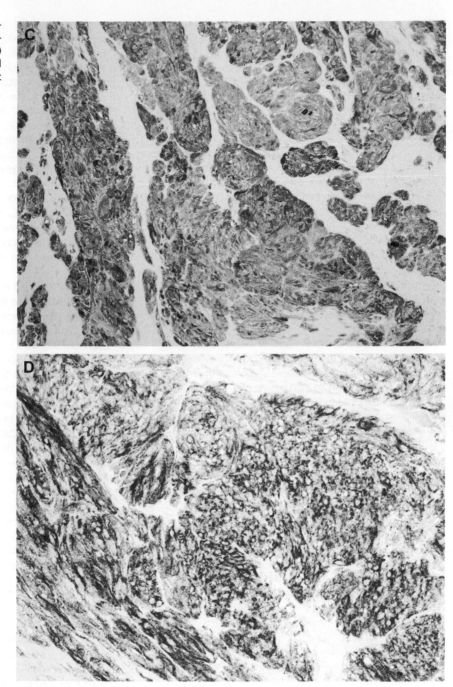

immunohistochemical overlap is sufficient enough that FISH to identify the *EWSR1* rearrangement of CCS is needed to exclude melanoma.

## SUMMARY

Over the past few years, insights into the genetic characterization of several different cutaneous mesenchymal neoplasms has allowed for the description of new tumor types, refinements in tumor classification, and the development of novel diagnostic markers, and therefore these insights have had significant diagnostic, therapeutic, and prognostic implications. Although the use of molecular diagnostic studies, such as FISH or RT-PCR, is relatively limited in the evaluation of cutaneous mesenchymal neoplasms, protein correlates of molecular alterations, such as FOSB,

CAMTA1, ALK, and PLAG1, are very useful diagnostic immunohistochemical markers in clinical practice. This review details important advances in the histologic and genetic classification of a diverse group of mesenchymal neoplasms of the skin along with their associated clinical and diagnostic implications.

## REFERENCES

1. Mirra JM, Kessler S, Bhuta S, et al. The fibroma-like variant of epithelioid sarcoma. A fibrohistiocytic/myoid cell lesion often confused with benign and malignant spindle cell tumors. Cancer 1992;69(6): 1382–95.
2. Hornick JL, Fletcher CD. Pseudomyogenic hemangioendothelioma: a distinctive, often multicentric tumor with indolent behavior. Am J Surg Pathol 2011; 35(2):190–201.
3. Mangham DC, Kindblom LG. Rarely metastasizing soft tissue tumours. Histopathology 2014;64(1): 88–100.
4. Hornick JL, Dal Cin P, Fletcher CD. Loss of INI1 expression is characteristic of both conventional and proximal-type epithelioid sarcoma. Am J Surg Pathol 2009;33(4):542–50.
5. Trombetta D, Magnusson L, von Steyern FV, et al. Translocation t(7;19)(q22;q13)—a recurrent chromosome aberration in pseudomyogenic hemangioendothelioma? Cancer Genet 2011;204(4):211–5.
6. Walther C, Tayebwa J, Lilljebjörn H, et al. A novel SERPINE1-FOSB fusion gene results in transcriptional up-regulation of FOSB in pseudomyogenic haemangioendothelioma. J Pathol 2014;232(5): 534–40.
7. Sugita S, Hirano H, Kikuchi N, et al. Diagnostic utility of FOSB immunohistochemistry in pseudomyogenic hemangioendothelioma and its histological mimics. Diagn Pathol 2016;11(1):75.
8. Hung YP, Fletcher CD, Hornick JL. FOSB is a useful diagnostic marker for pseudomyogenic hemangioendothelioma. Am J Surg Pathol 2016, [Epub ahead of print].
9. Simpson AJ, Booth NA, Moore NR, et al. Distribution of plasminogen activator inhibitor (PAI-1) in tissues. J Clin Pathol 1991;44(2):139–43.
10. Declerck PJ, Gils A. Three decades of research on plasminogen activator inhibitor-1: a multifaceted serpin. Semin Thromb Hemost 2013;39(4):356–64.
11. Milde-Langosch K. The Fos family of transcription factors and their role in tumourigenesis. Eur J Cancer 2005;41(16):2449–61.
12. Shaulian E. AP-1–The Jun proteins: Oncogenes or tumor suppressors in disguise? Cell Signal 2010; 22(6):894–9.
13. Sabatakos G, Sims NA, Chen J, et al. Overexpression of DeltaFosB transcription factor(s) increases bone formation and inhibits adipogenesis. Nat Med 2000;6(9):985–90.
14. Ohnishi YN, Sakumi K, Yamazaki K, et al. Antagonistic regulation of cell-matrix adhesion by FosB and DeltaFosB/Delta2DeltaFosB encoded by alternatively spliced forms of fosB transcripts. Mol Biol Cell 2008;19(11):4717–29.
15. Sabatakos G, Rowe GC, Kveiborg M, et al. Doubly truncated FosB isoform (Delta2DeltaFosB) induces osteosclerosis in transgenic mice and modulates expression and phosphorylation of Smads in osteoblasts independent of intrinsic AP-1 activity. J Bone Miner Res 2008;23(5):584–95.
16. Huang SC, Zhang L, Sung YS, et al. Frequent FOS gene rearrangements in epithelioid hemangioma: a molecular study of 58 cases with morphologic reappraisal. Am J Surg Pathol 2015;39(10): 1313–21.
17. Antonescu CR, Chen HW, Zhang L, et al. ZFP36-FOSB fusion defines a subset of epithelioid hemangioma with atypical features. Genes Chromosomes Cancer 2014;53(11):951–9.
18. Rosenberg AE. WHO classification of soft tissue and bone, fourth edition: summary and commentary. Curr Opin Oncol 2013;25(5):571–3.
19. Jo VY, Fletcher CD. WHO classification of soft tissue tumours: an update based on the 2013 (4th) edition. Pathology 2014;46(2):95–104.
20. Mentzel T, Beham A, Calonje E, et al. Epithelioid hemangioendothelioma of skin and soft tissues: clinicopathologic and immunohistochemical study of 30 cases. Am J Surg Pathol 1997;21(4):363–74.
21. Quante M, Patel NK, Hill S, et al. Epithelioid hemangioendothelioma presenting in the skin: a clinicopathologic study of eight cases. Am J Dermatopathol 1998;20(6):541–6.
22. Clarke LE, Lee R, Militello G, et al. Cutaneous epithelioid hemangioendothelioma. J Cutan Pathol 2008;35(2):236–40.
23. Weiss SW, Enzinger FM. Epithelioid hemangioendothelioma: a vascular tumor often mistaken for a carcinoma. Cancer 1982;50(5):970–81.
24. Deyrup AT, Tighiouart M, Montag AG, et al. Epithelioid hemangioendothelioma of soft tissue: a proposal for risk stratification based on 49 cases. Am J Surg Pathol 2008;32(6):924–7.
25. Folpe AL, Chand EM, Goldblum JR, et al. Expression of Fli-1, a nuclear transcription factor, distinguishes vascular neoplasms from potential mimics. Am J Surg Pathol 2001;25(8):1061–6.
26. Miettinen M, Wang ZF, Paetau A, et al. ERG transcription factor as an immunohistochemical marker for vascular endothelial tumors and prostatic carcinoma. Am J Surg Pathol 2011;35(3):432–41.
27. Kleer CG, Unni KK, McLeod RA. Epithelioid hemangioendothelioma of bone. Am J Surg Pathol 1996;20(11):1301–11.

28. Makhlouf HR, Ishak KG, Goodman ZD. Epithelioid hemangioendothelioma of the liver: a clinicopathologic study of 137 cases. Cancer 1999;85(3):562–82.

29. Miettinen M, Fetsch JF. Distribution of keratins in normal endothelial cells and a spectrum of vascular tumors: implications in tumor diagnosis. Hum Pathol 2000;31(9):1062–7.

30. Mendlick MR, Nelson M, Pickering D, et al. Translocation t(1;3)(p36.3;q25) is a nonrandom aberration in epithelioid hemangioendothelioma. Am J Surg Pathol 2001;25(5):684–7.

31. Tanas MR, Sboner A, Oliveira AM, et al. Identification of a disease-defining gene fusion in epithelioid hemangioendothelioma. Sci Transl Med 2011; 3(98):98ra82.

32. Errani C, Zhang L, Sung YS, et al. A novel WWTR1-CAMTA1 gene fusion is a consistent abnormality in epithelioid hemangioendothelioma of different anatomic sites. Genes Chromosomes Cancer 2011;50(8):644–53.

33. Patel NR, Salim AA, Sayeed H, et al. Molecular characterization of epithelioid haemangioendotheliomas identifies novel WWTR1-CAMTA1 fusion variants. Histopathology 2015;67(5): 699–708.

34. Chan SW, Lim CJ, Chen L, et al. The Hippo pathway in biological control and cancer development. J Cell Physiol 2011;226(4):928–39.

35. Chan SW, Lim CJ, Guo K, et al. A role for TAZ in migration, invasion, and tumorigenesis of breast cancer cells. Cancer Res 2008;68(8):2592–8.

36. Balasenthil S, Chen N, Lott ST, et al. A migration signature and plasma biomarker panel for pancreatic adenocarcinoma. Cancer Prev Res (Phila) 2011;4(1):137–49.

37. Lei QY, Zhang H, Zhao B, et al. TAZ promotes cell proliferation and epithelial-mesenchymal transition and is inhibited by the hippo pathway. Mol Cell Biol 2008;28(7):2426–36.

38. Bouche N, Scharlat A, Snedden W, et al. A novel family of calmodulin-binding transcription activators in multicellular organisms. J Biol Chem 2002; 277(24):21851–61.

39. Doyle LA, Fletcher CD, Hornick JL. Nuclear expression of CAMTA1 distinguishes epithelioid hemangioendothelioma from histologic mimics. Am J Surg Pathol 2016;40(1):94–102.

40. Antonescu CR, Le Loarer F, Mosquera JM, et al. Novel YAP1-TFE3 fusion defines a distinct subset of epithelioid hemangioendothelioma. Genes Chromosomes Cancer 2013;52(8):775–84.

41. Antonescu C. Malignant vascular tumors–an update. Mod Pathol 2014;27(Suppl 1):S30–8.

42. Sidhar SK, Clark J, Gill S, et al. The t(X;1)(p11.2;q21.2) translocation in papillary renal cell carcinoma fuses a novel gene PRCC to the TFE3 transcription factor gene. Hum Mol Genet 1996;5(9):1333–8.

43. Clark J, Lu YJ, Sidhar SK, et al. Fusion of splicing factor genes PSF and NonO (p54nrb) to the TFE3 gene in papillary renal cell carcinoma. Oncogene 1997;15(18):2233–9.

44. Argani P, Antonescu CR, Illei PB, et al. Primary renal neoplasms with the ASPL-TFE3 gene fusion of alveolar soft part sarcoma: a distinctive tumor entity previously included among renal cell carcinomas of children and adolescents. Am J Pathol 2001;159(1):179–92.

45. Argani P, Lui MY, Couturier J, et al. A novel CLTC-TFE3 gene fusion in pediatric renal adenocarcinoma with t(X;17)(p11.2;q23). Oncogene 2003; 22(34):5374–8.

46. Ladanyi M, Lui MY, Antonescu CR, et al. The der(17)t(X;17)(p11;q25) of human alveolar soft part sarcoma fuses the TFE3 transcription factor gene to ASPL, a novel gene at 17q25. Oncogene 2001;20(1):48–57.

47. Marshall-Taylor C, Fanburg-Smith JC. Hemosiderotic fibrohistiocytic lipomatous lesion: ten cases of a previously undescribed fatty lesion of the foot/ ankle. Mod Pathol 2000;13(11):1192–9.

48. Browne TJ, Fletcher CD. Haemosiderotic fibrolipomatous tumour (so-called haemosiderotic fibrohistiocytic lipomatous tumour): analysis of 13 new cases in support of a distinct entity. Histopathology 2006;48(4):453–61.

49. Hallor KH, Sciot R, Staaf J, et al. Two genetic pathways, t(1;10) and amplification of 3p11-12, in myxoinflammatory fibroblastic sarcoma, haemosiderotic fibrolipomatous tumour, and morphologically similar lesions. J Pathol 2009; 217(5):716–27.

50. Antonescu CR, Zhang L, Nielsen GP, et al. Consistent t(1;10) with rearrangements of TGFBR3 and MGEA5 in both myxoinflammatory fibroblastic sarcoma and hemosiderotic fibrolipomatous tumor. Genes Chromosomes Cancer 2011;50(10):757–64.

51. Cools J, Mentens N, Odero MD, et al. Evidence for position effects as a variant ETV6-mediated leukemogenic mechanism in myeloid leukemias with a t(4;12)(q11-q12;p13) or t(5;12)(q31;p13). Blood 2002;99(5):1776–84.

52. Thisse B, Thisse C. Functions and regulations of fibroblast growth factor signaling during embryonic development. Developmental Biol 2005;287(2): 390–402.

53. Valta MP, Hentunen T, Qu Q, et al. Regulation of osteoblast differentiation: a novel function for fibroblast growth factor 8. Endocrinology 2006;147(5): 2171–82.

54. Ishibe T, Nakayama T, Okamoto T, et al. Disruption of fibroblast growth factor signal pathway inhibits the growth of synovial sarcomas: potential application of signal inhibitors to molecular target therapy. Clin Cancer Res 2005;11(7):2702–12.

55. Tanaka A, Furuya A, Yamasaki M, et al. High frequency of fibroblast growth factor (FGF) 8 expression in clinical prostate cancers and breast tissues, immunohistochemically demonstrated by a newly established neutralizing monoclonal antibody against FGF 8. Cancer Res 1998;58(10):2053–6.

56. Mattila MM, Harkonen PL. Role of fibroblast growth factor 8 in growth and progression of hormonal cancer. Cytokine Growth Factor Rev 2007; 18(3–4):257–66.

57. Faucheux C, Naye F, Treguer K, et al. Vestigial like gene family expression in *Xenopus*: common and divergent features with other vertebrates. Int J Dev Biol 2010;54(8–9):1375–82.

58. Halperin DS, Pan C, Lusis AJ, et al. Vestigial-like 3 is an inhibitor of adipocyte differentiation. J Lipid Res 2013;54(2):473–81.

59. Carter JM, Sukov WR, Montgomery E, et al. TGFBR3 and MGEA5 rearrangements in pleomorphic hyalinizing angiectatic tumors and the spectrum of related neoplasms. Am J Surg Pathol 2014;38(9):1182–992.

60. Elco CP, Mariño-Enríquez A, Abraham JA, et al. Hybrid myxoinflammatory fibroblastic sarcoma/hemosiderotic fibrolipomatous tumor: report of a case providing further evidence for a pathogenetic link. Am J Surg Pathol 2010;34(11):1723–7.

61. Meis-Kindblom JM, Kindblom LG. Acral myxoinflammatory fibroblastic sarcoma: a low-grade tumor of the hands and feet. Am J Surg Pathol 1998;22(8):911–24.

62. Jurcic V, Zidar A, Montiel MD, et al. Myxoinflammatory fibroblastic sarcoma: a tumor not restricted to acral sites. Ann Diagn Pathol 2002;6(5):272–80.

63. Smith ME, Fisher C, Weiss SW. Pleomorphic hyalinizing angiectatic tumor of soft parts. A low-grade neoplasm resembling neurilemoma. Am J Surg Pathol 1996;20(1):21–9.

64. Folpe AL, Weiss SW. Pleomorphic hyalinizing angiectatic tumor: analysis of 41 cases supporting evolution from a distinctive precursor lesion. Am J Surg Pathol 2004;28(11):1417–25.

65. Płaszczyca A, Nilsson J, Magnusson L, et al. Fusions involving protein kinase C and membrane-associated proteins in benign fibrous histiocytoma. Int J Biochem Cell Biol 2014;53:475–81.

66. Walther C, Hofvander J, Nilsson J, et al. Gene fusion detection in formalin-fixed paraffin-embedded benign fibrous histiocytomas using fluorescence in situ hybridization and RNA sequencing. Lab Invest 2015;95(9):1071–6.

67. Zeng L, Webster SV, Newton PM. The biology of protein kinase C. Adv Exp Med Biol 2012;740: 639–61.

68. Jones EW, Cerio R, Smith NP. Epithelioid cell histiocytoma: a new entity. Br J Dermatol 1989;120(2). 185–95.

69. Doyle LA, Mariño-Enriquez A, Fletcher CD, et al. ALK rearrangement and overexpression in epithelioid fibrous histiocytoma. Mod Pathol 2015;28(7): 904–12.

70. Szablewski V, Laurent-Roussel S, Rethers L, et al. Atypical fibrous histiocytoma of the skin with CD30 and p80/ALK1 positivity and ALK gene rearrangement. J Cutan Pathol 2014;41(9):715–9.

71. Jedrych J, Nikiforova M, Kennedy TF, et al. Epithelioid cell histiocytoma of the skin with clonal ALK gene rearrangement resulting in VCL-ALK and SQSTM1-ALK gene fusions. Br J Dermatol 2015; 172(5):1427–9.

72. Singh Gomez C, Calonje E, Fletcher CD. Epithelioid benign fibrous histiocytoma of skin: clinico-pathological analysis of 20 cases of a poorly known variant. Histopathology 1994;24(2):123–9.

73. Doyle LA, Fletcher CD. Metastasizing "benign" cutaneous fibrous histiocytoma: a clinicopathologic analysis of 16 cases. Am J Surg Pathol 2013;37(4): 484–95.

74. Glusac EJ, Barr RJ, Everett MA, et al. Epithelioid cell histiocytoma. A report of 10 cases including a new cellular variant. Am J Surg Pathol 1994;18(6): 583–90.

75. Doyle LA, Fletcher CDM. EMA positivity in epithelioid fibrous histiocytoma: a potential diagnostic pitfall. J Cutan Pathol 2011;38(9):697–703.

76. Glusac EJ, McNiff JM. Epithelioid cell histiocytoma: a simulant of vascular and melanocytic neoplasms. Am J Dermatopathol 1999;21(1):1–7.

77. Volpicelli ER, Fletcher CD. Desmin and CD34 positivity in cellular fibrous histiocytoma: an immuno-histochemical analysis of 100 cases. J Cutan Pathol 2012;39(8):747–52.

78. Soini Y. Cell differentiation in benign cutaneous fibrous histiocytomas. An immunohistochemical study with antibodies to histiomonocytic cells and intermediate filament proteins. Am J Dermatopathol 1990;12(2):134–40.

79. Wiesner T, He J, Yelensky R, et al. Kinase fusions are frequent in Spitz tumours and spitzoid melanomas. Nat Commun 2014;5:3116.

80. Morris SW, Kirstein MN, Valentine MB, et al. Fusion of a kinase gene, ALK, to a nucleolar protein gene, NPM, in non-Hodgkin's lymphoma. Science 1994; 263(5151):1281–4.

81. Lawrence B, Perez-Atayde A, Hibbard MK, et al. TPM3-ALK and TPM4-ALK oncogenes in inflammatory myofibroblastic tumors. Am J Pathol 2000; 157(2):377–84.

82. George RE, Sanda T, Hanna M, et al. Activating mutations in ALK provide a therapeutic target in neuroblastoma. Nature 2008;455(7215):975–8.

83. Chen Y, Takita J, Choi YL, et al. Oncogenic mutations of ALK kinase in neuroblastoma. Nature 2008;455(7215):971–4.

84. Janoueix-Lerosey I, Lequin D, Brugieres L, et al. Somatic and germline activating mutations of the ALK kinase receptor in neuroblastoma. Nature 2008;455(7215):967–70.

85. Mosse YP, Laudenslager M, Longo L, et al. Identification of ALK as a major familial neuroblastoma predisposition gene. Nature 2008;455(7215): 930–5.

86. Kilpatrick SE, Hitchcock MG, Kraus MD, et al. Mixed tumors and myoepitheliomas of soft tissue: a clinicopathologic study of 19 cases with a unifying concept. Am J Surg Pathol 1997;21(1):13–22.

87. Hornick JL, Fletcher CD. Myoepithelial tumors of soft tissue: a clinicopathologic and immunohistochemical study of 101 cases with evaluation of prognostic parameters. Am J Surg Pathol 2003; 27(9):1183–96.

88. Antonescu CR, Zhang L, Shao SY, et al. Frequent PLAG1 gene rearrangements in skin and soft tissue myoepithelioma with ductal differentiation. Genes Chromosomes Cancer 2013;52(7):675–82.

89. Bahrami A, Dalton JD, Krane JF, et al. A subset of cutaneous and soft tissue mixed tumors are genetically linked to their salivary gland counterpart. Genes Chromosomes Cancer 2012;51(2):140–8.

90. Matsuyama A, Hisaoka M, Hashimoto H. PLAG1 expression in cutaneous mixed tumors: an immunohistochemical and molecular genetic study. Virchows Arch 2011;459(5):539–45.

91. Hornick JL, Fletcher CD. Cutaneous myoepithelioma: a clinicopathologic and immunohistochemical study of 14 cases. Hum Pathol 2004;35(1): 14–24.

92. Jo VY, Antonescu CR, Zhang L, et al. Cutaneous syncytial myoepithelioma: clinicopathologic characterization in a series of 38 cases. Am J Surg Pathol 2013;37(5):710–8.

93. Kawai A, Hosono A, Nakayama R, et al. Clear cell sarcoma of tendons and aponeuroses: a study of 75 patients. Cancer 2007;109(1):109–16.

94. Enzinger FM. Clear-cell sarcoma of tendons and aponeuroses. An analysis of 21 cases. Cancer 1965;18:1163–74.

95. Hoffman GJ, Carter D. Clear cell sarcoma of tendons and aponeuroses with melanin. Arch Pathol 1973;95(1):22–5.

96. Ekfors TO, Rantakokko V. Clear cell sarcoma of tendons and aponeuroses: malignant melanoma of soft tissues? Report of four cases. Pathol Res Pract 1979;165(4):422–8.

97. Chung EB, Enzinger FM. Malignant melanoma of soft parts. A reassessment of clear cell sarcoma. Am J Surg Pathol 1983;7(5):405–13.

98. Bearman RM, Noe J, Kempson RL. Clear cell sarcoma with melanin pigment. Cancer 1975;36(3): 977–84.

99. Hisaoka M, Ishida T, Kuo TT, et al. Clear cell sarcoma of soft tissue: a clinicopathologic, immunohistochemical, and molecular analysis of 33 cases. Am J Surg Pathol 2008;32(3):452–60.

100. Granter SR, Weilbaecher KN, Quigley C, et al. Clear cell sarcoma shows immunoreactivity for microphthalmia transcription factor: further evidence for melanocytic differentiation. Mod Pathol 2001; 14(1):6–9.

101. Panagopoulos I, Mertens F, Debiec-Rychter M, et al. Molecular genetic characterization of the EWS/ATF1 fusion gene in clear cell sarcoma of tendons and aponeuroses. Int J Cancer 2002;99(4): 560–7.

102. Coindre JM, Hostein I, Terrier P, et al. Diagnosis of clear cell sarcoma by real-time reverse transcriptase-polymerase chain reaction analysis of paraffin embedded tissues: clinicopathologic and molecular analysis of 44 patients from the French sarcoma group. Cancer 2006;107(5):1055–64.

103. Antonescu CR, Tschernyavsky SJ, Woodruff JM, et al. Molecular diagnosis of clear cell sarcoma: detection of EWS-ATF1 and MITF-M transcripts and histopathological and ultrastructural analysis of 12 cases. J Mol Diagn 2002;4(1):44–52.

104. Wang WL, Mayordomo E, Zhang W, et al. Detection and characterization of EWSR1/ATF1 and EWSR1/CREB1 chimeric transcripts in clear cell sarcoma (melanoma of soft parts). Mod Pathol 2009;22(9): 1201–9.

# Atypical Fibroxanthoma Revisited

Thomas Mentzel, MD[a],*, Luis Requena, MD[b], Thomas Brenn, MD, PhD[c]

## KEYWORDS

- Atypical fibroxanthoma • Pleomorphic dermal sarcoma • Mesenchymal neoplasms
- Immunohistochemistry • Differential diagnosis

## Key Points

- Atypical fibroxanthoma is a rare dermal-based mesenchymal neoplasm occurring almost exclusively in sun-damaged skin of elderly patients (men are more frequently affected), especially in the head and neck area.

- Atypical fibroxanthoma is characterized by an exophytic growth and represents a well-circumscribed pleomorphic neoplasm with increased proliferative activity, but lacks tumor necrosis and an infiltrative growth.

- The diagnosis of atypical fibroxanthoma is a diagnosis of exclusion, should never made on a superficial biopsy only, and includes a panel of immunohistochemical antibodies.

- The morphologic spectrum of atypical fibroxanthoma is broad and includes a number of variants.

- If strict diagnostic criteria are applied, the clinical behavior of atypical fibroxanthoma is benign.

- The relationship of atypical fibroxanthoma and pleomorphic dermal sarcoma is still under debate.

## ABSTRACT

Atypical fibroxanthoma (AFX) represents a rare mesenchymal neoplasm arising predominantly in the head and neck area of elderly patients. Clinically, the neoplasm is characterized by a rapid and exophytic growth with frequent ulceration of the epidermis. Histopathologically, AFX represents a well-circumscribed, dermal-based neoplasm composed of a variable admixture of large histiocytoid cells, enlarged spindled and epithelioid tumor cells, and multinucleated tumor giant cells with bizarre and pleomorphic nuclei. If strict diagnostic criteria are applied, the clinical behavior of AFX is benign in most cases, and complete excision represents the treatment of choice.

## OVERVIEW

Atypical fibroxanthoma (AFX) is defined in the World Health Organization classification of tumors of soft tissue and bone as a benign, dermal neoplasm of uncertain line of differentiation.[1] The term AFX was used in the 1960s and 1970s to describe a morphologically pleomorphic and proliferative active dermal neoplasm that is characterized clinically by an almost always benign clinical course despite worrisome morphologic features.[2,3] AFX has been regarded as a so-called fibrohistiocytic tumor and the cutaneous counterpart of "malignant fibrous histiocytoma" of deep soft tissues ("MFH"). However, given the rather nonspecific electron microscopic and immunohistochemical findings, the fibrohistiocytic

Statements: The authors declare that the study was done according to the ethical standards, there is no funding, and the authors have no conflict of interest.
[a] Dermatopathology, Bodensee, Siemensstrasse 6/1, Friedrichshafen D-88048, Germany; [b] Department of Dermatology, Fundacion Jimenez Diaz, Madrid, Spain; [c] Department of Pathology, University of Edinburgh, United Kingdom
* Corresponding author.
E-mail address: mentzel@dermpath.de

Surgical Pathology 10 (2017) 319–335
http://dx.doi.org/10.1016/j.path.2017.01.007

line of differentiation has been questioned in AFX and "MFH,"[4] and it became obvious that the diagnosis of AFX is a diagnosis of exclusion. Although AFX has been studied in detail over more than 50 years, there is an ongoing debate about its exact relationship to sarcomatoid squamous cell carcinoma and pleomorphic dermal sarcoma (PDS). It has been even suggested recently that AFX, PDS, and sarcomalike tumors with immunohistochemical evidence of epithelial differentiation are related, and the term "sarcomalike tumor" was used for these neoplasms.[5] The clinicopathological and immunohistochemical features of AFX are described in this review, and the differential diagnosis with special emphasis to PDS is discussed.

## CLINICAL FEATURES

AFX is a classic tumor of elderly patients, and most neoplasms occur in the sun-exposed head and neck area with chronic sun-damaged skin, especially in elderly male patients. The upper extremities and the back of the hands are only rarely affected, and cases arising in children with xeroderma pigmentosum are exceedingly rare.[6] Clinically, cases of AFX are described as fast-growing, exophytic, dome-shaped, solid nodules that are often ulcerated. The size of the neoplasms rarely exceeds 2 cm in diameter (Fig. 1). In contrast, PDS is often rather asymmetrical and larger; however, the clinical picture does not allow a reliable distinction (Fig. 2).

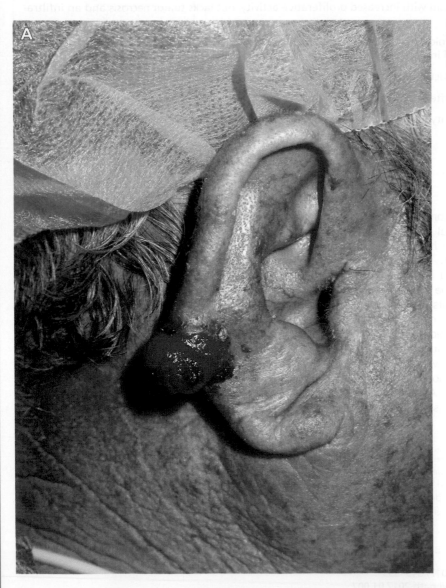

Fig. 1. Clinically, AFX is characterized as a small, exophytic growing lesion, which is often ulcerated (A, B).

*Fig. 1.* (*continued*).

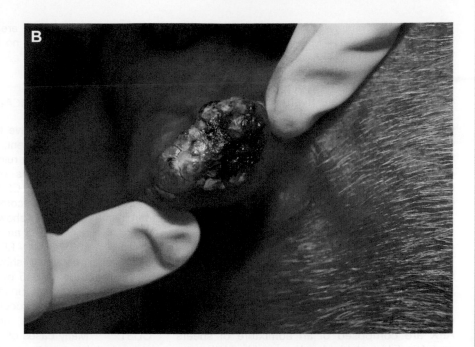

Cases of reported AFX arising in young patients in non–sun-exposed areas most likely represent cases of atypical dermatofibroma. In a recent review of almost 3000 cases of AFX, rare cases arising at the trunk and the limbs have been mentioned; however, old cases with no or limited immunohistochemical stainings were included in this review as well, which represents a bias.[7]

Applying strict diagnostic criteria, most cases of AFX show a benign clinical behavior, local recurrences are rare, and distant metastases exceptional.[8] Cases of AFX with documented metastases may have no or only limited study by immunohistochemistry and may show invasion, tumor necrosis, and/or lymphovascular and perineurial infiltration. Complete excision is regarded as the treatment of choice.

*Fig. 2.* A case of PDS presenting as a rather ill-defined, nodular lesion.

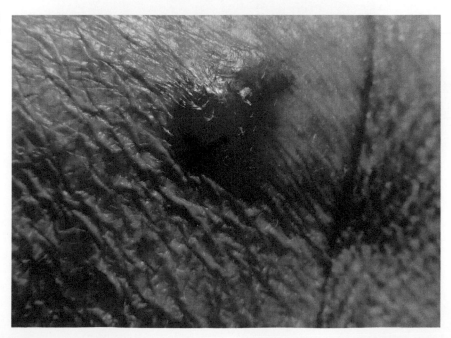

## HISTOPATHOLOGICAL FEATURES

The histopathological criteria for the diagnosis of AFX must be used very strictly to avoid misdiagnosis of a more or less aggressive neoplasm, resulting in inadequate treatment of the patient. Given the problematic distinction of cellular dermatofibroma, PDS, malignant melanoma, poorly differentiated sarcomatous carcinoma, and sarcomas of other lines of differentiation, the diagnosis of AFX should never be made on a small biopsy only, or without the use of a panel of immunohistochemical antibodies. Typically, AFX represents a dermal-based mesenchymal neoplasm that is characterized by an exophytic growth and a nodular or polypoid configuration. The neoplasm is often ulcerated and a collaret formation of the lateral epidermis is frequently seen. The symmetric and well-circumscribed tumor shows no diffuse infiltration of the subcutis or deeper structures (**Fig. 3**). Typical cases of AFX are composed of an admixture of sheets and fascicles of highly pleomorphic histiocyte-like cells, atypical multinucleated tumor giant cells, a variable number of enlarged and atypical spindled and epithelioid cells, and associated inflammatory cells. Tumor cells contain enlarged and vesicular or hyperchromatic nuclei and numerous mitoses, including atypical mitotic figures, are present (**Fig. 4**). Despite worrisome morphologic features and an increased proliferative activity, no areas of tumor necrosis are noted and there is no lymphovascular and/or perineural invasion.

## IMMUNOHISTOCHEMICAL FEATURES

Unfortunately, no positive immunohistochemical marker for AFX is present, and a panel of antibodies must be used in ruling out the differential diagnoses. Tumor cells of classic AFX stain positively for vimentin, CD10, and p53 (**Fig. 5**); however, cases of sarcomatoid squamous cell carcinoma also may show these results.[9] By definition, cases of AFX are negative for pancytokeratin, S-100, CD34, ERG, desmin, and h-caldesmon, but may show an expression of Melan-A and/or HMB45 by multinucleated giant cells, as well as an unspecific expression of MiTF1, factor XIIIa, procollagen 1, EMA, p63, CD99, CD68, and a granular positivity of CD31.[10–15] Many cases of AFX show an expression of alpha-smooth muscle actin[16,17] (**Fig. 6**) and calponin,[18] suggestive of fibroblastic/myofibroblastic differentiation. The presence of scattered S-100 positive dendritic cells in cases of AFX should not be misdiagnosed as a melanocytic differentiation. Given that cases of poorly differentiated sarcomatoid carcinoma may show a loss of cytokeratin expression, multiple keratin antibodies should be used.

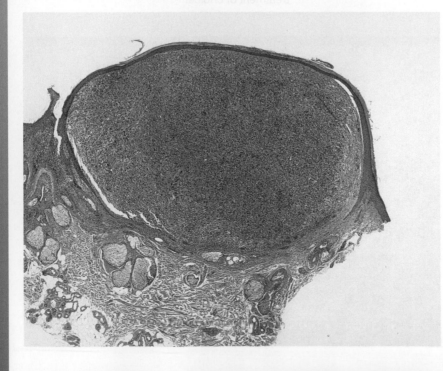

**Fig. 3.** Low-power view of an AFX shows a nodular and well-circumscribed neoplasm. Note the collaret formation of the hyperplastic epidermis.

*Fig. 4.* A cellular neoplasm composed of sheets of enlarged and pleomorphic histiocytoid cells seen (*A*). This AFX shows an admixture of enlarged and pleomorphic spindled, round and multinucleated cells. Numerous mitoses are detected (*B*).

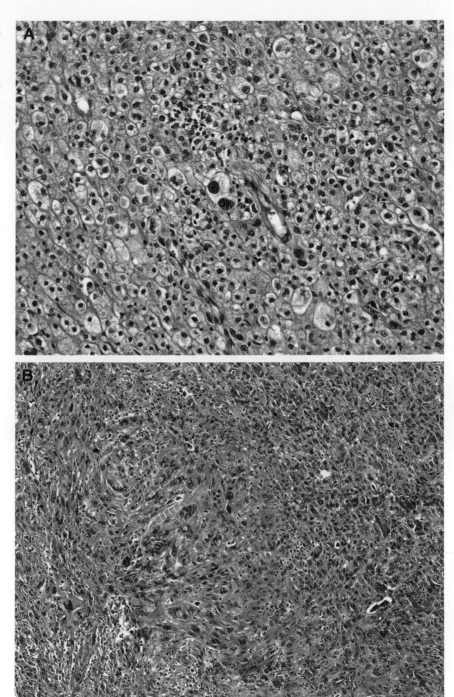

## MOLECULAR FEATURES

Sun-exposed skin represents the most frequent site of occurrence of AFX but also of squamous cell carcinoma, basal cell carcinoma, and malignant melanoma. UV radiation induces DNA mutations and an inactivation and mutation of the p53 tumor suppressor gene.[19] It has been shown convincingly that cases of AFX show an abnormal accumulation of p53 with strong nuclear immunopositivity and a characteristic p53 mutation pattern different from that of undifferentiated pleomorphic sarcoma of soft tissues, emphasizing also on this level that AFX/PDS are biologically different neoplasms.[20] In addition, it has been shown that cases of AFX show a rather diploid distribution of

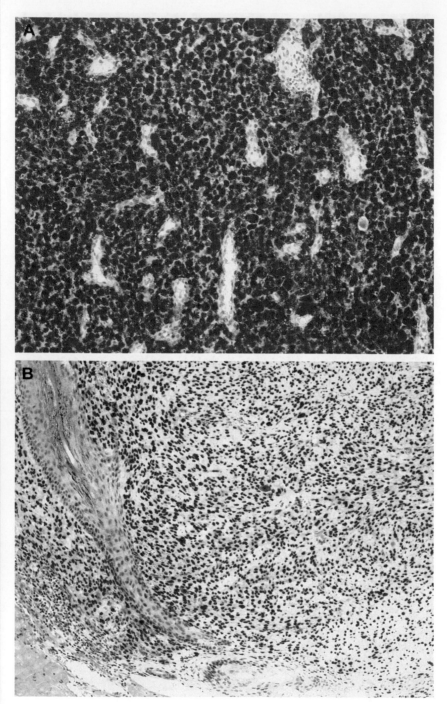

*Fig. 5.* Immunohistochemically, a homogeneous expression of CD10 (*A*), and a nuclear expression of p53 (*B*) are seen in cases of AFX.

nuclear DNA in contrast to so-called malignant fibrous histiocytoma (undifferentiated pleomorphic sarcoma),[21] and that H-*ras* and K-*ras* gene mutations were detected in so-called malignant fibrous histiocytoma (undifferentiated pleomorphic sarcoma), but not in cases of AFX.[22] On the other hand, *TERT* promotor mutations with a UV signature that allows tumor cells to proliferate continuously were found in both AFX and PDS.[23]

## DIFFERENTIAL DIAGNOSIS

Dermatofibroma (fibrous histiocytoma) occurs only rarely on the face, and in contrast to AFX as an

*Fig. 6.* The atypical spindle-shaped tumor cells in AFX often stain positively for alpha-smooth muscle actin.

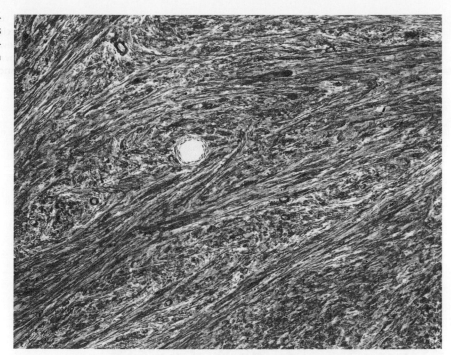

exophytic growing and well-circumscribed neoplasm, cases of dermatofibroma in this anatomic location are rather ill-defined and tend to infiltrate deeper structures early, resulting in an increased number of local recurrences.[24] Histopathologically, dermatofibroma shows less atypia of neoplastic cells and a lower proliferative activity. Atypical (pseudosarcomatous) dermatofibroma, characterized by the presence of enlarged and atypical tumor cells with pleomorphic nuclei, tends to occur at the extremities of younger patients, and shows a low proliferative activity with no atypical mitotic figures. The most important differential diagnoses include sarcomatoid and spindle-cell carcinoma, poorly differentiated, spindle-cell malignant melanoma, and poorly differentiated leiomyosarcoma and angiosarcoma. Sarcomatoid and spindle-cell carcinoma represents an ill-defined and infiltrative neoplasm that shows at least focally an expression of pancytokeratin by neoplastic cells (**Fig. 7**). Poorly differentiated, spindle-cell malignant melanoma arising in the head and neck area may contain a junctional component visible best with Melan-A and MiTF1 antibodies, may show desmoplasia and neural invasion, and is composed of tumor cells staining homogeneously positive for S-100 protein, SOX10, and p75 (**Fig. 8**). Cases of poorly differentiated superficial leiomyosarcoma are infiltrative and poorly circumscribed neoplasms composed of bundles of plump spindled eosinophilic tumor cells staining positively for desmin and h-caldesmon. Poorly differentiated cutaneous angiosarcoma shows, at

least focally, vasoformative structures, and neoplastic cells stain positively for CD31 and especially for ERG. The most problematic issue represents the distinction of AFX and PDS (see later in this article). According to the literature, cases of PDS are, in contrast to AFX, often larger, ill-defined, and infiltrative, and may show areas of tumor necrosis and lymphovascular or perineural invasion. Whereas cases of AFX, if strict diagnostic criteria are applied, show a benign clinical course, PDS may recur locally and metastasize in a number of cases.[25,26]

## MORPHOLOGIC VARIANTS

Several morphologic variants of AFX have been described during the past years, and knowledge of them is important to avoid misdiagnosis of a more or less aggressive neoplasm.

## SPINDLE-CELL NONPLEOMORPHIC ATYPICAL FIBROXANTHOMA

First described in 1993,[27] spindle-cell nonpleomorphic AFX shows all clinicopathological features of classic AFX but is composed of relatively monomorphic, palely eosinophilic spindle-shaped tumor cells arranged in bundles and fascicles. Tumor cells lack prominent pleomorphism and contain enlarged and vesicular nuclei, and numerous mitoses, including atypical mitotic figures, are found (**Fig. 9**).

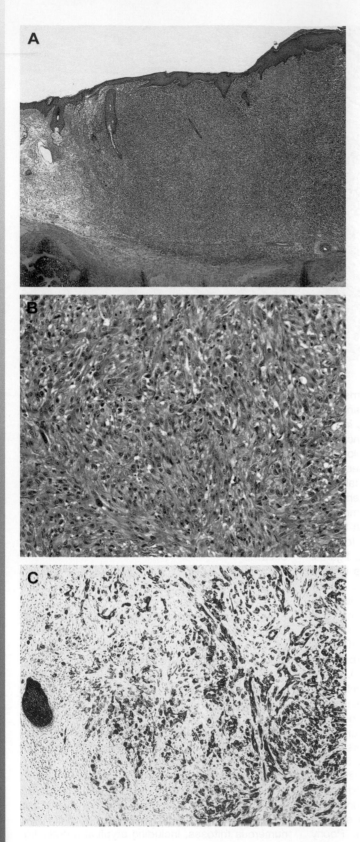

*Fig. 7.* A case of poorly differentiated sarcomatoid carcinoma (*A*) that shows on high-power view features comparable with AFX (*B*). However, neoplastic cells stain positively for pancytokeratin (AE1/3) (*C*).

*Fig. 8.* Nodular malignant melanoma composed of atypical, spindled tumor cells (*A*, *B*), which stain positively for S-100 protein (*C*).

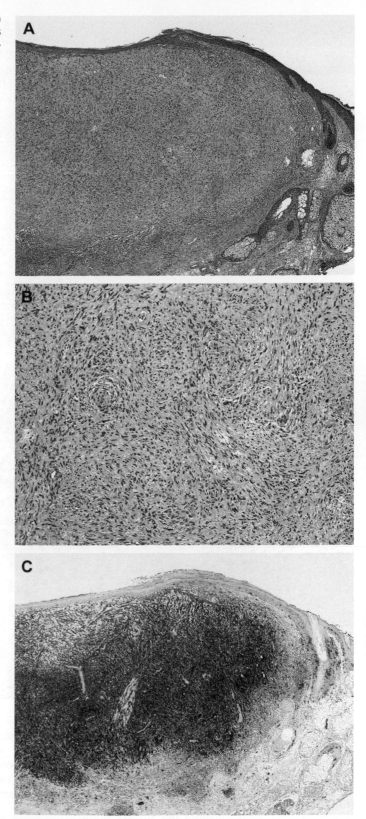

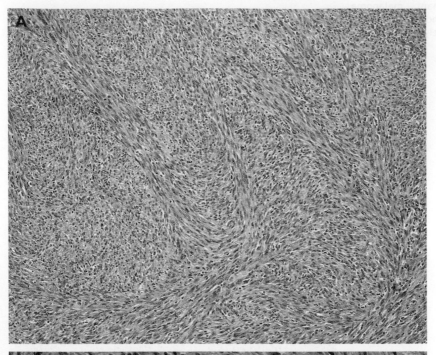

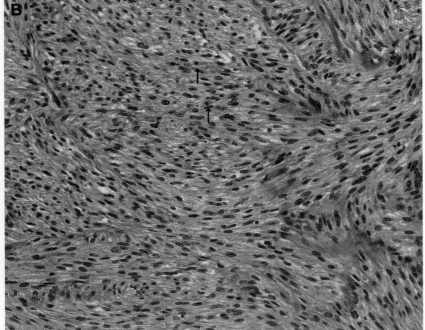

*Fig. 9.* Spindle-cell non-pleomorphic AFX is composed of atypical spindled tumor cells arranged in bundles and fascicles (*A*). Note numerous mitoses (*arrow*) (*B*).

## CLEAR-CELL ATYPICAL FIBROXANTHOMA

In rare cases, AFX is composed of pleomorphic clear tumor cells with foamy and clear cytoplasm and enlarged and hyperchromatic nuclei (**Fig. 10**), and needs to be distinguished from xanthoma and xanthogranuloma (no bizarre hyperchromatic multinucleated tumor giant cells and no atypical mitoses are present), balloon cell malignant melanoma (expression of melanocytic immunohistochemical markers), sebaceous carcinoma, clear-cell carcinoma, metastatic clear-cell carcinoma of the kidney (expression of cytokeratins),[28,29] signet ring cutaneous angiosarcoma (expression of endothelial markers),[30] and clear-cell cutaneous PEComa (HMB-45 positive).[31]

*Fig. 10.* Clear cell AFX is composed of sheets of enlarged and atypical tumor cells containing abundant clear cytoplasm.

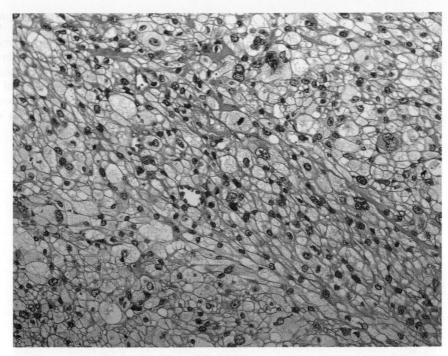

## PIGMENTED ATYPICAL FIBROXANTHOMA

Cases of pigmented (probably better named hemosiderotic) AFX resemble clinically and histologically malignant melanoma and are characterized by abundant intratumoral hemorrhages with blood-filled pseudocystic spaces (**Fig. 11**) and may contain osteoclastlike giant cells as well. The pleomorphic neoplastic cells show a variable degree of erythrophagocytosis, and intracellular deposition of hemosiderin pigment, as well as intracytoplasmic collections of eosinophilic

*Fig. 11.* Pigmented (hemosiderotic) AFX shows abundant intratumoral hemorrhages and fibrin depositions.

globules representing most likely degenerated erythrocytes, similar to those seen in vascular neoplasms, are present.[32] Immunohistochemical antibodies are helpful in the distinction of malignant melanoma and spitzoid melanocytic neoplasms, whereas aneurysmal dermatofibroma occurs only rarely on the face and lacks prominent atypia and numerous mitoses.

## MYXOID ATYPICAL FIBROXANTHOMA

Prominent myxoid stromal changes are a relatively frequent finding in benign and malignant mesenchymal tumors and led to the characterization of a number of entities and variants. Rarely, cases of otherwise typical AFX show a prominent myxomatous stroma[33] (**Fig. 12**) and

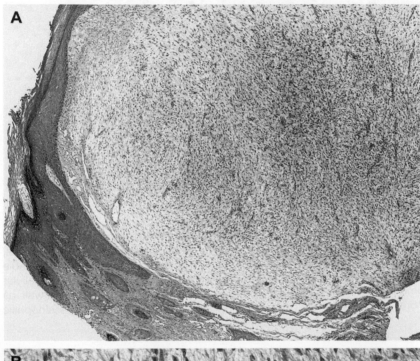

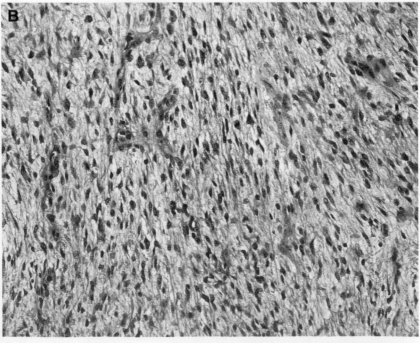

*Fig. 12.* A rare case of myxoid AFX presenting as a well-circumscribed, nodular neoplasm with abundant myxomatous stroma (*A*), composed of atypical spindled tumor cells with enlarged, hyperchromatic nuclei (*B*).

need to be distinguished from carcinomas and malignant melanomas with myxoid changes, as well as from myxoid mesenchymal neoplasms, including high-grade myxofibrosarcoma, myxoinflammatory fibroblastic tumor, and myxoid leiomyosarcoma.

## OSTEOCLAST-LIKE GIANT-CELL RICH ATYPICAL FIBROXANTHOMA

In rare cases, AFX may contain numerous osteoclast-like giant cells lacking prominent atypia and increased proliferative activity and stain strongly positive for CD68[34] (Fig. 13). These neoplasms

*Fig. 13.* Numerous osteoclast-like giant cells with abundant eosinophilic cytoplasm and small, bland nuclei are seen in this AFX (*A*). Strong expression of CD68 by osteoclastlike giant cells (*B*).

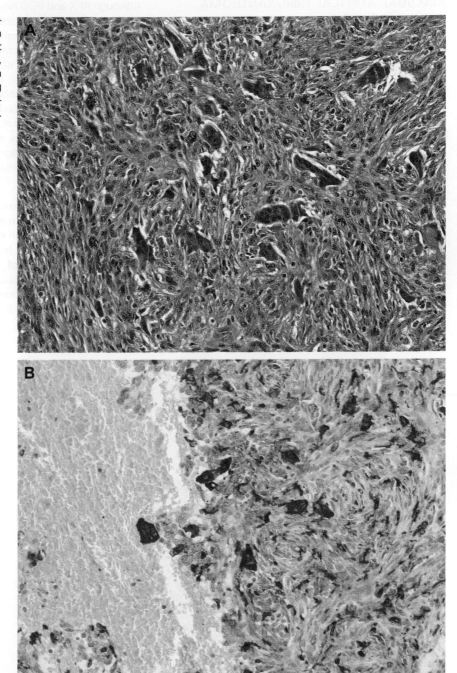

must be distinguished from giant-cell tumor of soft tissues (occurs often at the extremities and is characterized by a multinodular growth without prominent atypia), leiomyosarcoma with prominent osteoclastlike giant cells (evidence of myogenic differentiation by immunohistochemistry), and dermatofibroma with osteoclast-like giant cells (lacks prominent atypia and atypical mitoses).

## KELOIDAL ATYPICAL FIBROXANTHOMA

Occasionally, AFX may show features of regression and contain thick bundles of hyalinized collagen masking nuclear atypia and worrisome morphologic features. These neoplasms are composed of enlarged and atypical cells set in a prominent collagenous stroma with keloidlike changes (**Fig. 14**) and perivascular sclerotic collagen depositions are found. These neoplasms must be distinguished from a keloid and from keloidal dermatofibroma.[35]

## GRANULAR CELL ATYPICAL FIBROXANTHOMA

Rarely AFX is composed of enlarged and pleomorphic tumor cells with abundant granular cytoplasm and irregular, hyperchromatic nuclei. The tumor cells stain positively for CD68 and NKIC3, but are negative for S-100 protein, pancytokeratin, and actins (**Fig. 15**). Degenerative cellular changes

explain the morphology of granular cell AFX that needs to be distinguished from granular cell tumor, non-neural granular cell tumor, and other neoplasms with granular cell changes.[36,37]

## PROBLEMATIC RELATIONSHIP OF ATYPICAL FIBROXANTHOMA AND PLEOMORPHIC DERMAL SARCOMA

Although AFX and PDS have been studied in detail over the past years, there is an ongoing debate about the exact relationship of these neoplasms. Whereas the cellular components of AFX and PDS are identical and no reliable immunohistochemical and molecular differences are known, cases of well-circumscribed AFX are characterized by an exophytic growth, but PDS is by definition an ill-defined, infiltrative neoplasm that may show tumor necrosis as well as lymphovascular and/or perineurial invasion. Despite these distinguishing diagnostic criteria, a number of questions may be raised.

1. As in other neoplasms, sampling errors may occur and lead to a misinterpretation. Most of a given neoplasm can show features of a well-circumscribed AFX; however, if a peripheral diffuse infiltration of deeper structures is evident, the diagnosis of PDS has to be made.
2. If it is impossible to excise a case of a typical AFX on time and if the lesion can grow

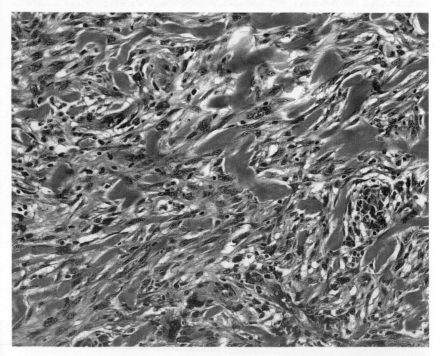

**Fig. 14.** Thick bundles of hyalinized collagen are seen in this example of keloidal AFX.

*Fig. 15.* Granular cell AFX is composed of enlarged tumor cells containing abundant granular cytoplasm and enlarged nuclei (*A*). Immunohistochemically, a strong expression of NKIC3 is noted (*B*).

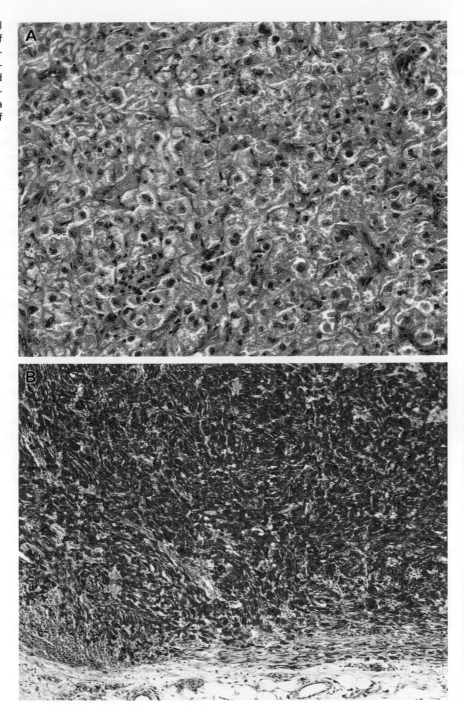

continuously, is there probably a change of the growth to an infiltrative neoplasm comparable with the diagnosis of a PDS?

3. Rarely, documented cases of AFX show an infiltration of deeper structures in the local recurrence[7]: does it represent a transition from AFX to PDS?

4. Do the reported cases of metastatic AFX with minimal or no subcutaneous involvement[8] represent misdiagnoses?

5. May AFX show a time-dependent progression to PDS?

6. Are AFX and PDS morphologic points of a spectrum of a single clinicopathological entity

in which the prognosis is strongly dependent on the depth of the neoplasm (as is the case in atypical smooth muscle tumor of the dermis and well-differentiated pilar leiomyosarcoma)?

In summary, AFX represents a biologically interesting mesenchymal neoplasm in which the exact relationship to PDS is still unclear. The diagnosis of AFX should never made on a small biopsy only and without a panel of immunohistochemical antibodies, and knowledge of the morphologic variants is mandatory to avoid misdiagnosis and overtreatment or undertreatment of patients.

## REFERENCES

1. Calonje JE, Brenn T, Komminoth P. Atypical fibroxanthoma. In: Fletcher CDM, Bridge JA, Hogendoorn PCW, et al, editors. WHO classification of tumours of soft tissue and bone. 4th edition. Lyon (France): International Agency for Research on Cancer; 2013. p. 202–3.
2. Kempson RI, McGavran MH. Atypical fibroxanthomas of the skin. Cancer 1964;176:1463–71.
3. Fretzin DF, Helwig EB. Atypical fibroxanthoma of the skin. A clinicopathologic study of 140 cases. Cancer 1973;31:1541–52.
4. Fletcher CDM. Pleomorphic malignant fibrous histiocytoma: fact or fiction? A critical reappraisal based on 159 tumors diagnosed as pleomorphic sarcomas. Am J Surg Pathol 1992;16:213–28.
5. Nonaka D, Bishop PW. Sarcoma-like tumor of head and neck skin. Am J Surg Pathol 2014;38:956–65.
6. Chappell AG, Chase EP, Chang B, et al. Atypical fibroxanthoma in a 13-year-old Guatemalan girl with xeroderma pigmentosum. Pediatr Dermatol 2016;33:228–9.
7. Koch M, Freundl AJ, Agaimy A, et al. Atypical fibroxanthoma–histological diagnosis, immunohistochemical markers and concepts of therapy. Anticancer Res 2015;35:5717–35.
8. Wang WL, Torres-Cabala C, Curry JL, et al. Metastatic atypical fibroxanthoma: a series of 11 cases including with minimal and no subcutaneous involvement. Am J Dermatopathol 2015;37:455–61.
9. Hall JM, Saenger JS, Fadare O. Diagnostic utility of p63 and CD10 in distinguishing cutaneous spindle cell/sarcomatoid squamous carcinoma and atypical fibroxanthomas. Int J Clin Exp Pathol 2008;7:524–30.
10. Thum C, Hollowood K, Birch J, et al. Aberrant Melan-A expression in atypical fibroxanthoma and undifferentiated pleomorphic sarcoma of the skin. J Cutan Pathol 2011;38:954–60.
11. Tallon B, Beer TW. MITF positivity in atypical fibroxanthoma: a diagnostic pitfall. Am J Dermatopathol 2014;36:888 91.
12. Luzar B, Calonje E. Morphological and immunohistochemical characteristics of atypical fibroxanthoma with a special emphasis on potential diagnostic pitfalls: a review. J Cutan Pathol 2010;37:301–9.
13. de Feraudy S, Mar N, McCalmont TH. Evaluation of CD10 and procollagen 1 expression in atypical fibroxanthoma and dermatofibroma. Am J Surg Pathol 2008;32:1111–22.
14. Longacre TA, Smoller BR, Rouse RV. Atypical fibroxanthoma. Multiple immunohistologic profiles. Am J Surg Pathol 1993;17:1199–209.
15. Monteagudo C, Calduch L, Navarro S, et al. CD99 immunoreactivity in atypical fibroxanthoma. A common feature of diagnostic value. Am J Clin Pathol 2002;117:126–31.
16. Ma CK, Zarbo RJ, Gown AM. Immunohistochemical characterization of atypical fibroxanthoma and dermatofibrosarcoma protuberans. Am J Clin Pathol 1992;97:478–83.
17. Beer TW, Drury P, Heenan PJ. Atypical fibroxanthoma: a histological and immunohistochemical review of 171 cases. Am J Dermatopathol 2010;32:533–40.
18. Sakamoto A, Oda Y, Yamamoto H, et al. Calponin and h-caldesmon expression in atypical fibroxanthoma and superficial leiomyosarcoma. Virchows Arch 2002;440:404–9.
19. Vogelstein B, Kinzler KM. Carcinogens leave fingerprints. Nature 1992;355:209–10.
20. Dei Tos AP, Maestro R, Doglioni C, et al. Ultraviolet-induced p53 mutations in atypical fibroxanthoma. Am J Pathol 1994;145:11–7.
21. Worrell JT, Ansari MQ, Ansari SJ, et al. Atypical fibroxanthoma: DNA ploidy analysis of 14 cases with possible histogenetic implications. J Cutan Pathol 1993;20:211–5.
22. Sakamoto A, Oda Y, Itakura E, et al. H-, K-, and N-ras gene mutation in atypical fibroxanthoma and malignant fibrous histiocytoma. Hum Pathol 2001;32:1225–31.
23. Griewank KG, Schilling B, Murali R, et al. TERT promotor mutations are frequent in atypical fibroxanthoma and pleomorphic dermal sarcoma. Mod Pathol 2014;27:502–8.
24. Mentzel T, Kutzner H, Rütten A, et al. Benign fibrous histiocytoma (dermatofibroma) of the face: clinicopathologic and immunohistochemical study of 34 cases associated with an aggressive clinical course. Am J Dermatopathol 2001;23:419–26.
25. Miller K, Goodlad JR, Brenn T. Pleomorphic dermal sarcoma. Adverse histologic features predict aggressive behavior and allow distinction from atypical fibroxanthoma. Am J Surg Pathol 2012;36:1317–26.
26. Tardio JC, Pinedo F, Aramburu JA, et al. Pleomorphic dermal sarcoma: a more aggressive neoplasm than previously estimated. J Cutan Pathol 2015;43:101–12.
27. Calonje E, Wadden C, Wilson-Jones E, et al. Spindle-cell non-pleomorphic atypical fibroxanthoma: analysis of a series and delineation of a distinctive variant. Histopathology 1993;22:247–54.

28. Crowson AN, Carlson-Sweet K, Macinnis C, et al. Clear cell atypical fibroxanthoma: a clinicopathologic study. J Cutan Pathol 2002;29:374–81.

29. Tardio JC, Pinedo F, Aramburu JA, et al. Clear cell atypical fibroxanthoma: clinicopathological study of 6 cases and review of the literature with special emphasis on the differential diagnosis. Am J Dermatopathol 2016;38:586–92.

30. Wood A, Mentzel T, van Gorp J, et al. The spectrum of rare morphological variants of cutaneous epithelioid angiosarcoma. Histopathology 2015;66:856–63.

31. Mentzel T, Reisshauer S, Rütten A, et al. Cutaneous clear cell myomelanocytic tumour: a new member of the growing family of perivascular epithelioid cell tumours (PEComas). Clinicopathological and immunohistochemical analysis of seven cases. Histopathology 2005;46:498–504.

32. Diaz-Cascajo C, Weyers W, Borghi S. Pigmented atypical fibroxanthoma. A tumor that may be easily mistaken for malignant melanoma. Am J Dermatopathol 2003;25:1–5.

33. Patton A, Page R, Googe PB, et al. Myxoid atypical fibroxanthoma: a previously undescribed variant. J Cutan Pathol 2009;36:1177–84.

34. Tomaszewski MM, Lupton GP. Atypical fibroxanthoma. An unusual variant with osteoclast-like giant cells. Am J Surg Pathol 1997;21:213–8.

35. Kim J, McNiff JM. Keloidal atypical fibroxanthoma: a case series. J Cutan Pathol 2009;36:535–9.

36. Rudisaile SN, Hurt MA, Santa Cruz DJ. Granular cell atypical fibroxanthoma. J Cutan Pathol 2005;32:314–7.

37. Rios-Martin JJ, Delgado MD, Moreno-Ramirez D, et al. Granular cell atypical fibroxanthoma: report of two cases. Am J Dermatopathol 2007;29:84–7.

# Cutaneous Malignant Peripheral Nerve Sheath Tumor

Boštjan Luzar, MD, PhD[a],*, Giovanni Falconieri, MD[b]

## KEYWORDS

- Malignant peripheral nerve sheath tumor • Superficial/cutaneous • Conventional variant
- Epithelioid variant

## Key Points

- Cutaneous malignant peripheral nerve sheath tumors (MPNSTs) are rare sarcomas of neuroectodermal origin arising in the dermis and/or subcutis.

- In contrast with their deep soft tissue and visceral counterparts, cutaneous MPNSTs are rarely associated with neurofibromatosis type 1.

- Two main subtypes of cutaneous MPNST can be distinguished histologically: conventional (ie, spindle cell) and epithelioid MPNST.

- The 2 subtypes also differ in predilection for deep versus superficial locations, association with preexistent benign peripheral nerve sheath tumors and S100 immunohistochemistry.

- Herein, we review current knowledge of cutaneous MPNST and discuss its differential diagnosis.

## ABSTRACT

Cutaneous malignant peripheral nerve sheath tumors (MPNSTs) are rare sarcomas of neuroectodermal origin arising in the dermis and/or subcutis. In contrast with their deep soft tissue and visceral counterparts, cutaneous MPNSTs are rarely associated with neurofibromatosis type 1. Two main subtypes of cutaneous MPNST can be distinguished histologically: conventional (ie, spindle cell) and epithelioid MPNST. The 2 subtypes also differ in predilection for deep versus superficial locations, association with preexistent benign peripheral nerve sheath tumors and S100 immunohistochemistry. Herein, we review current knowledge of cutaneous MPNST and discuss its differential diagnosis.

## OVERVIEW

Malignant peripheral nerve sheath tumor is a malignant soft tissue tumor featuring a neuroectodermal line of differentiation similar to the normal peripheral nerve sheath.[1,2] Defined as such, the cellular composition of MPNST can be fairly heterogeneous, but Schwann cells and perineural fibroblasts generally predominate.[1] Representing from 5% to 10% of all soft tissue sarcomas,[3] the development of MPNSTs is strongly related to neurofibromatosis type 1 (NF-1), in which the lifetime risk of MPNST is estimated to be from 2% to 10%.[2,4,5] In addition, MPNST can also develop in a sporadic setting, either de novo or from a preexisting benign peripheral nerve sheath tumor, most commonly from neurofibroma.[1] The ratio between NF-1–related

The authors have no conflict of interest to declare and there are no financial or commercial conflicts to disclose.
[a] Institute of Pathology, Medical Faculty University of Ljubljana, Korytkova 2, Ljubljana 1000, Slovenia;
[b] Department of Pathology, University of Trieste School of Medicine, Strada di Fiume 449, Trieste 34149, Italy
* Corresponding author.
*E-mail address:* bostjan.luzar@mf.uni-lj.si

Surgical Pathology 10 (2017) 337–343
http://dx.doi.org/10.1016/j.path.2017.01.008
1875-9181/17/© 2017 Elsevier Inc. All rights reserved.

and sporadic MPNSTs seems to be approximately equal.[2] In the past, about 10% of MPNSTs occurred at sites of previous irradiation, usually in patients with a history of radiation treatment for neurofibroma, a practice that has been discontinued.[6,7] Clinically, MPNST displays a strong predilection for the deep soft tissues of the proximal lower extremities[8] and the trunk.[1] Although age at presentation is usually within a broad range, most case series have recorded a predominance for the fourth and fifth decades of life for sporadic MPNSTs.[8] However, MPNST patients with NF-1 are usually younger, tumors can already develop during adolescence, and are slightly more frequent in females.[1] MPNSTs pursue an unfavorable clinical course, with an overall poor prognosis owing to a high risk of local recurrence, distant metastases, and poor response to treatment.[3] As such, NF-1 patients with MPNST have a reported 5-year survival rate of 16%, compared with the 53% seen in those without NF-1.[1] Advances in molecular genetics of these neoplasms have demonstrated complex clonal abnormalities, with significant chromosome gain(s) and deletion(s) in the majority of cases,[3] the most important being *NF1* mutations and *CDKN2A* inactivation.[9,10] The latter is considered to be an early event in the onset of MPNST, resulting in loss of H3K27me3 (ie, trimethylation at lysine 27 of histone H3), which may have potential targeting implications for MPNST patients.[11]

## CUTANEOUS MALIGNANT PERIPHERAL NERVE SHEATH TUMOR

Primary occurrence of MPNST in the skin is rare. Cutaneous MPNST is defined as an MPNST predominantly localized in the dermis and/or subcutis.[3] Although phenotypically comparable with their deep soft tissue counterpart, they exhibit a number of distinctive features, including a rare association with NF-1 and potential surgical resectability owing to their superficial location.[3,12] Microscopically, cutaneous MPNSTs segregate into 2 major categories: conventional (spindle cell) and epithelioid subtypes. In this paper, we review current knowledge of cutaneous MPNST and discuss its differential diagnosis.

## CUTANEOUS CONVENTIONAL MALIGNANT PERIPHERAL NERVE SHEATH TUMOR

### Clinical Features

Cutaneous conventional MPNST (CC-MPNST) accounts for about 2% of MPNSTs[13]; males are affected slightly more often.[3] Commonly reported sites of occurrence include the head and neck[14,15] or the limbs.[3] These tumors typically arise in association with a preexisting neurofibroma or a peripheral nerve[15,16] and are characterized by a relatively long period of slow growth followed by a sudden growth acceleration. As a distinguishing feature, the association of CC-MPNST with NF1 is less strong than for deep-seated MPNSTs (23% vs 31%, respectively,[3]). Complete surgical resection with wide clear margins remains the mainstay of treatment.[3] The prognosis of CC-MPNST seems to be less favorable than with other sarcomas arising at superficial locations.[15–17] A compilation study by Allison and colleagues[15] including 27 patients with a mean follow-up of 3.3 years revealed that 62% of patients were alive at this time, 8% alive with disease, and 8% died of the tumor. A study by Dabski and colleagues[18] revealed an overall 4-year survival rate of 66% for superficial CC-MPNST. In the most recent paper by Feng and colleagues,[3] the 5-year survival rate was 64.2% for these tumors.

### Pathologic Features

Macroscopically, CC-MPNSTs appear as firm, poorly circumscribed tan masses with a whorled appearance on cut section; necrotic and pseudocystic areas may be noted.[15,19] On histology, CC-MPNSTs are usually fairly cellular spindle cell proliferations, growing in long fascicles with occasional storiform arrangements (**Fig. 1**). Low-power magnification often reveals a so-called marbled growth pattern characterized by alternating hypocellular and hypercellular areas with distinct perivascular accentuation. Tumor cells often feature wavy or comma-shaped nuclei reminiscent of those seen in neurofibromas, and they may be arranged in a palisading pattern. A focal epithelioid morphology of tumor cells is not uncommon, especially in high-grade tumors, but epithelioid cells do not predominate. The cytoplasm of tumor cells is usually scant, eosinophilic, and can be barely discerned in tumors with packed cellularity. Brisk mitotic activity is easily recognized and may range from just a few mitotic figures up to more than 50 per 10 high-power fields.[15] Tumor necrosis, when present, is focal and rarely exceeds 5% of the neoplastic tissue.[15] A prominent delicate vascular network of thin-walled vessels is often seen. A herniation or invagination of tumor cells into the vascular channels has been reported as a characteristic feature of MPNST.[20] Myxoid and sclerotic changes of the stroma can be present to a variable extent. A wide range of heterologous components reflecting divergent differentiation has been reported, including

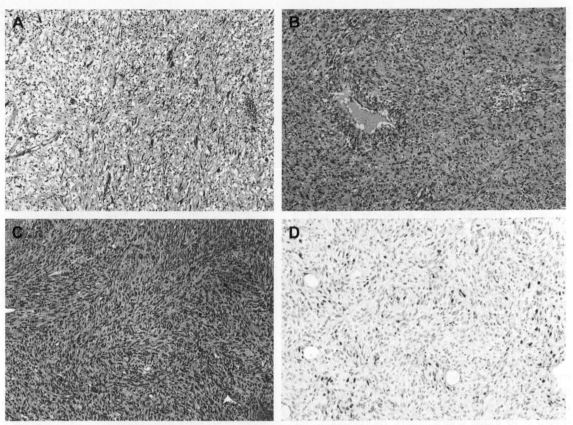

*Fig. 1.* Conventional malignant peripheral nerve sheath tumor (MPNST). (*A*) This low-grade malignant tumor developed in the background of a diffuse neurofibroma. Three mitoses per 10 high-power fields were found in the most cellular areas. (*B*) Another example of an MPNST with more cellular spindle cells proliferation with characteristic perivascular accentuation. (*C*) Tumor with high-grade morphology cannot be distinguished from other high-grade sarcomas on morphologic grounds alone. Note the presence of tumoral necrosis in upper left corner. (*D*) About 50% of conventional MPSTs reveal patchy S100 positivity.

chondrosarcomatous, osteosarcomatous, leiosarcomatous, or angiosarcomatous phenotypes.[15] Rhabdoid differentiation (malignant triton tumors[21]) has also been reported, as in ordinary MPNST.[21,22] Although the number of reports is very limited, the presence of rhabdoid differentiation in CC-MPNST seems to be an additional unfavorable prognostic factor.[15,23]

## Immunohistochemical Features

In MPNST, immunohistochemistry has a limited role in the diagnosis owing to often inconsistent staining patterns against various antigens, including S100 protein, CD34, GFAP, EMA, and CD34.[2] As such, immunohistochemistry is applied mainly to exclude potential histologic mimickers.[2] In fact, staining for S100 protein generally reveals only focal positivity, but can also be entirely negative in about one-half of cases. Recently, however, the loss of H3K27me3 has been investigated by means of immunohistochemistry and has been

proven to be a highly specific marker of MPNST, although its sensitivity is still not superior to S100 protein.[11]

## Differential Diagnosis

CC-MPNST raises a broad differential diagnosis. In addition to morphologic assessment and judicious application of immunostains, clinicopathologic correlation is crucial.[24]

Spindle cell melanoma can be difficult or sometimes impossible to distinguish from CC-MPNST on morphologic grounds alone, bearing in mind that a junctional component may be focal or absent in primary cutaneous melanomas. Furthermore, immunohistochemistry for various second-line melanoma antigens, including HMB45, melan A, or thyrosinase, is often negative[25] However, the strong and diffuse immunoreaction to S100 protein seen in melanoma is unexpected in spindle cell MPNST.

Monophasic synovial sarcoma enters into the differential diagnosis of CC-MPNST because the

2 tumors share several architectural, cytologic, and some immunohistochemical features. Furthermore, although primary cutaneous synovial sarcoma is exceedingly rare in the skin,[26] metastases to the skin from primary tumors elsewhere have been reported.[27] By immunohistochemistry, about one-third of monophasic synovial sarcomas display focal S100 positivity.[2] In addition, they often show focal or patchy cytokeratin positivity, in particular CK7 and CK19, a reaction pattern rarely detected in CC-MPNST.[8,28] Although monophasic synovial sarcoma is characteristically positive for blc2, calponin, H-caldesmon, and CD99, these markers are not specific to the entity.[29,30] Recently, transducin-like enhancer of split 1 (TLE1) has been introduced as a valuable marker in the differential diagnosis of malignant spindle cell proliferations. In particular, most synovial sarcomas display strong and diffuse nuclear TLE1 positivity, as opposed to CC-MPNST with a focal and weak staining pattern.[31] Nevertheless, demonstration of translocation t(x;18) and/or SYT-SSX fusion transcripts is diagnostic of synovial sarcoma.[32]

Defining histological features of cutaneous leiomyosarcoma include tumor fascicles composed of cells with cigar-shaped nuclei with blunt ends and distinctive brightly eosinophilic cytoplasm. In addition to these characteristic morphologic features, leiomyosarcoma is usually strongly and diffusely positive for desmin,[24] whereas strong positivity for desmin in genuine CC-MPNST suggests heterologous rhabdomyoblastic differentiation (eg, malignant Triton tumor).[15,23,33]

Fibrosarcomatous dermatofibrosarcoma protuberans can display morphologic overlap with CC-MPNST. Furthermore, CD34 expression is frequently lost in this morphologic variant of dermatofibrosarcoma protuberans.[34] In problematic examples, a confirmation of t(17;22) is diagnostic of dermatofibrosarcoma protuberans.[8,24]

Atypical neurofibroma (also designated cellular neurofibroma with atypia) displays increased cellularity, with tumor cells arranged in haphazard fascicles, hyperchromatic nuclei, nuclear enlargement, and absent or very limited mitotic activity (about 1 per 50 high-power fields), raising concern about malignant transformation.[35] For practical purposes, any degree of mitotic activity associated with increased cellularity, and nuclear atypia(s) with nuclear hyperchromasia in a neurofibroma would suggest the possibility of malignancy.[2]

Cellular schwannoma poses similar interpretive challenges. However, despite increased cellularity, cellular schwannoma lacks the degree of nuclear pleomorphism expected for CC-MPNST,[2] and is typically encapsulated.[8] Furthermore, cellular schwannoma is strongly and uniformly positive for S100 protein, as opposed to the focal and inconsistent staining in CC-MPNST.[2] The perineurial capsule of schwannoma is EMA positive, whereas such a feature is generally lacking in CC-MPNSTs.[8]

## CUTANEOUS EPITHELIOID MALIGNANT PERIPHERAL NERVE SHEATH TUMOR

Cutaneous epithelioid MPNST (CE-MPNST) is a variant of MPNST occurring in the dermis and/or subcutis, composed predominantly (at least 50%) or exclusively of epithelioid tumor cells, generally displaying diffuse and at least moderate degrees of cytologic atypia.[36,37] Epithelioid MPNSTs represent up to 5% of all MPNSTs and have a much greater propensity to arise at superficial locations than in the deep soft tissues, in contrast with conventional MPNST.[14,37]

### Clinical Features

CE-MPNST has a wide age distribution and most commonly affects patient in their fifth decade of life, with a slight male predominance.[36] Occurrence in infancy and childhood is most uncommon.[36,37] Predilection sites include the lower extremities and trunk, although various sites of occurrence have been reported.[38] Clinical presentation is not distinctive, with painful or nontender discrete nodule(s) or plaques of variable duration.[15,37] Alternatively, an increase in size in a preexistent benign peripheral nerve sheath tumor is observed. In contrast with conventional MPNST, association of CE-MPNST with NF1 or neurofibroma is rare.[36,37] Interestingly, 14% of epithelioid MPNSTs develop in association with a preexistent schwannoma, an otherwise exceptional event in conventional MPNSTs.[36] Complete excision of the tumor is the basis of treatment. Local recurrences have been observed in roughly 20% of cases.[37] Although a recent study demonstrated a low risk of recurrence and metastatic spread for cutaneous and deep epithelioid MPNST,[36] CE-MPNST has, nevertheless, the potential to pursue an aggressive clinical course. A study specifically addressing the prognosis of CE-MPNSTs reported death owing to disseminated disease in one third of patients (33%) in a follow-up period from 24 to 100 months.[37] Unfortunately, no clinicopathologic features have been found to predict the biological behavior of CE-MPNST.[37]

### Pathologic Features

CE-MPNSTs are generally much smaller in size than their deep soft tissue counterparts, with a reported median size of 1.6 and 5 cm, respectively,[37,39] although tumors measuring as large as 8 cm in the greatest diameter have also been reported at superficial locations.[38] Microscopically, CE-MPNST is distinguished by a predominance of polygonal epithelioid cells, displaying a nodular/multinodular and less often an infiltrative growth pattern, frequently admixed with variable proportions of spindled tumor cells, the latter representing a minor cell component (**Fig. 2**).[36,37] Tumor cells tend to grow in cords, strands, nests, or sheets and are surrounded by hyalinized or myxoid stroma. Epithelioid tumor cells have round to oval nuclei, vesicular chromatin, variably prominent basophilic nucleoli, and abundant eosinophilic or amphophylic cytoplasm with well-defined cell borders.[37] Nuclear atypia is generally widespread and at least moderate. Mitotic activity is often pronounced (mean number of 7 mitoses per 10 high-power fields), reflecting the degree of nuclear atypia.[37] Divergent heterologous differentiation can be observed, albeit less frequently than in ordinary or CC-MPNST.[40]

## Immunohistochemical Features

In contrast with conventional MPNST, CE-MPNST displays consistent, strong, and diffuse positivity for S100 protein. S100 staining is much less frequently focal and patchy. Staining for second-line melanoma markers (including HMB45, melan A, tyrosinase, and MITF) and vascular markers is usually negative. Nevertheless, a focal positivity for melan and HMB45 has been detected in isolated cases of CE-MPNST, representing a potential diagnostic pitfall.[37,41,42] Focal positivity for cytokeratins and EMA has occasionally been reported.[2,36] About 50% to 67% of CE-MPNSTs show loss of nuclear integrase interactor 1 (INI1) staining.[36,43,44]

## Differential Diagnosis

The differential diagnosis of CE-MPNST includes other tumors with an epithelioid morphology. Only the most common mimickers occurring in

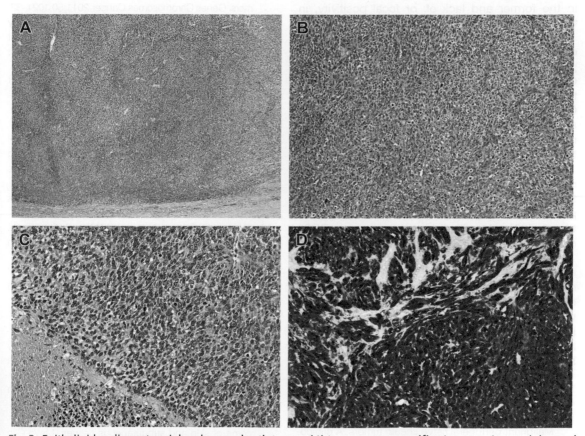

*Fig. 2.* Epithelioid malignant peripheral nerve sheath tumor. (*A*) Low-power magnification reveals a nodular and high cellular proliferation composed of tumor cells with an epithelioid morphology. (*B*) Epithelioid tumor cells with confluent atypia and pronounced mitotic activity. (*C*) Higher magnification also depicting an area of confluent necroses within the epithelioid tumor cell population. (*D*) Diffuse S100 positivity is typical of an epithelioid malignant peripheral nerve sheath tumor.

the skin are discussed herein, such as melanoma (primary and metastatic), metastatic poorly differentiated carcinoma, myoepithelial carcinoma, epithelioid sarcoma, and epithelioid schwannoma.

Melanoma can feature a remarkable epithelioid phenotype, making distinction from CE-MPNST difficult or impossible on histologic grounds alone. The presence of an atypical junctional component or melanin pigment strongly favors melanoma. Obtaining an accurate clinical history is equally of crucial importance to exclude a possible history of melanoma elsewhere. Both melanoma and CE-MPNST have the same S100 protein reaction pattern, with a strong, diffuse nuclear and cytoplasmic positivity. Nevertheless, the second-line melanocytic markers (eg, melan A, HMB45, MITF) are usually positive in melanomas with an epithelioid morphology.[2] Furthermore, loss of INI1 nuclear expression is not seen in melanoma, in contrast with CE-MPNST.[36,43]

Metastatic poorly differentiated carcinoma can be distinguished from CE-MPNST by consistent (usually diffuse and strong) cytokeratin positivity in the former and lack of, or focal positivity, in the latter.[2,37]

Myoepithelial carcinoma can share morphologic overlap with CE-MPNST, especially if composed predominantly of epithelioid cells. In contrast with CE-MPNST, myoepithelial carcinoma is positive for various cytokeratins, including CK-AE1/AE3, CAM 5.2, and/or EMA.[36] Importantly, however, strong and multifocal S100 positivity is not uncommon in myoepithelial carcinoma and up to 40% of these tumors show loss of INI1 expression.[45]

Epithelioid sarcoma should be distinguished readily from CE-MPNST by the use of immunohistochemistry, revealing consistent cytokeratin positivity and negativity for S100.[36,46] In addition, about 50% of epithelioid sarcomas are CD34 positive.[36,46,47]

Among benign conditions, epithelioid schwannoma deserves mention. Helpful discriminant morphologic features favoring epithelioid schwannoma over CE-MPNST are good circumscription with encapsulation and a lack of diffuse and significant nuclear atypia/pleomorphism, as well as the absence of prominent nucleoli, atypical mitoses, and tumor necrosis.[36,48]

## REFERENCES

1. Ducatman BS, Scheithauer BW, Piepgras DG, et al. Malignant peripheral nerve sheath tumors. A clinicopathologic study of 120 cases. Cancer 1986;57: 2006–21.
2. Marino-Enriquez A, Guillou L, Hornick JL. Spindle cell tumors of adults. In: Hornick JL, editor. Practical soft tissue pathology: a diagnostic approach. Philadelphia: Elsevier Saunders; 2013. p. 14–93.
3. Feng CJ, Ma H, Liao WC. Superficial or cutaneous malignant peripheral nerve sheath tumor–clinical experience at Taipei Veterans General Hospital. Ann Plast Surg 2015;74(Suppl 2):S85–8.
4. Sorensen SA, Mulvihill JJ, Nielsen A. Long-term follow-up of von Recklinghausen neurofibromatosis. Survival and malignant neoplasms. N Engl J Med 1986;314:1010–5.
5. Woodruff JM. Pathology of tumors of the peripheral nerve sheath in type 1 neurofibromatosis. Am J Med Genet 1999;89:23–30.
6. Ducatman BS, Scheithauer BW. Postirradiation neurofibrosarcoma. Cancer 1983;51:1028–33.
7. Foley KM, Woodruff JM, Ellis FT, et al. Radiation-induced malignant and atypical peripheral nerve sheath tumors. Ann Neurol 1980;7:311–8.
8. Miettinen M. Modern soft tissue pathology: tumors and non-neoplastic conditions. Cambridge (United Kingdom): Cambridge University Press; 2010.
9. Beert E, Brems H, Daniels B, et al. Atypical neurofibromas in neurofibromatosis type 1 are premalignant tumors. Genes Chromosomes Cancer 2011;50:1021–32.
10. Lee W, Teckie S, Wiesner T, et al. PRC2 is recurrently inactivated through EED or SUZ12 loss in malignant peripheral nerve sheath tumors. Nat Genet 2014;46: 1227–32.
11. Schaefer IM, Fletcher CD, Hornick JL. Loss of H3K27 trimethylation distinguishes malignant peripheral nerve sheath tumors from histologic mimics. Mod Pathol 2016;29:4–13.
12. Inoue T, Kuwashiro M, Misago N, et al. Superficial malignant peripheral nerve sheath tumor arising from diffuse neurofibroma in a neurofibromatosis type 1 patient. J Dermatol 2014;41:631–3.
13. Wick MR. Malignant peripheral nerve sheath tumors of the skin. Mayo Clin Proc 1990;65:279–82.
14. Thomas C, Somani N, Owen LG, et al. Cutaneous malignant peripheral nerve sheath tumors. J Cutan Pathol 2009;36:896–900.
15. Allison KH, Patel RM, Goldblum JR, et al. Superficial malignant peripheral nerve sheath tumor: a rare and challenging diagnosis. Am J Clin Pathol 2005;124: 685–92.
16. Evans HL. Sporadic superficial diffuse neurofibromas with repeated local recurrence over many years and a tendency toward malignant change: a report of 3 cases. Am J Surg Pathol 2013;37:987–94.
17. Fields JP, Helwig EB. Leiomyosarcoma of the skin and subcutaneous tissue. Cancer 1981;47:156–69.
18. Dabski C, Reiman HM Jr, Muller SA. Neurofibrosarcoma of skin and subcutaneous tissues. Mayo Clin Proc 1990;65:164–72.
19. Sangueza OP, Requena L. Neoplasms with neural differentiation: a review. Part II: malignant neoplasms. Am J Dermatopathol 1998;20:89–102.

20. Fanburg-Smith JC. Nerve sheath and neuroectodermal tumors. In: Folpe AL, Inwards CY, editors. Bone and soft tissue pathology. Philadelphia: Churchill-Livingstone; 2010. p. 193–238.

21. Woodruff JM, Chernik NL, Smith MC, et al. Peripheral nerve tumors with rhabdomyosarcomatous differentiation (malignant "Triton" tumors). Cancer 1973;32:426–39.

22. Stasik CJ, Tawfik O. Malignant peripheral nerve sheath tumor with rhabdomyosarcomatous differentiation (malignant triton tumor). Arch Pathol Lab Med 2006;130:1878–81.

23. Mae K, Kato Y, Usui K, et al. A case of malignant peripheral nerve sheath tumor with rhabdomyoblastic differentiation: malignant triton tumor. Case Rep Dermatol 2013;5:373–8.

24. Brenn T, Hornick JL. Cutaneous mesenchymal tumors. In: Hornick JL, editor. Practical soft tissue pathology: a diagnostic approach. Philadelphia: Elsevier Saunders; 2013. p. 387–436.

25. Plaza JA, Bonneau P, Prieto V, et al. Desmoplastic melanoma: an updated immunohistochemical analysis of 40 cases with a proposal for an additional panel of stains for diagnosis. J Cutan Pathol 2016;43:313–23.

26. Flieder DB, Moran CA. Primary cutaneous synovial sarcoma: a case report. Am J Dermatopathol 1998;20:509–12.

27. Achtman JC, Pavlidakey PG, Zhang PJ, et al. Synovial sarcoma with cutaneous metastasis. J Cutan Pathol 2016;43:85–7.

28. Smith TA, Machen SK, Fisher C, et al. Usefulness of cytokeratin subsets for distinguishing monophasic synovial sarcoma from malignant peripheral nerve sheath tumor. Am J Clin Pathol 1999;112:641–8.

29. Fisher C. Synovial sarcoma. Ann Diagn Pathol 1998;2:401–21.

30. Fisher C, Montgomery E, Healy V. Calponin and h-caldesmon expression in synovial sarcoma; the use of calponin in diagnosis. Histopathology 2003;42:588–93.

31. Kosemehmetoglu K, Vrana JA, Folpe AL. TLE1 expression is not specific for synovial sarcoma: a whole section study of 163 soft tissue and bone neoplasms. Mod Pathol 2009;22:872–8.

32. Thway K, Fisher C. Synovial sarcoma: defining features and diagnostic evolution. Ann Diagn Pathol 2014;18:369–80.

33. Dewit L, Albus-Lutter CE, de Jong AS, et al. Malignant schwannoma with a rhabdomyoblastic component, a so-called triton tumor. A clinicopathologic study. Cancer 1986;58:1350–6.

34. Mentzel T, Beham A, Katenkamp D, et al. Fibrosarcomatous ("high-grade") dermatofibrosarcoma protuberans: clinicopathologic and immunohistochemical study of a series of 41 cases with emphasis on prognostic significance. Am J Surg Pathol 1998;22:576–87.

35. Jokinen CH, Argenyi ZB. Atypical neurofibroma of the skin and subcutaneous tissue: clinicopathologic analysis of 11 cases. J Cutan Pathol 2010;37:35–42.

36. Jo VY, Fletcher CD. Epithelioid malignant peripheral nerve sheath tumor: clinicopathologic analysis of 63 cases. Am J Surg Pathol 2015;39:673–82.

37. Luzar B, Shanesmith R, Ramakrishnan R, et al. Cutaneous epithelioid malignant peripheral nerve sheath tumour: a clinicopathological analysis of 11 cases. Histopathology 2016;68:286–96.

38. Manganoni AM, Farisoglio C, Lonati A, et al. Cutaneous epithelioid malignant schwannoma: review of the literature and case report. J Plast Reconstr Aesthet Surg 2009;62:e318–21.

39. Laskin WB, Weiss SW, Bratthauer GL. Epithelioid variant of malignant peripheral nerve sheath tumor (malignant epithelioid schwannoma). Am J Surg Pathol 1991;15:1136–45.

40. Yamamoto T, Minami R, Ohbayashi C. Subcutaneous malignant epithelioid schwannoma with cartilaginous differentiation. J Cutan Pathol 2001;28:486–91.

41. Shimizu S, Teraki Y, Ishiko A, et al. Malignant epithelioid schwannoma of the skin showing partial HMB-45 positivity. Am J Dermatopathol 1993;15:378–84.

42. Thewes M, Jungfer-Weber B, Wiebecke B, et al. Malignant epithelioid schwannoma with melanocytic differentiation: a rare tumour with an unusual feature. Acta Derm Venereol 1997;77:493–4.

43. Hornick JL, Dal Cin P, Fletcher CD. Loss of INI1 expression is characteristic of both conventional and proximal-type epithelioid sarcoma. Am J Surg Pathol 2009;33:542–50.

44. Carter JM, O'Hara C, Dundas G, et al. Epithelioid malignant peripheral nerve sheath tumor arising in a schwannoma, in a patient with "neuroblastoma-like" schwannomatosis and a novel germline SMARCB1 mutation. Am J Surg Pathol 2012;36:154–60.

45. Gleason BC, Fletcher CD. Myoepithelial carcinoma of soft tissue in children: an aggressive neoplasm analyzed in a series of 29 cases. Am J Surg Pathol 2007;31:1813–24.

46. Fisher C. Epithelioid sarcoma of Enzinger. Adv Anat Pathol 2006;13:114–21.

47. Laskin WB, Miettinen M. Epithelioid sarcoma: new insights based on an extended immunohistochemical analysis. Arch Pathol Lab Med 2003;127:1161–8.

48. McMenamin ME, Fletcher CD. Expanding the spectrum of malignant change in schwannomas: epithelioid malignant change, epithelioid malignant peripheral nerve sheath tumor, and epithelioid angiosarcoma: a study of 17 cases. Am J Surg Pathol 2001;25:13–25.

# Histopathology of Spindle Cell Vascular Tumors

Zlatko Marušić, MD, PhD[a], Steven D. Billings, MD[b],*

## KEYWORDS

- Spindle cell hemangioma • Acquired tufted angioma • Angioblastoma of Nakagawa
- Kaposiform hemangioendothelioma • Kaposi sarcoma • Angiosarcoma

## ABSTRACT

Vascular tumors with a spindled morphology represent a diagnostic challenge in soft tissue pathology. It may be difficult to distinguish certain benign entities in this category from spindled vascular tumors of intermediate malignancy or even spindled variants of angiosarcoma. This article focuses on vascular tumors characterized by a predominantly spindled morphology, including spindle cell hemangioma, acquired tufted angioma (angioblastoma of Nakagawa), kaposiform hemangioendothelioma, Kaposi sarcoma, and spindle cell variants of angiosarcoma.

angioblastoma of Nakagawa and kaposiform hemangioendothelioma, Kaposi sarcoma, and spindled examples of angiosarcoma.

## OVERVIEW

Vascular tumors with a predominantly spindled morphology can pose a diagnostic challenge. It may be difficult to discern the vascular nature of certain tumors in this group by morphology alone. Therefore, many other soft tissue tumors with spindled cells enter the differential diagnosis. Another potential caveat is that there can be a degree of morphologic overlap between different spindle cell vascular tumors of varying malignant potential. However, the combination of clinical findings, histologic features, and, in some cases, immunohistochemical markers allows accurate diagnosis. This article discusses the most salient histopathologic, clinical, and pathogenetic features of vascular tumors with a spindled morphology, including spindle cell hemangioma, the related entities acquired tufted angioma/

## SPINDLE CELL HEMANGIOMA

Spindle cell hemangioma, originally described in 1986 as spindle cell hemangioendothelioma, was initially considered a vascular tumor of intermediate malignancy because of its propensity for local recurrence and 1 case in the original series that metastasized.[1] Ten years after its original description, its malignant potential was reassessed by one of the original investigators.[2] Based on this analysis of a larger series, spindle cell hemangioendothelioma was reclassified as spindle cell hemangioma, owing to the lack of metastasis, although local recurrence was still an issue.

Clinically, spindle cell hemangioma is a superficial, subcutaneous or dermal erythematous to violaceous nodule with a predilection for the distal extremities of young adults, especially the hands. It has a slow rate of growth and usually reaches 1 to 2 cm. In some cases, spindle cell hemangioma presents as multiple smaller nodules. There is an equal sex distribution or a very slight female predominance.[3,4] Rare cases presenting in the oral cavity have also been described.[5,6]

In a subset of cases, spindle cell hemangiomas are associated with Maffucci syndrome,[2,7,8] a rare mesodermal dysplasia characterized by multiple spindle cell hemangiomas, enchondromas, and an increased risk for the development of chondrosarcoma (or rarely angiosarcoma).[9] Maffucci

Disclosure: The authors have nothing to disclose.
[a] Department of Pathology, University Hospital Center Zagreb, Kišpatićeva 12, Zagreb 10 000, Croatia;
[b] Department of Pathology, Cleveland Clinic, 9500 Euclid Avenue, L25, Cleveland, OH 44195, USA
* Corresponding author.
E-mail address: billins@ccf.org

surgpath.theclinics.com

syndrome is associated with somatic mutations of isocitrate dehydrogenase. Recent studies have shown that most sporadic spindle cell hemangiomas not associated with Maffucci syndrome also harbor mutations in isocitrate dehydrogenase, usually isocitrate dehydrogenase-1, but with a minority harboring mutations in isocitrate dehydrogenase-2.[10] This mutation seems to be unique to spindle cell hemangioma, because a wide range of other vascular tumors that have been studied lack mutations in isocitrate dehydrogenase.

Microscopically, spindle cell hemangiomas are circumscribed, subcutaneous or dermal tumors (Fig. 1). About half are at least partially intravascular (Fig. 2). Spindle cell hemangiomas have a biphasic composition; one component consists of cavernous vascular spaces lined by bland, flattened endothelial cells and the other consists of more solid spindle cell areas (Fig. 3). The cavernous vessels may contain phleboliths (organized and hyalinized thrombi). The solid spindled areas are composed of bland spindled cells with tapered ends that frequently contain slitlike vascular spaces. Spindled cells are also evident in the cavernous vessel septa, which appear more cellular than the septa of cavernous hemangiomas. The spindle cell component also contains rounded epithelioid endothelial cells with cytoplasmic vacuoles; so-called blister cells (Fig. 4). In cases with pronounced vacuolization, these cells can be mistaken for adipocytes. Focal cytoplasmic vacuolization can also be seen in the endothelial lining of cavernous vessels. Mitotic activity and atypia are generally low within both components.

The intravascular nature of spindle cell hemangiomas may explain the high rate of local recurrence with propagation of the tumor within the affected vessel. In the periphery of the nodule, there are often clearly abnormal thick-walled vessels with fibrointimal thickening, which has led to speculation that spindle cell hemangioma may be a reactive tumor, rather than a neoplasm.[11] However, the fact that spindle cell hemangioma harbors a recurrent mutation confirms the neoplastic nature of spindle cell hemangioma.

By immunohistochemistry, the endothelial and vacuolated cells are positive for CD31 and other endothelial markers, whereas the spindle cell component is positive only for vimentin and in a smaller percentage for smooth muscle actin and/or desmin.[12]

Cavernous hemangioma, nodular Kaposi sarcoma, and kaposiform hemangioendothelioma enter the differential diagnosis. Cavernous hemangioma has less cellular vascular septa and lacks solid spindled areas. Nodular Kaposi sarcoma lacks the cavernous spaces of spindle cell hemangioma, shows intracytoplasmic hyaline globules in spindle cells, lacks epithelioid vacuolated cells, and is invariably positive for human herpesvirus 8 (HHV-8) latent nuclear antigen, unlike spindle cell hemangioma. Kaposiform hemangioendotheliomas occur in children primarily. Although kaposiform hemangioendothelioma

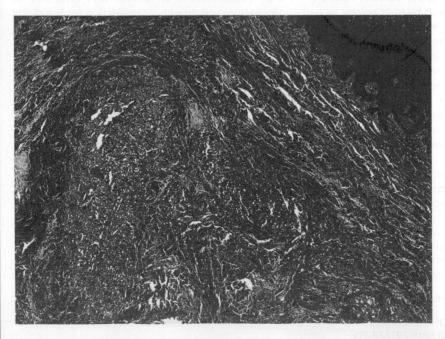

Fig. 1. Low-power view of spindle cell hemangioma.

**Fig. 2.** Spindle cell hemangioma arising in a pre-existing vessel.

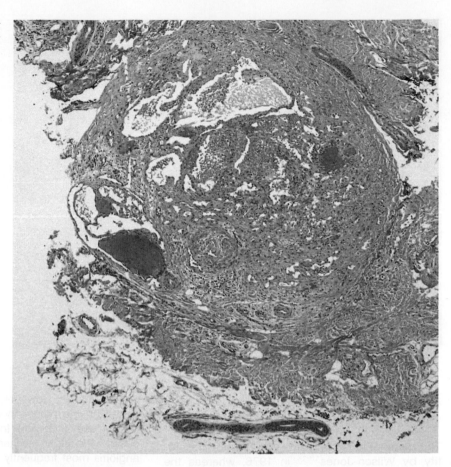

may have ectatic vascular spaces, they are at the periphery of spindle cell nodules that lack vacuolated endothelial cells. The ectatic vascular spaces of kaposiform hemangioendothelioma lack phleboliths.

Approximately 60% of spindle cell hemangiomas recur, usually in the form of multiple regional nodules. The local recurrence is likely related to local intravascular propagation of tumor. There has been no convincing evidence of metastatic spread.[2]

| Spindle Cell Hemangioma vs | Helpful Distinguishing Features |
|---|---|
| Cavernous hemangioma | • Less cellular vascular septa<br>• Lacks solid spindled areas |
| Kaposiform hemangio-endothelioma | • Lacks vacuolated endothelial cells<br>• Ectatic vascular spaces only at the periphery of spindle cell nodules and lacks phleboliths<br>• Occur in children primarily |
| Nodular Kaposi sarcoma | • Lacks cavernous spaces and epithelioid vacuolated cells<br>• Shows intracytoplasmic hyaline globules in spindle cells<br>• Invariably positive for HHV-8 |

---

**⚠ Pitfalls**

**SPINDLE CELL HEMANGIOMA**

! In cases with pronounced vacuolization, so-called blister cells can be mistaken for adipocytes or vacuolated endothelial cells of epithelioid hemangioendothelioma

! Bland spindled areas may be reminiscent of Kaposi sarcoma

! May be multifocal

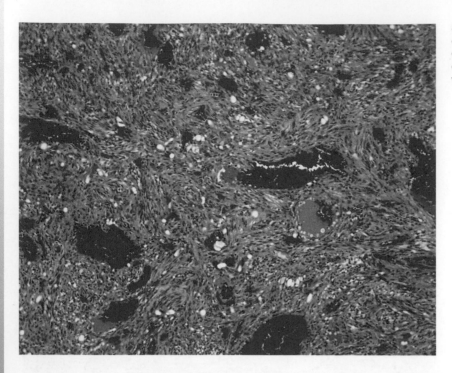

*Fig. 3.* Spindle cell hemangiomas are composed of a combination of spindled cells and ectatic vascular spaces.

## ACQUIRED TUFTED ANGIOMA (ANGIOBLASTOMA OF NAKAGAWA)

The name of tufted angioma was given to this entity by Wilson-Jones[13,14] in 1976, whereas the term acquired tufted angioma was introduced a decade later.[15] However, both terms were preceded by the name angioblastoma, which had been in use since 1949 for histologically identical cases in the Japanese literature.[16] Acquired tufted angioma most frequently presents in early childhood as a progressively enlarging cutaneous

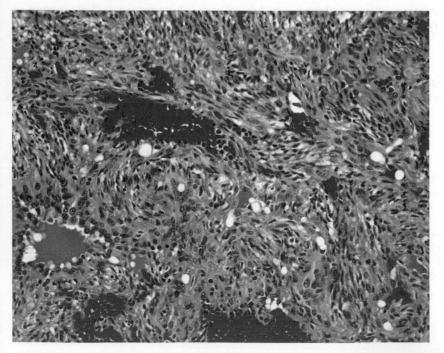

*Fig. 4.* Higher power view of spindle cell hemangioma showing ectatic vascular spaces, spindled cells, and vacuolated endothelial cells.

macule in the head and neck region. There is no gender predilection.[4] Rare cases can be encountered in older adults, whereas congenital cases are rare.[17,18] Multifocality is exceptional.[19,20] Cases associated with severe consumptive coagulopathy (Kasabach-Merritt syndrome) have been described, but less frequently than in kaposiform hemangioendothelioma.[21]

On histology, the tumor is situated in the dermis or subcutis, and presents with the so-called cannonball pattern of scattered, spherical, well-demarcated lobules of tightly packed, poorly canalized capillaries containing few if any erythrocytes (**Fig. 5**). At the periphery of some lobules, there are slightly dilated, crescent-shaped lymphatic channels (**Fig. 6**). The capillary lumina are lined by a single, bland endothelial cell layer and surrounded by bland-looking smooth muscle actin (SMA)-positive pericytes, which can be prominent and impart a spindled appearance to the lesion (**Fig. 7**). Besides highlighting the lymphatic channels, immunostains for podoplanin (D2-40) may also show partial staining within the capillary network.[22]

Features of acquired tufted angioma show an extensive overlap with those of kaposiform hemangioendothelioma.[2] Both tumors are usually encountered in children and share association with the Kasabach-Merritt syndrome as well as similar histologic features, to the extent that many of them cannot be distinguished based on published photomicrographs. There are several reports that include features of both entities in the same lesion; that is, a transformation between one lesion and the other.[23,24] Acquired tufted angioma has recently been shown to have a familial component, involving 3 potential genes (*EDR, ENG, and FLT4*),[25] whereas such an association has not yet been reported in kaposiform hemangioendothelioma. However, they likely represent a spectrum of the same tumor. It may be reasonable to retain the terminology of acquired tufted angioma for small, superficial lesions, especially those presenting in adult patients, reserving the diagnosis of kaposiform hemangioendothelioma for the more extensive and deeper childhood lesions associated with consumptive coagulopathy.

The differential diagnosis includes nodular Kaposi sarcoma and kaposiform hemangioendothelioma (if there is reason to distinguish the tufted angioma from kaposiform hemangioendothelioma). Nodular Kaposi sarcoma lacks the cannonball pattern, has a much more confluent spindle

*Fig. 5.* Low-power view of acquired tufted angioma showing cannonball pattern of the vascular proliferation in the dermis.

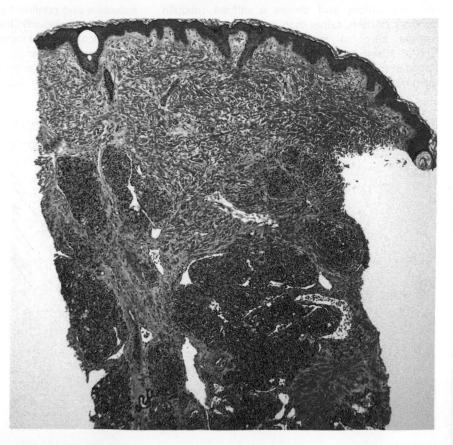

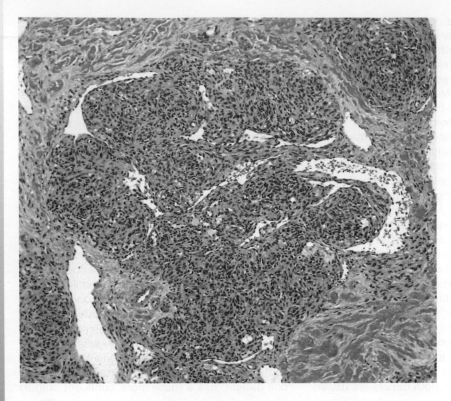

*Fig. 6.* Acquired tufted angioma is characterized by nodules of spindled cells with slitlike vascular spaces and surrounding ectatic vessels.

cell population, and shows a diffuse reticulin network pattern, rather than a vasoformative one. Kaposi sarcoma shows immunoreactivity for HHV-8 latent nuclear antigen, whereas acquired tufted angioma does not. Classic cases of kaposiform hemangioendothelioma tend to show a more extensive and confluent growth, even though, as mentioned previously, they are likely to be ends of a spectrum of the same tumor.

Acquired tufted angioma follows a benign clinical course. Some have been shown to regress spontaneously.[26,27] Rare, unresectable cases

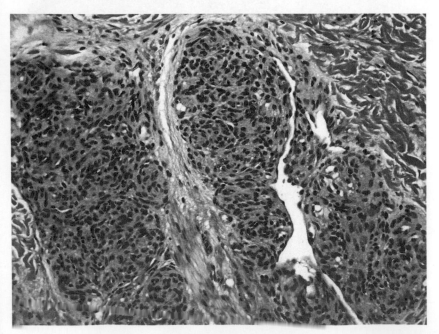

*Fig. 7.* High-power view of a vascular nodule of acquired tufted angioma.

with Kasabach-Merritt syndrome are better classified as kaposiform hemangioendotheliomas. In this setting, chemotherapeutic options with vincristine, prednisolone, or propranolol can be successful.[28]

> **Pitfalls**
> TUFTED ANGIOMA
>
> ! Shows considerable overlap with kaposiform hemangioendothelioma
>
> ! The term tufted angioma should probably be reserved for small cutaneous lesions in adults

| Acquired Tufted Angioma vs | Helpful Distinguishing Features |
|---|---|
| Kaposiform hemangioendothelioma | • Likely a spectrum of the same tumor<br>• More extensive and confluent growth<br>• More frequent Kasabach-Merritt syndrome |
| Nodular Kaposi sarcoma | • Lacks the cannonball pattern<br>• More confluent spindle cell population and diffuse reticulin network pattern<br>• Invariably positive for HHV-8 |

## KAPOSIFORM HEMANGIOENDOTHELIOMA

The term hemangioendothelioma is used for vascular tumors with biological behavior intermediate between hemangioma and angiosarcoma. Hemangioendotheliomas tend to produce local recurrences and some have the potential to metastasize, but at a far reduced level compared with angiosarcoma.[2]

Kaposiform hemangioendothelioma was first described in the retroperitoneum on autopsy cases under 2 different names.[29,30] Subsequently, it was reported by Zukerberg and colleagues[31] in a larger series and given its current name. It is a very rare tumor of infancy and childhood, occurring most frequently as multinodular lesions in peripheral soft tissue or skin, followed by the retroperitoneum (**Fig. 8**).[32] Strictly cutaneous cases frequently present as a poorly defined violaceous plaque.[33] A subset of cases is associated with lymphangiomatosis.[34] There is no sex predilection and most of the patients are in the first 2 years of life; however, it has been reported in adults as well.[35]

Microscopically, the tumor forms a plexiform mass of lobules separated by fibrous septa (**Fig. 9**). The lobules consist of capillary hemangioma-like areas alternating with spindled areas reminiscent of Kaposi sarcoma (**Fig. 10**). Spindle cells are separated by slitlike lumina containing erythrocytes and show a mild degree of atypia with few mitoses (**Fig. 11**). Glomeruloid structures are a specific feature of this tumor. They are composed of small vessels surrounded by pericytes and hyaline globules, erythrocytes, and often fine granular hemosiderin (**Fig. 12**). The hyaline globules represent erythrocyte fragments and small thrombi. This condition is a morphologic manifestation of what can result in the development of consumptive coagulopathy (Kasabach-Merritt syndrome). Some hyaline globules can also be seen in the spindled cells. The periphery of the lobules can show a striking lymphatic proliferation, with ectatic vascular spaces partially surrounding the spindle cell nodules (**Fig. 13**).

Immunohistochemical properties of kaposiform hemangioendothelioma reflect its cellular components: most of the cells express CD31, CD34, and ERG, whereas pericytes are highlighted by SMA stains, especially within the glomeruloid structures. Lymphatic markers vascular endothelial growth factor (VEGF)-3 and podoplanin are positive in both the lymphatic channels at the lobule periphery and the spindled cells, and so is Prox1, a lymphatic endothelial nuclear transcription factor. The juvenile hemangioma-associated marker glucose transporter 1 (GLUT1) is negative.[36–39]

As mentioned previously, acquired tufted angioma and kaposiform hemangioendothelioma represent different spectral parts of the same entity. Both tumors show histologic overlap and a similar immunohistochemical profile. However, lesions reported as acquired tufted angiomas are described as having more of a cannonball pattern and superficial involvement of peripheral soft tissue, whereas kaposiform hemangioendothelioma is deeper and more extensive. Acquired tufted angiomas also show lower propensity for the induction of Kasabach-Merritt syndrome, but this may simply be a reflection of small tumor size in entities diagnosed as acquired tufted angioma.[2]

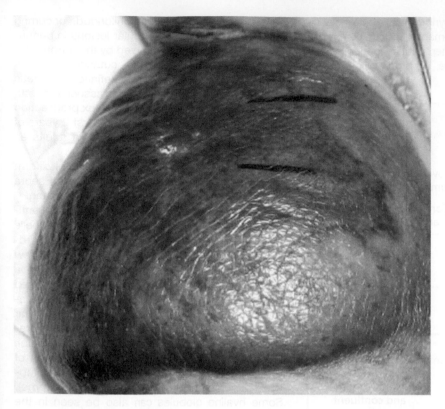

*Fig. 8.* Clinical view of kaposiform hemangioendothelioma in an infant.

Juvenile capillary hemangioma does not feature spindling of the cells, lacks glomeruloid structures, and is negative for Prox1. The spindled areas of kaposiform hemangioendothelioma can be indistinguishable from Kaposi sarcoma.

However, Kaposi sarcoma is vanishingly rare in children, except for the endemic lymphadenopathy type of African Kaposi sarcoma. It is more uniformly spindled, and lacks the lobular structure of kaposiform hemangioendothelioma. In addition,

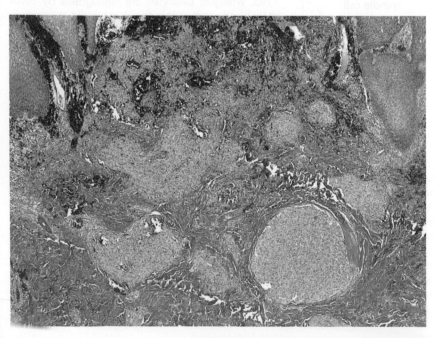

*Fig. 9.* Kaposiform hemangioendothelioma with nodules of spindled cells separated by collagenous stroma.

*Fig. 10.* Portions of the kaposiform hemangioendothelioma are reminiscent of a capillary hemangioma, whereas other areas resemble the spindle cell proliferation of tumor-stage Kaposi sarcoma.

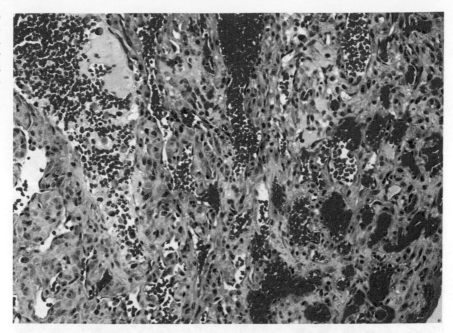

the two can be readily distinguished by immunohistochemical stains for HHV-8, which is characteristic for Kaposi sarcoma.

Kaposiform hemangioendothelioma may show regional perinodal soft tissue involvement,[34] but has not been reported to produce distant metastasis. Instead, they can be infiltrative, and retroperitoneal cases tend to extensively infiltrate surrounding organs. In the original description,

the tumors had invaded the kidneys, pancreas, adrenal glands, and gastrointestinal tract in both cases.[29] As mentioned previously, kaposiform hemangioendothelioma may induce the Kasabach-Merritt syndrome,[40] characterized by thrombocytopenia and consumption coagulopathy. The consumptive coagulopathy is related to tumor size and location. Large intrathoracic or retroperitoneal tumors are associated with

*Fig. 11.* High-power view of Kaposi sarcoma–like area of kaposiform hemangioendothelioma.

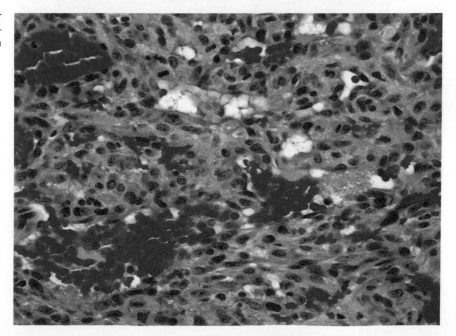

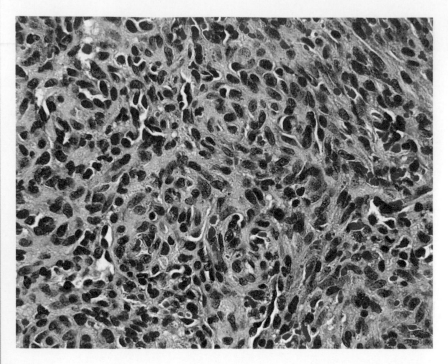

*Fig. 12.* Glomeruloid-like area in kaposiform hemangioendothelioma.

Kasabach-Merritt syndrome in close to 100% of cases, whereas it is less common in tumors confined to the skin or superficial soft tissue.[41]

Up to 10% of kaposiform hemangioendotheliomas carry a lethal outcome, usually secondary to complications of Kasabach-Merritt syndrome. In unresectable cases complicated by coagulopathy, patients undergo a multimodality treatment using vincristine, prednisolone, β-blockers, or sirolimus.[42,43]

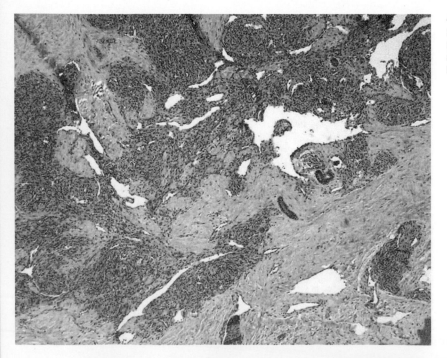

*Fig. 13.* Ectatic lymphatic vessels at periphery of spindle cell nodules in kaposiform hemangioendothelioma.

## Pitfalls
### Kaposiform Hemangioendothelioma

! May be associated with lymphangiomatosis

! Spindled areas may be morphologically indistinguishable from Kaposi sarcoma

! Can have areas resembling juvenile hemangioma

| Kaposiform Hemangioendothelioma vs | Helpful Distinguishing Features |
| --- | --- |
| Acquired tufted angioma | • Likely a spectrum of the same tumor<br>• Cannonball pattern and superficial involvement<br>• Lower propensity for the induction of Kasabach-Merritt syndrome |
| Juvenile hemangioma | • No spindling of the cells<br>• Lacks glomeruloid structures<br>• Negative for Prox1 |
| Nodular Kaposi sarcoma | • Vanishingly rare in children<br>• Uniformly spindled, lacks the lobular structure<br>• Invariably positive for HHV-8 |

## KAPOSI SARCOMA

In 1872, an Austro-Hungarian dermatologist by the name of Moritz Kaposi[44] first described the classic form of disease in 5 patients (4 elderly men and one child) as "idiopathic multiple pigmented sarcoma."[44] Interestingly and presciently, Dr Kaposi[44] thought that the multifocal nature of the disease represented a systemic disease rather than metastatic disease from a single neoplasm. Early in the twentieth century, there was significant debate in the literature as to whether this disease truly represented a sarcoma.[45,46]

In the mid–twentieth century, a tumor with similar presentation and histologic features was discovered in sub-Saharan Africa.[47] With the advent of the acquired immunodeficiency syndrome (AIDS) epidemic in the 1980s, it became clear that both previously observed forms were related to the new, progressive, and fulminant form of disease encountered mostly in male homosexual patients with AIDS.[48,49] The single most important subsequent discovery regarding Kaposi sarcoma was of its causative relationship with HHV-8.[50–52]

There are 4 clinical forms of Kaposi sarcoma. The first is the classic form described by Kaposi,[44] typically presenting as purple to reddish skin lesions in the lower extremities of men, usually more than 60 years of age. This form is more frequent in certain populations, such as those

inhabiting the Mediterranean region and parts of Eastern Europe. It is characterized by multiple recurrences, but the disease typically follows an indolent course. However, it is frequently accompanied by a second malignancy.[53]

The endemic African form of Kaposi sarcoma is encountered in sub-Saharan Africa. It can present as the classic form or as a progressive form, which is frequently encountered in children and characterized by generalized lymph node involvement, whereas some other subtypes of the progressive form resemble AIDS-related Kaposi sarcoma.[54]

Kaposi sarcoma occurred in as many as 30% of patients with AIDS before the advent of highly effective antiretroviral therapy, earning this form of disease the designation of epidemic Kaposi sarcoma. In this form, cutaneous lesions do not follow the typical clinical presentation as a tumor of the lower extremity, but are distributed more diffusely throughout the skin and in mucosal sites. Involvement of internal organs is common, including various sites, such as the lung, gastrointestinal tract, spleen, and lymph nodes.[55]

The iatrogenic form of Kaposi sarcoma is encountered in patients under immunosuppression, especially in renal transplant recipients. It has predilection for the involvement of skin, mucosal sites, and internal organs.[56]

There are 3 clinical stages of cutaneous lesions: patch, plaque, and nodular stages. They show respective histologic patterns with a certain degree of overlap. The patch stage is characterized by a proliferation of small and irregular, jagged, complex vascular channels within the superficial reticular dermis, whose endothelium shows mild atypia without multilayering of endothelial cells (**Fig. 14**). The proliferation is often oriented parallel to the surface. The neoplastic vessels often dissect around preexisting vascular and adnexal structures, resulting in the promontory sign, in which the neoplastic vessels surround normal blood vessels and adnexal structures (**Fig. 15**). The vessels can be surrounded by a slightly more atypical spindle cell component, hemosiderin granules, perivascular lymphocytes and plasma cells, and rare hyaline globules.[57] Plaque stage is clinically slightly elevated and may be viewed as an exaggerated version of the patch stage with a more substantial spindle cell component, more hemosiderin, and more easily visible hyaline globules (**Fig. 16**). It frequently involves the entire dermis, sometimes spreading into the subcutis. Nodular Kaposi sarcoma is a well-circumscribed violaceous nodule situated in the dermis, composed of sheets and fascicles of uniform spindle cells with little cytologic atypia and frequent mitotic activity. There are numerous slit-like vascular spaces between spindle cells, containing erythrocytes (**Fig. 17**). Eosinophilic hyaline globules are typically present. These PAS-positive structures situated within and outside vessels represent lysosomes with partially digested erythrocytes.[58]

Not all presentations of Kaposi sarcoma have the identical set of features described earlier. Even though cytologic characteristics of Kaposi sarcoma include mild atypia, cases with significant pleomorphism or even anaplastic transformation have been described and are suggested to present most frequently among African patients.[59,60] Another variant is the so-called lymphangiomatous Kaposi sarcoma, characterized by ectatic vessels resembling vascular spaces of lymphangioma (**Fig. 18**).[61,62] Cases with histologic overlap with pyogenic granuloma may also occur (**Fig. 19**).[63,64] These lesions have a polypoid silhouette, an epidermal collarette, and areas with more well-formed vascular channels in addition to the spindled endothelial cells more typical of Kaposi sarcoma.

Involvement of lymph nodes starts in the subcapsular sinuses and may be subtle at first, mimicking the condition called vascular transformation of sinuses, caused by lymph node obstruction. More advanced cases of lymph node Kaposi sarcoma are easier to detect because of their more solid spindle cell component accompanied by partial or complete effacement of the lymph node. In patients with AIDS, a mycobacterial pseudotumor should enter the differential diagnosis, because pseudotumors may present within lymph nodes in this setting.[65]

By immunohistochemistry, Kaposi sarcoma is positive for CD31, CD34, ERG, podoplanin, and VEGF-3.[66–68] HHV-8 latency–associated nuclear antigen (LANA-1) is expressed in tissues infected by HHV-8 and represents a highly sensitive and specific marker for Kaposi sarcoma, both in the endothelia of early lesions and in the spindle cells of the more advanced stages (**Fig. 20**).[69]

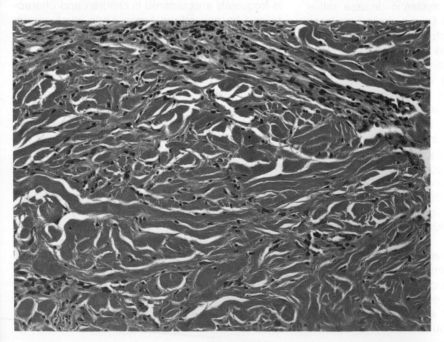

*Fig. 14.* In patch-stage Kaposi sarcoma there is a proliferation of thin-walled vessels lined by small hyperchromatic endothelial cells infiltrating through the dermal collagen.

*Fig. 15.* The vessels of Kaposi sarcoma often dissect around preexisting dermal structures, resulting in the promontory sign.

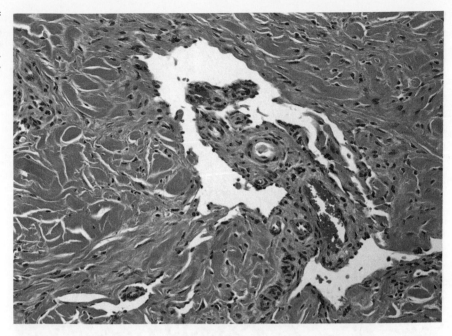

The list of Kaposi sarcoma differential diagnoses is extensive. It includes other vascular tumors such as spindle cell hemangioma, acquired tufted angioma, kaposiform hemangioendothelioma, and cutaneous angiosarcoma. Some of the differential diagnoses were discussed previously in this article. Cutaneous angiosarcoma shows more cytologic atypia and endothelial multilayering. Microvenular hemangioma can be confused with the patch stage of Kaposi sarcoma, but microvenular hemangioma is not associated with immunosuppression and consists of a dermal vascular proliferation with a conspicuous pericyte layer that can be highlighted with stains for SMA.[70] Unlike all of the other tumors in the differential diagnosis, only Kaposi sarcoma is positive for HHV-8 latent nuclear antigen.

Nonvascular tumors that could be considered in the differential diagnosis include fibrosarcomatous

*Fig. 16.* In plaque stage, the neoplastic vessels may be associated with an increased number of spindled cells, plasma cells, and hemosiderin deposition.

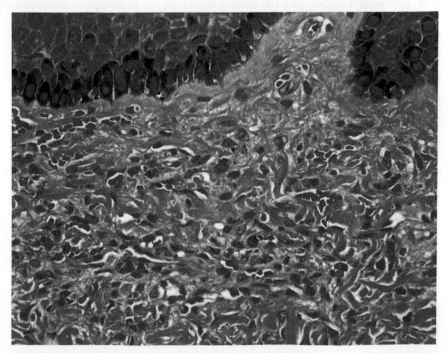

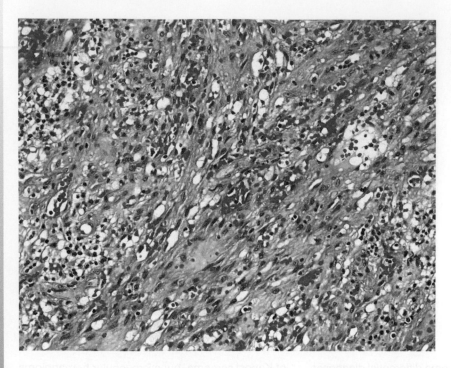

*Fig. 17.* The nodular or tumor phase of Kaposi sarcoma is composed of spindled cells with slitlike lumens and extravasated erythrocytes.

dermatofibrosarcoma protuberans, but the fibrosarcomatous component has a herringbone pattern, more nuclear atypia, and lacks slitlike vascular channels, hemorrhage, and immunoreactivity for HHV-8.[71,72] Aneurysmal dermatofibroma is more polymorphous, usually contains some foamy histiocytes, and lacks slitlike spaces.[73,74] A host of other smooth muscle, myofibroblastic, and epithelial tumors can be distinguished by lack of Kaposi sarcoma staining for actin, desmin, keratins, and epithelial membrane antigen (EMA).[75]

Acroangiodermatitis (pseudo-Kaposi sarcoma) has a similar clinical and histologic presentation as patch-stage lesions in classic Kaposi sarcoma. Clinically, it is most often associated with chronic venous insufficiency, arteriovenous malformation, or iatrogenic arteriovenous shunt. Microscopically,

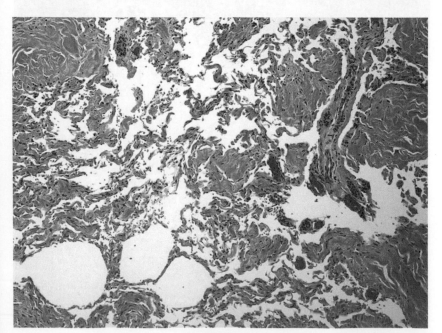

*Fig. 18.* In some cases the vascular proliferation of Kaposi sarcoma can be reminiscent of lymphangioma.

**Fig. 19.** Some cases of Kaposi sarcoma are well circumscribed with an epidermal collarette resembling pyogenic granuloma.

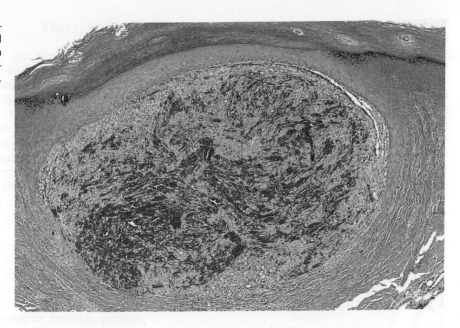

there is a superficial proliferation of small vessels, but, in contrast with patch-stage Kaposi sarcoma, the inflammatory infiltrate is lacking and the vessels are smaller and less irregular.[76–79]

Some aspects of the behavior of Kaposi sarcoma have been mentioned previously. Briefly, the prognosis depends on the form, the stage at presentation, involvement of internal organs, and presence of opportunistic infections. In classic form, the mortality is 10% to 20%, but development of a second malignancy in these patients accounts for an equal, if not a higher, percentage of lethal outcomes.[3] The endemic African form is heterogeneous in behavior, as is the clinical presentation. The lymphadenopathic form in young children follows a progressive course. In patients with AIDS, Kaposi sarcoma was once a common contributor to mortality, but effective antiretroviral therapy has reduced the occurrence and lethality of Kaposi sarcoma.[80] In addition, the prognosis in the iatrogenic form depends on whether there is involvement of the internal organs and whether

**Fig. 20.** Nuclear immunoreactivity for HHV-8 latent nuclear antigen in Kaposi sarcoma.

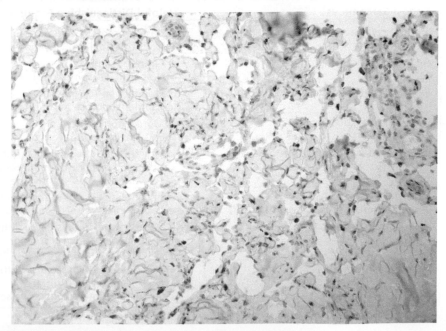

the patient can tolerate reduction of immunosuppression dosage. In some patients, tumors may regress with withdrawal of immunosuppressive medications.[81,82]

The behavior of Kaposi sarcoma can be altered by antiretroviral medication or withdrawal of immunosuppressive medications, which calls into question whether this disease should be considered a sarcoma. Doubts as to the nature of the behavior of Kaposi sarcoma have existed since the early twentieth century.[45,46] More recently, it has been found that patients with multiple different lesions frequently have different HHV-8 clones, arguing that Kaposi sarcoma should be considered a reactive vascular proliferation related to an underlying viral infection rather than a true sarcoma.[83]

## ANGIOSARCOMA

The entire clinical and histologic spectrum of angiosarcoma is very broad and beyond the scope of this article. Most cutaneous angiosarcomas occur in heavily sun-damaged skin of the head and neck of older patients, with a second population of patients who develop angiosarcoma in the setting of radiation therapy or chronic lymphedema. Although in most patients there are obvious, atypical vasoformative channels, the authors have encountered cases of cutaneous angiosarcoma that have a solid spindle cell growth pattern with little evidence of vascular channel formation (**Fig. 21A**).

In clinical settings at risk for angiosarcoma (eg, sun-damaged skin of the head and neck), clinicians should keep a high index of suspicion for angiosarcoma in cases with intratumoral hemorrhage, especially if the tumors infiltrate around preexisting adnexal structures (**Fig. 22**). In such cases, more obvious neoplastic vessels may be present at the periphery of the tumor and careful scrutiny of the tumor is recommended (**Fig. 21B**). In small biopsy specimens in which the periphery of the tumor is not well-visualized, the differential diagnosis can include atypical fibroxanthoma and pleomorphic dermal sarcoma, spindle cell squamous cell carcinoma, and spindle cell melanoma. In general, the nuclei of atypical fibroxanthoma, pleomorphic dermal sarcoma, and

### Pitfalls
#### KAPOSI SARCOMA

! Atypical variants: anaplastic, lymphangiomatous, and pyogenic granulomalike

! Differential diagnosis includes both vascular and nonvascular tumors

! If in doubt, immunohistochemical stains for HHV-8 should be performed

| Kaposi Sarcoma vs | Helpful Distinguishing Features[a] |
|---|---|
| Spindle cell hemangioma | • Has cavernous spaces and epithelioid vacuolated cells<br>• No intracytoplasmic hyaline globules in spindle cells |
| Acquired tufted angioma | • Cannonball pattern<br>• No confluent spindle cell population |
| Kaposiform hemangioendothelioma | • Predilection for children<br>• Lobular structure, not uniformly spindled |
| Cutaneous angiosarcoma | • More cytologic atypia<br>• Endothelial multilayering |
| Microvenular hemangioma | • May be confused with patch stage of Kaposi sarcoma<br>• Not associated with immunosuppression<br>• Conspicuous SMA-positive pericyte layer |
| Fibrosarcomatous dermatofibrosarcoma protuberans | • Herringbone pattern, more nuclear atypia<br>• Lacks slitlike vessels and hemorrhage |
| Aneurysmal dermatofibroma | • More polymorphous, lacks slitlike spaces<br>• Peripheral collagen trapping<br>• Usually contains some foamy histiocytes |
| Acroangiodermatitis | • Associated with vascular insufficiency<br>• No inflammatory infiltrate<br>• Smaller and more regular vessels |

[a] All of these entities are negative for the HHV-8 latent nuclear antigen.

*Fig. 21.* (*A*) Angiosarcoma predominantly composed of solid fascicles of spindled cells. (*B*) At the periphery of the tumor, there were vessels with multilayering of atypical endothelial cells.

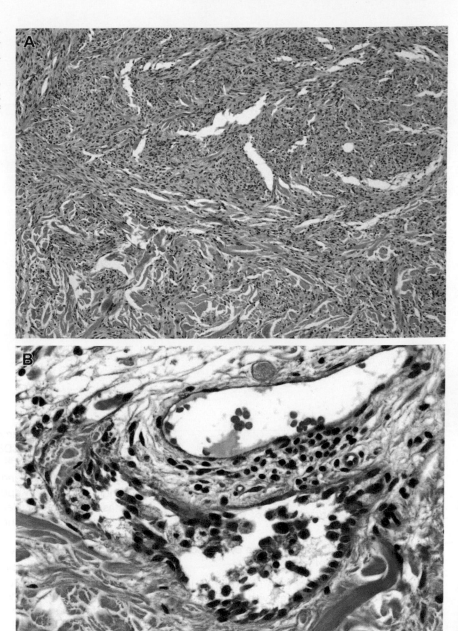

spindle cell squamous cell carcinoma show more nuclear pleomorphism. Angiosarcomas have nuclear atypia, but the nuclei generally do not vary much in morphology. However, atypical fibroxanthomas and pleomorphic dermal sarcomas may have pseudoangiomatous features.[84]

Melanomas usually have a coexisting junctional component and areas with a nested pattern.

Immunohistochemistry allows accurate diagnosis in the setting of a small biopsies. The authors recommend immunohistochemical stains in any tumor that has significant intratumoral hemorrhage in atypical spindle cell tumors from sun-damaged skin of the head and neck. We prefer immunostains for ERG, because of the specificity of this marker compared with CD31 or CD34.[67] If stains for ERG are not available, it has been our personal experience that CD34 may be superior to CD31 in the spindled forms of angiosarcoma. It should be pointed out that atypical fibroxanthoma and

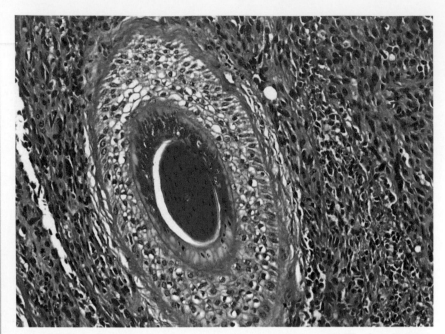

*Fig. 22.* Spindled cell angiosarcoma infiltrating around a hair follicle. There is subtle intratumoral hemorrhage.

**Pitfalls**

ANGIOSARCOMA

! High index of suspicion should be kept for all tumors in sun-damaged skin of the head and neck

! Vasoformative channels may be evident only at the periphery of lesion

! Immunohistochemistry is recommended, especially in small biopsies with hemorrhage: ERG>CD34>CD31

pleomorphic dermal sarcomas may show some immunoreactivity for CD31, possibly related to intratumoral histiocytes.[85,86]

Spindled forms of angiosarcoma need to be distinguished from Kaposi sarcoma. Angiosarcomas have more nuclear atypia and are negative for HHV-8 latent nuclear antigen by immunohistochemistry.

In summary, a variety of vascular tumors may have a predominantly spindled morphology spanning the range of benign, intermediate malignancy, to fully malignant tumors. Careful attention to histologic features in the correct clinical context generally allows accurate diagnosis (**Table 1**).

| Spindled Angiosarcoma vs | Helpful Distinguishing Features |
| --- | --- |
| Pseudoangiomatous atypical fibroxanthoma/pleomorphic dermal sarcoma | • Lack true vascular spaces<br>• Use of immunohistochemistry recommended;<br>• ERG negative, CD34 negative |
| Kaposi sarcoma | • Less nuclear atypia<br>• Positive for HHV-8 |

**Table 1**
Summary of spindle cell vascular tumors

| | SCH | TA | KHE | KS | AS |
|---|---|---|---|---|---|
| Gross features | Sometimes intravascular and multinodular | Enlarging cutaneous macule | Poorly defined violaceous plaque | Patch, plaque, or nodular | Ill-defined erythematous to violaceous patch, plaque, or nodule |
| Growth pattern | Cavernous vessels and solid spindled areas | Cannonball pattern | Plexiform, cavernous, and solid spindled areas | Small vessels or solid spindled areas | Some vessel formation, can have solid spindled areas |
| Nuclei | Uniform, open chromatin; small nucleolus | Uniform, open chromatin; small nucleolus | Mild atypia | Mild, rarely moderate atypia | Moderate to severe atypia |
| Immunophenotype | CD31+, CD34+, ERG+ in endothelial cells spindle cells SMA+, HHV-8– | CD31+, CD34+, ERG+, D2-40+/–, HHV-8–, SMA+ in pericytes | CD31+, CD34+, ERG+, Prox1+, Glut-1–, HHV-8– | CD31+, CD34+, ERG+, D2-40+, HHV-8+ | ERG+, CD34+, CD31+, HHV-8– |

*Abbreviations:* AS, angiosarcoma; KHE, kaposiform hemangioendothelioma; KS, Kaposi sarcoma; SCH, spindle cell hemangioma; TA, tufted angioma.

## REFERENCES

1. Weiss SW, Enzinger FM. Spindle cell hemangioendothelioma. A low-grade angiosarcoma resembling a cavernous hemangioma and Kaposi's sarcoma. Am J Surg Pathol 1986;10(8):521–30.
2. Perkins P, Weiss SW. Spindle cell hemangioendothelioma. An analysis of 78 cases with reassessment of its pathogenesis and biologic behavior. Am J Surg Pathol 1996;20(10):1196–204.
3. Enzinger and Weiss's soft tissue tumors. In: Goldblum JR, Folpe AL, Weiss SW, editors. Malignant vascular tumors. 6th edition. Philadelphia: Mosby; 2014. p. 703–32.
4. Modern soft tissue pathology: tumors and non-neoplastic conditions. In: Miettinen M, editor. Hemangiomas, lymphangiomas, and reactive vascular proliferations. New York: Cambridge University Press; 2010. p. 574–612.
5. Sheehan M, Roumpf SO, Summerlin DJ, et al. Spindle cell hemangioma: report of a case presenting in the oral cavity. J Cutan Pathol 2007;34(10):797–800.
6. Tosios K, Koutlas IG, Kapranos N, et al. Spindle-cell hemangioendothelioma of the oral cavity. A case report. J Oral Pathol Med 1995;24(8):379–82.
7. Maffucci A. Di un caso di encondroma ed angioma multipleo. Movimento Medico-Chirurico 1881;3:399.
8. Carleton A, Elkington J, Greenfield J, et al. Maffucci's syndrome (dyschondroplasia with hemangiomata). Quart J Med 1942;11(1):203.
9. Fanburg JC, Meis-Kindblom JM, Rosenberg AE. Multiple enchondromas associated with spindle cell hemangioendotheliomas: an overlooked variant of Maffucci's syndrome. Am J Surg Pathol 1995;19(9):1029–38.
10. Kurek KC, Pansuriya TC, van Ruler MA, et al. R132C IDH1 mutations are found in spindle cell hemangiomas and not in other vascular tumors or malformations. Am J Pathol 2013;182(5):1494–500.
11. Fletcher CD. The non-neoplastic nature of spindle cell hemangioendothelioma. Am J Clin Pathol 1992;98(5):545–6.
12. Fukunaga M, Ushigome S, Nikaido T, et al. Spindle cell hemangioendothelioma: an immunohistochemical and flow cytometric study of six cases. Pathol Int 1995;45(8):589–95.
13. Wilson-Jones E. Dowling oration. Malignant vascular tumours. Clin Exp Dermatol 1976;1(4):287–312.
14. Wilson-Jones E, Orkin M. Tufted angioma (angioblastoma). A benign progressive angioma, not to be confused with Kaposi's sarcoma or low-grade angiosarcoma. J Am Acad Dermatol 1989;20(2 Pt 1):214–25.
15. Padilla RS, Orkin M, Rosai J. Acquired "tufted" angioma (progressive capillary hemangioma): A distinctive clinicopathologic entity related to lobular capillary hemangioma. Am J Dermatopathol 1987;9(4):292–300.
16. Cho KH, Kim SH, Park KC, et al. Angioblastoma (Nakagawa) – is it the same as tufted angioma? Clin Exp Dermatol 1991;16(2):110–3.
17. Satter EK, Graham BS, Gibbs NF. Congenital tufted angioma. Pediatr Dermatol 2002;19(5):445–7.
18. Osio A, Fraitag S, Hadi-Rabia S, et al. Clinical spectrum of tufted angioma in childhood: report of 13 cases and a review of the literature. Arch Dermatol 2010;146(7):758–63.
19. Maronn M, Chamlin S, Metry D. Multifocal tufted angiomas in 2 infants. Arch Dermatol 2009;145(7):847–8.
20. Wang L, Liu L, Wang G, et al. Congenital disseminated tufted angioma. J Cutan Pathol 2013;40(4):405–8.
21. Seo SK, Suh JC, Na GY, et al. Kasabach-Merritt syndrome: identification of platelet trapping in a tufted angioma by immunohistochemistry technique using monoclonal antibody to CD61. Pediatr Dermatol 1999;16(5):392–4.
22. Sadeghpour M, Antaya RJ, Lazova R, et al. Dilated lymphatic vessels in tufted angioma: a potential source of diagnostic confusion. Am J Dermatopathol 2012;34(4):400–3.
23. Brasanac D, Janic D, Boricic I, et al. Retroperitoneal kaposiform hemangioendothelioma with tufted angioma-like features in an infant with Kasabach-Merritt syndrome. Pathol Int 2003;53(9):627–31.
24. Chu CY, Hsiao CH, Chiu HC. Transformation between kaposiform hemangioendothelioma and tufted angioma. Dermatology 2003;206(4):334–7.
25. Tille JC, Morris MA, Brundler MA, et al. Familial predisposition to tufted angioma: identification of blood and lymphatic vascular components. Clin Genet 2003;63(5):393–9.
26. Miyamoto T, Mihara M, Mishima E, et al. Acquired tufted angioma showing spontaneous regression. Br J Dermatol 1992;127(6):645–8.
27. Lam WY, Mac-Moune Lai F, Look CN, et al. Tufted angioma with complete regression. J Cutan Pathol 1994;21(5):461–6.
28. Chiu YE, Drolet BA, Blei F, et al. Variable response to propranolol treatment of kaposiform hemangioendothelioma, tufted angioma, and Kasabach-Merritt phenomenon. Pediatr Blood Cancer 2012;59(5):934–8.
29. Niedt GW, Greco MA, Wieczorek R, et al. Hemangioma with Kaposi's sarcoma-like features: report of 2 cases. Pediatr Pathol 1989;9(5):567–75.
30. Tsang WYW, Chan JKC. Kaposi-like infantile hemangioendothelioma: a distinctive vascular neoplasm of the retroperitoneum. Am J Surg Pathol 1991;15(10):982–9.

31. Zukerberg LR, Nickoloff BJ, Weiss SW. Kaposiform hemangioendothelioma of infancy and childhood: an aggressive neoplasm associated with Kasabach-Merritt syndrome and lymphangiomatosis. Am J Surg Pathol 1993;17(4):321–8.

32. Tsang WYW, Chan JKC, Fletcher CDM. Recently characterized vascular tumours of skin and soft tissues. Histopathology 1991;19(6):489–501.

33. Lai FMM, Choi PCL, Leung PC, et al. Kaposiform hemangioendothelioma: five patients with cutaneous lesions and long follow-up. Mod Pathol 2001; 14(11):1087–92.

34. Lyons LL, North PE, Mac-Moune Lai F, et al. Kaposiform hemangioendothelioma: a study of 33 cases emphasizing its pathologic, immunophenotypic, and biologic uniqueness from juvenile hemangiomas. Am J Surg Pathol 2004;28(5):559–68.

35. Mentzel T, Mazzoleni G, Dei Tos AP, et al. Kaposiform hemangioendothelioma in adults. Clinicopathologic and immunohistochemical analysis of three cases. Am J Clin Pathol 1997;108(4):450–5.

36. Liu Q, Jiang L, Wu D, et al. Clinicopathological features of Kaposiform hemangioendothelioma. Int J Clin Exp Pathol 2015;8(10):13711–8.

37. Folpe AL, Veikkola T, Valtola R, et al. Vascular endothelial growth factor receptor-3 (VEGFR-3): a marker of vascular tumors with presumed lymphatic differentiation, including Kaposi's sarcoma, kaposiform and Dabska-type hemangioendotheliomas, and a subset of angiosarcomas. Mod Pathol 2000;13(2):180–5.

38. Debelenko LV, Perez-Atayde AR, Mulliken JB, et al. D2–40 immunohistochemical analysis of pediatric vascular tumors reveals positivity in Kaposiform hemangioendothelioma. Mod Pathol 2005;18(11): 1454–60.

39. Le Huu AR, Jokinen CH, Rubin BP, et al. Expression of prox1, lymphatic endothelial nuclear transcription factor, in Kaposiform hemangioendothelioma and tufted angioma. Am J Surg Pathol 2010;34(11): 1563–73.

40. Kasabach HH, Merritt KK. Capillary hemangioma with extensive purpura: report of a case. Am J Dis Child 1940;59(5):1063–70.

41. Croteau SE, Liang MG, Kozakewich HP, et al. Kaposiform hemangioendothelioma: atypical features and risks of Kasabach-Merritt phenomenon in 107 referrals. J Pediatr 2013;162(1):142–7.

42. Kai L, Wang Z, Yao W, et al. Sirolimus, a promising treatment for refractory Kaposiform hemangioendothelioma. J Cancer Res Clin Oncol 2014;140(3): 471–6.

43. Wang Z, Li K, Dong K, et al. Successful treatment of Kasabach-Merritt phenomenon arising from Kaposiform hemangioendothelioma by sirolimus. J Pediatr Hematol Oncol 2015;37(1):72–3.

44. Kaposi M. Idiopathisches multiples Pigmentsarkom der Haut. Arch Dermatol Syph 1872;4(2):265–73.

45. Sequeira JH. So-called multiple idiopathic pigment sarcoma (Kaposi). Proc R Soc Med 1921; 14(Dermatol Sect):86.

46. Sequeira JH. Case of so-called multiple idiopathic pigment sarcoma of Kaposi. Proc R Soc Med 1918;11(Dermatol Sect):20–1.

47. Kestens L, Melbye M, Biggar RJ, et al. Endemic African Kaposi's sarcoma is not associated with immunodeficiency. Int J Cancer 1985;36(1):49–54.

48. Marmor M, Friedman-Kien AE, Laubenstein L, et al. Risk factors for Kaposi's sarcoma in homosexual men. Lancet 1982;1(8281):1083–7.

49. Bayley AC, Downing RG, Cheingsong-Popov R, et al. HTLV-III serology distinguishes atypical and endemic Kaposi's sarcoma in Africa. Lancet 1985; 1(8425):359–61.

50. Chang Y, Cesarman E, Pessin MS, et al. Identification of herpesvirus-like DNA sequences in AIDS-associated Kaposi sarcoma. Science 1994; 266(5192):1865–9.

51. Li JJ, Huang YQ, Cockrell CJ, et al. Localization of human herpes-like virus type 8 in vascular endothelial cells and perivascular spindle-shaped cells of Kaposi sarcoma lesions by in situ hybridization. Am J Pathol 1996;148(6):1741–8.

52. Flore O, Rafii S, Ely S, et al. Transformation of primary human endothelial cells by Kaposi sarcoma-associated herpes virus. Nature 1998;394(6693): 588–92.

53. Safai B, Mike V, Giraldo G, et al. Association of Kaposi sarcoma with second primary malignancies: possible etiopathogenic implications. Cancer 1980; 45(6):1472–9.

54. Moskowitz LB, Hensley GT, Gould EW, et al. Frequency and anatomic distribution of lymphadenopathic Kaposi's sarcoma in the acquired immunodeficiency syndrome. Hum Pathol 1985;16(5):447–56.

55. Lemlich G, Schwam L, Lebwohl M. Kaposi's sarcoma and acquired immunodeficiency syndrome: postmortem findings in twenty-four cases. J Am Acad Dermatol 1987;16(2 Pt 1):319–25.

56. Penn I. Kaposi's sarcoma in transplant recipients. Transplantation 1997;64(5):669–73.

57. Ackerman AB. Subtle clues to diagnosis by conventional microscopy: the patch stage of Kaposi's sarcoma. Am J Dermatopathol 1979;1(2):165–72.

58. Kao G, Johnson FB, Sulica VI. The nature of hyaline (eosinophilic) globules and vascular slits in Kaposi's sarcoma. Am J Dermatopathol 1990;12(3):256–67.

59. Cox FH, Helwig EB. Kaposi sarcoma. Cancer 1959; 12(2):289–98.

60. Satta R, Cossu S, Massarelli G, et al. Anaplastic transformation of classic Kaposi's sarcoma: clinicopathological study of five cases. Br J Dermatol 2001;145(5):847–9.

61. Cossu S, Satta R, Cottoni F, et al. Lymphangioma-like variant of Kaposi sarcoma: clinicopathologic

study of seven cases with review of the literature. Am J Dermatopathol 1997;19(1):16–22.

62. Gange RW, Wilson-Jones E. Lymphangioma-like Kaposi sarcoma: a report of 3 cases. Br J Dermatol 1979;100(3):327–34.

63. McClain CM, Haws AL, Galfione SK, et al. Pyogenic granuloma-like Kaposi's sarcoma. J Cutan Pathol 2016;43(6):549–51.

64. Cabibi D, Cacciatore M, Viviano E, et al. 'Pyogenic granuloma-like Kaposi's sarcoma' on the hands: immunohistochemistry and human herpesvirus-8 detection. J Eur Acad Dermatol Venereol 2009; 23(5):587–9.

65. Logani S, Lucas DR, Cheng JD, et al. Spindle cell tumors associated with mycobacteria in lymph node of HIV-positive patients: "Kaposi sarcoma with mycobacteria" and "mycobacterial pseudotumor." Am J Surg Pathol 1999;23(6):656–61.

66. Traweek ST, Kandalaft PL, Mehta P, et al. The human hematopoietic progenitor cell antigen (CD34) in vascular neoplasia. Am J Clin Pathol 1991;96(1): 25–31.

67. Miettinen M, Wang ZF, Paetau A, et al. ERG transcription factor as an immunohistochemical marker for vascular endothelial tumors and prostatic carcinoma. Am J Surg Pathol 2011;35(3):432–41.

68. Weninger W, Partanen TA, Breiteneder-Geleff S, et al. Expression of vascular endothelial growth factor receptor-3 and podoplanin suggests a lymphatic endothelial cell origin of Kaposi's sarcoma tumor cells. Lab Invest 1999;79(2):243–51.

69. Patel RM, Goldblum JR, Hsi ED. Immunohistochemical detection of human herpes virus-8 latent nuclear antigen-1 is useful in the diagnosis of Kaposi sarcoma. Mod Pathol 2004;17(4):456–60.

70. Napekoski KM, Fernandez AP, Billings SD. Microvenular hemangioma: a clinicopathologic review of 13 cases. J Cutan Pathol 2014;41(11):816–22.

71. Llombart B, Serra-Guillén C, Monteagudo C, et al. Dermatofibrosarcoma protuberans: a comprehensive review and update on diagnosis and management. Semin Diagn Pathol 2013;30(1):13–28.

72. Kuzel P, Mahmood MN, Metelitsa AI, et al. A clinicopathologic review of a case series of dermatofibrosarcoma protuberans with fibrosarcomatous differentiation. J Cutan Med Surg 2015;19(1): 28–34.

73. Shin JW, Park HS, Kim BK, et al. Aneurysmal benign fibrous histiocytoma with atrophic features. Ann Dermatol 2009;21(1):42–5.

74. Santa Cruz DJ, Kyriakos M. Aneurysmal ("angiomatoid") fibrous histiocytoma of the skin. Cancer 1981; 47(8):2053–61.

75. Chor PJ, Santa-Cruz DJ. Kaposi's sarcoma: a clinicopathologic review and differential diagnosis. J Cutan Pathol 1992;19(1):6–20.

76. Marshall ME, Hatfield ST, Hatfield DR. Arteriovenous malformation simulating Kaposi sarcoma (pseudo Kaposi sarcoma). Arch Dermatol 1985;121(1):99–101.

77. Huguen J, Bonsang B, Lemasson G, et al. Acroangiodermatitis or pseudo-Kaposi sarcoma: two cases in patients with paralyzed legs. Br J Dermatol 2016; 174(6):e84.

78. Pimentel MI, Cuzzi T, Azeredo-Coutinho RB, et al. Acroangiodermatitis (pseudo-Kaposi sarcoma): a rarely-recognized condition. A case on the plantar aspect of the foot associated with chronic venous insufficiency. An Bras Dermatol 2011;86(4 Suppl 1):S13–6.

79. Sbano P, Miracco C, Risulo M, et al. Acroangiodermatitis (pseudo-Kaposi sarcoma) associated with verrucous hyperplasia induced by suction-socket lower limb prosthesis. J Cutan Pathol 2005;32(6):429–32.

80. Chu KM, Mahlangeni G, Swannet S, et al. AIDS-associated Kaposi's sarcoma is linked to advanced disease and high mortality in a primary care HIV programme in South Africa. J Int AIDS Soc 2010; 8(13):23.

81. Nagy S, Gyulai R, Kemeny L, et al. Iatrogenic Kaposi's sarcoma: HHV8 positivity persists but the tumors regress almost completely without immunosuppressive therapy. Transplantation 2000;69(10):2230–1.

82. Montagnino G, Bencini PL, Tarantino A, et al. Clinical features and course of Kaposi's sarcoma in kidney transplant patients: report of 13 cases. Am J Nephrol 1994;14(2):121.

83. Duprez R, Lacoste V, Brière J, et al. Evidence for a multiclonal origin of multicentric advanced lesions of Kaposi sarcoma. J Natl Cancer Inst 2007; 99(14):1086–94.

84. Thum C, Husain EA, Mulholland K, et al. Atypical fibroxanthoma with pseudoangiomatous features: a histological and immunohistochemical mimic of cutaneous angiosarcoma. Ann Diagn Pathol 2013; 17(6):502–7.

85. Brenn T. Pleomorphic dermal neoplasms: a review. Adv Anat Pathol 2014;21(2):108–30.

86. McKenney JK, Weiss SW, Folpe AL. CD31 expression in intratumoral macrophages: a potential diagnostic pitfall. Am J Surg Pathol 2001;25(9):1167–73.

# Sebaceous Neoplasms

Katharina Flux, MD[a,b,*]

## KEYWORDS

- Sebaceous skin tumor • Sebaceous carcinoma • Sebaceoma • Muir-Torre syndrome

## ABSTRACT

Sebaceous skin tumors are classified into sebaceous adenoma, sebaceoma, and sebaceous carcinoma. An additional group of cystic sebaceous tumors indicate the Muir-Torre syndrome (MTS). Cystic sebaceous tumors are considered as morphologic variants of the 3 main categories. Multilineage adnexal tumors with partly sebaceous differentiation may pose a challenge to categorize. Sebaceous hyperplasia and nevus sebaceus are not considered as true sebaceous tumor entities. Recently, attention has been drawn to morphologic clues of sebaceous differentiation. Immunohistochemistry using the mismatch repair proteins and/or genetic microsatellite instability testing should be performed on sebaceous neoplasms to diagnose MTS as early as possible.

## OVERVIEW

True sebaceous neoplasms (sebaceous adenoma, sebaceoma, and sebaceous carcinoma) are rare skin tumors, in contrast with sebaceous gland hyperplasia, which is encountered frequently in the general population, especially in sun-exposed skin.[1–3] Sebaceous tumors may occur at any age during adulthood, but usually they affect elderly people. Clinically, sebaceous tumors are often mistaken for more common skin tumors, such as basal cell carcinoma and squamous cell carcinoma, and consequently the diagnosis is made by histopathologists.

Predilection sites of sebaceous tumors are the head and neck area, but they may occur on any region of the body. The clinical presentation is heterogeneous and ranges from small, flesh-colored, umbilicated papules, to ulcerated or crusted lesions, to subcutaneous nodules or tumors with exophytic growth.[4,5] In most cases, sebaceous tumors are solitary, except in patients with Muir-Torre syndrome (MTS). Patients with MTS may present with numerous sebaceous tumors and/or keratoacanthomas that may be located at atypical body sites (outside the head and neck area). Patients with MTS may manifest sebaceous skin tumors at a younger age. The peak onset of sebaceous tumors in patients with MTS is 53 years of age (range, 21–88 years of age).[6]

## PATHOGENESIS AND GENETIC ASPECTS OF SEBACEOUS TUMORS

Little is known about the pathogenesis of sebaceous tumors and their genetic profile. A history of irradiation, immunosuppression, or familial retinoblastoma seem to be risk factors for the development of sebaceous carcinoma.[7] Apart from the microsatellite instability caused by mutations in the mismatch repair proteins relevant to MTS, it is accepted that the Wnt/beta-catenin signaling pathway is altered and plays an important role in the development of sebaceous tumors. Transgenic mice expressing a defective beta-catenin binding site in the transcription factor lymphoid enhancer-binding factor (LEF-1) spontaneously develop sebaceous skin tumors. Sebaceomas and sebaceous adenomas show mutations of the LEF-1 gene, whereas sebaceous carcinomas may show a complete silencing of the LEF-1 gene.[8–10] In addition, mutational inactivation of p53, a common tumor suppressor gene, was found in sporadic sebaceous carcinoma[11] as well as dysregulations of nuclear factor-kappaB, transforming growth factor-beta, and PTEN.[12] A recent study identified increased copy numbers of HER2 in a subset of eyelid sebaceous carcinomas, which needs to be further investigated as a possible target for treatment.[13] So far no ultraviolet light signature

[a] Department of Dermatology, University of Heidelberg, Im Neuenheimer Feld 440, 69120 Heidelberg, Germany; [b] Labor für Dermatohistologie und Oralpathologie, Bayerstrasse 69, 80335 München, Munich, Germany
* Labor für Dermatohistologie und Oralpathologie, Munich, Germany.
E-mail address: katharina.flux@o2online.de

Surgical Pathology 10 (2017) 367–382
http://dx.doi.org/10.1016/j.path.2017.01.009
1875-9181/17/© 2017 Elsevier Inc. All rights reserved.

mutations in the telomerase reverse transcriptase (TERT) gene promotor were found in sebaceous carcinomas, in contrast with basal cell carcinomas, squamous cell carcinomas, and melanomas.[14]

Nevus sebaceous represents an epidermal nevus or hamartoma and shows a somatic mosaicism with activating Ras mutations in HRAS (GTPase HRas) or KRAS (GTPase V-Ki-ras2 Kirsten rat sarcoma viral oncogene homolog) in lesional keratinocytes (but not in adjacent nonlesional skin or dermal fibroblasts) that undermines the difference of the pathogenesis compared with sebaceous adenoma, sebaceoma, and sebaceous carcinoma. Rarely, secondary sebaceous neoplasms develop within nevus sebaceus, but, to date, the second-hit mutations in these tumors have not been studied.[15,16]

## MORPHOLOGIC CLUES AND IMMUNOHISTOCHEMICAL MARKERS OF SEBACEOUS DIFFERENTIATION

The morphologic identification of sebaceous tumors is unproblematic if the neoplastic sebocytes are well differentiated. Mature sebocytes are easily spotted by their centrally located nucleus indented by numerous lipid vacuoles. Neoplastic sebocytes may show few or 1 lipid vacuole only and a roundish nucleus, and may resemble clear cells of squamous epithelial neoplasms.[17] They may produce a signet-ring appearance. The intracytoplasmic lipids of sebocytes can be confirmed immunohistochemically. Oil red O and Sudan black are stains for the use of fresh frozen tissue only, whereas adipophilin and perilipin are available for formalin-fixed paraffin-embedded tissue. Of these, adipophilin is the most commonly used marker; this is a monoclonal antibody against a protein on the surface of intracellular lipid droplets. It also shows reactivity with xanthomatous cells (ie, xanthelasma). In addition, mature sebocytes are immunohistochemically positive for epithelial membrane antigen (EMA), cytokeratin 7, CAM 5.2, and androgen receptors, but all these markers are unspecific.[18–20] Nuclear factor XIIIa; lipid synthesis; and processing proteins ABHD5 (1-acylglycerol-3-phosphate O-acyltransferase ABHD5), PGRMC1 (Progesterone receptor membrane component 1), and squalene synthase have been discussed as new sensitive and specific markers to discriminate sebaceous proliferations from basal cell carcinoma and clear cell neoplasms in small case studies, but further investigations are necessary to establish these markers.[21–23]

Immature neoplastic sebocytes appear as small, undifferentiated basophilic cells. Sebaceomas and sebaceous carcinomas may be mainly composed of immature sebocytes and therefore are a challenge to recognize and are easily confused with other basophilic/basaloid tumors. A specific immunohistochemical marker for immature sebocytes does not yet exist. Adipophilin and other lipid stains may be negative in immature sebocytes; EMA and androgen receptor can remain positive. Mature and immature sebocytes are usually negative for BerEp4, in contrast with basal cell carcinoma and trichoblastoma, which are important differential diagnoses.[17,18]

A clue for the sebaceous differentiation of tumors composed mainly of immature sebocytes may be the formation of neoplastic sebaceous ducts. Differentiation of neoplastic cells toward sebaceous ducts is recapitulated by irregular or cystic ductal spaces with a crenulated, eosinophilic inner lining, with or without sebaceous secretion material within the lumina (**Fig. 1**). In addition, immature neoplastic sebocytes have the ability to manifest distinct (organoid) growth patterns, such as the rippled, labyrinthine/sinusoidal, and carcinoidlike growth patterns. The rippled pattern shows the arrangement of neoplastic cells in parallel rows resembling Verocay bodies in schwannoma (**Fig. 2**). Basal cell carcinomas and trichoblastomas may also show this feature. The labyrinthine/sinusoidal pattern manifests as a mazelike arrangement of neoplastic cells with sinuslike spaces in between (see **Fig. 2**). In the carcinoidlike pattern the neoplastic cells form trabeculae, ribbons, rosettes, and pseudorosettes. Although these growth patterns are unspecific, the recognition of 1 or more of these growth patterns within a basaloid (blue-cell) tumor together with the identification of sebaceous ductal structures suggests a sebaceous tumor, even if typical mature sebocytes are rare or absent.[24–36]

Multilineage differentiation (additional tubular structures, apocrine glands, follicular germs, infundibulocystic structures) and squamous metaplasia have been described in sebaceous tumors, especially in sebaceomas[37–39] (**Figs. 3 and 4**). The phenomenon of multidirectional differentiation in 1 tumor entity is well known in adnexal neoplasms because of the embryologic derivation of the sebaceous glands, hair follicles, and apocrine glands from the common folliculosebaceous-apocrine unit. In this context, examples of basophilic tumors with multilineage differentiation include basal cell carcinoma and trichoblastoma with partial sebaceous differentiation, both being important differential diagnoses for sebaceoma and sebaceous carcinoma.[40–45]

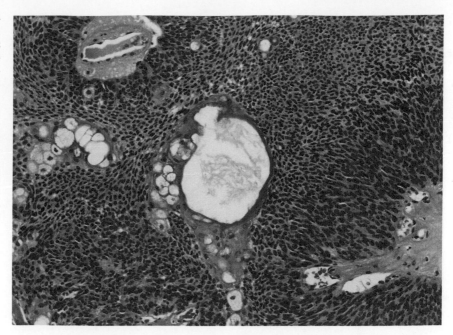

**Fig. 1.** Clue for sebaceous differentiation: the neoplastic sebaceous duct, a cystic ductal space with a crenulated, eosinophilic inner lining, and with sebaceous secretion material within the lumen. The duct is surrounded by immature and some more mature sebocytes with typically indented nuclei and foamy white or eosinophilic cytoplasm (H&E, original magnification ×10).

## SEBACEOUS SKIN TUMORS AS MARKER LESIONS OF MUIR-TORRE SYNDROME I AND II

Sebaceous adenoma, sebaceoma, and sebaceous carcinoma may all indicate MTS (OMIM [Online Mendelian Inheritance in Man] 158320). Sebaceous adenoma is by far the most common sebaceous tumor developing in association with MTS (**Fig. 5**). MTS I is a phenotypic variant of hereditary nonpolyposis colorectal cancer syndrome (Lynch syndrome) caused by dominantly inherited mutations in the DNA mismatch repair (MMR) genes and defined by the coincidence of at least 1 cutaneous sebaceous neoplasm and at least 1 internal malignancy.[46,47] In most cases germline mutations have been detected in mutator S homologue (MSH) 2 (approximately 90%), mutator L homologue (MLH) 1, MSH6, and postmeiotic

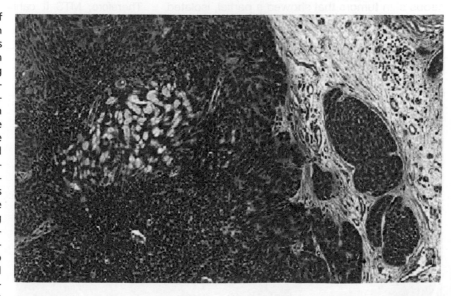

**Fig. 2.** Combination of the rippled growth pattern of immature sebocytes (arrangement of cells in parallel rows resembling Verocay bodies in schwannoma) and the labyrinthine/sinusoidal growth pattern in sebaceoma. The rippled pattern may be encountered in basal cell carcinoma and trichoblastoma as well, but in combination with sebaceous ducts and sparse mature sebocytes it is a strong hint to a tumor with primary sebaceous differentiation. There is no palisading of peripheral cells as in basal cell carcinoma or trichoblastoma (H&E, original magnification ×10).

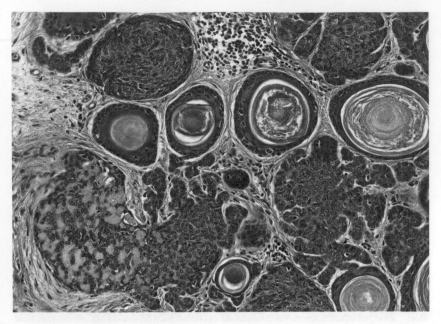

Fig. 3. Infundibulocystic structures in sebaceoma: the tumor is mainly composed of small basaloid cells forming small cysts suggesting a tumor with follicular differentiation (ie, trichoadenoma or trichoblastoma), but the surrounding basaloid cells are BerEp4 negative and form a labyrinthine/sinusoidal growth pattern; very sparse mature sebocytes are found. Note that the cysts are different from neoplastic sebaceous ducts (compare Fig. 1) (H&E, original magnification ×10).

segregation increased (PMS) 2. Any sebaceous neoplasm needs to be checked for a loss of MMR proteins routinely. The 4 MMR proteins mentioned earlier are commercially available as immunohistochemical markers. Immunohistochemistry (IHC) staining for MMR proteins has an approximately 80% sensitivity for MTS I. Antibodies against MLH1 and MSH2 may be more valuable than those against PMS2 and MSH6, because MLH1 forms a dimer with PMS2 and MSH2 does the same with MSH6. However, the author has experienced several cases of sebaceous skin tumors that showed a partial, isolated loss of MSH6, and therefore recommend a minimum IHC panel consisting of MLH1, MSH2, and MSH6. If IHC staining for MMR markers is positive (meaning no loss of MMR proteins), a genetic microsatellite instability analysis is recommended.[48–52]

MTS II is a recently described subtype of MTS that is inherited recessively and shows lower penetrance. MTS II is defined by biallelic inactivation of a base excision repair gene (MYH [a A/G mismatch-nicking endonuclease]) and, interestingly, is accompanied by microsatellite stability. Therefore, MTS II cannot be detected by IHC

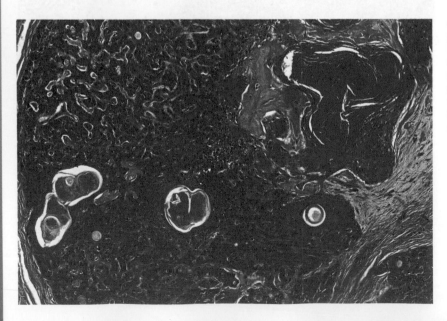

Fig. 4. Squamous metaplasia in sebaceoma: basaloid immature sebocytes merge with more eosinophilic cells and areas of squamoid tissue with irregular centers of compact keratin (H&E, original magnification ×10).

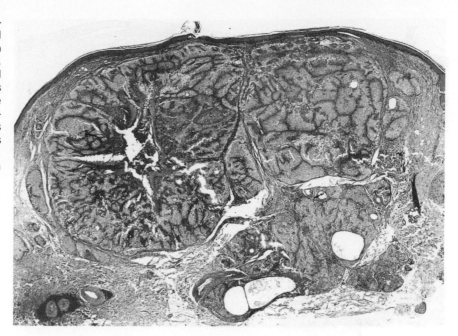

*Fig. 5.* Sebaceous adenoma: the tumor is well circumscribed, grows in a lobular organoid fashion, and is mainly composed of mature sebocytes (<50% of tumor cells are basaloid [immature sebocytes]). Cellular atypia is mild or absent. Mitoses may be frequent (H&E, original magnification ×2).

with the common MMR staining panel, or with microsatellite instability analysis.[53]

There are rare cases of sebaceous neoplasms that show a loss of MMR proteins by IHC and still are not associated with any type of MTS. In these cases, inactivation of MMR genes is usually caused by gene hypermethylation.[53]

## SEBACEOUS ADENOMA AND SEBACEOUS HYPERPLASIA

Sebaceous adenoma is considered as a benign neoplasm showing a multilobular organoid tumor growth still showing strong resemblance to a normal sebaceous gland. Sebaceous adenomas are well-circumscribed tumors with a plump silhouette that are usually located in the upper dermis. Clinically (similar to sebaceous hyperplasia) they usually develop in the head and neck area and appear as small, erythematous or yellowish, sometimes crusted or umbilicated lesions. They are multilobular tumors, mainly composed of mature sebocytes that are directly connected to the upper epidermis. The tumor lobules of sebaceous adenoma show variable layers of germinative, immature sebocytes in the periphery. These sebocytes show mitotic activity but no marked cell atypia (see **Fig. 5**; **Figs. 6** and **7**). A commonly used criterion for distinguishing sebaceous hyperplasia from sebaceous adenoma is the number of germinative cell layers in the periphery of the lobules.[5,54] More than 2 germinative cell layers indicate sebaceous adenoma. In the

literature, different opinions exist about the percentage of immature sebocytes that there can be in sebaceous adenoma.[54] Most investigators suggest that the basaloid layers may make up to 50% of the tumor but not more. In contrast with sebaceous hyperplasia, sebaceous adenoma is not supposed to show any fully developed hair follicles associated with the sebaceous lobules. However, sebaceous hyperplasia may be the result of an epithelial induction process (eg, dermatofibromas), in which it also may present without any associated hair follicles.[55,56] Some investigators claim that mature sebocytes in true neoplastic processes present with a more eosinophilic cytoplasm compared with normal sebocytes and that the nucleus may be found in the periphery of the cells instead of being centered.[54] These cytologic hints may be helpful in some cases, but do not prove to be reproducible or reliable in every individual. Sebaceous hyperplasia is usually small and measures 1 to 3 mm (although cases up to 1 cm have been described), and sebaceous adenoma is about 5 mm in diameter in general (although much smaller and larger sizes are found in the literature), which means that distinction by size is not possible either.[5] It becomes evident that, in some cases, the distinction between sebaceous adenoma and sebaceous hyperplasia is not clear-cut, especially if the histopathologist has to deal with shave biopsies or incomplete excisions. This situation is a dilemma because sebaceous hyperplasia is not associated with MTS, whereas sebaceous adenoma is the most common

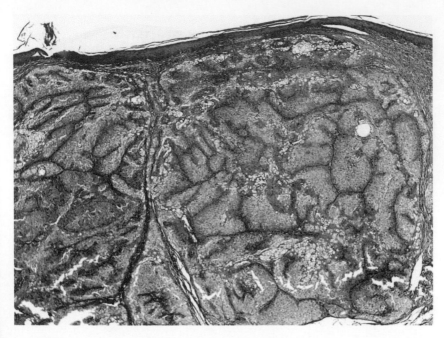

**Fig. 6.** Sebaceous adenoma: the tumor is well circumscribed, multilobular, and mainly composed of mature sebocytes (>50%). Frequent mitoses are usually found in the periphery of tumor lobules, but cytologic atypia is very mild. Necroses are not found. Sebaceous adenoma is the most common sebaceous tumor in patients with MTS (H&E, original magnification ×4).

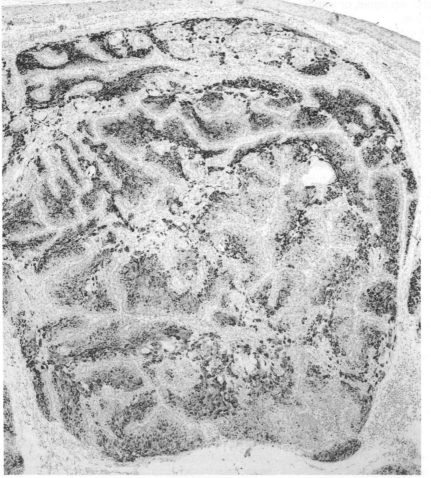

**Fig. 7.** Sebaceous adenoma, adipophilin stain. Adipophilin highlights the lipid droplets in the cytoplasm of sebocytes. Neoplastic sebocytes with few or no lipid vacuoles are weakly positive or negative for adipophilin. A specific immunohistochemical marker for immature sebocytes does not yet exist (Adipophilin ×4).

sebaceous tumor in MTS and should be screened routinely for the loss of MMR proteins.[52,53]

In rare cases, well-differentiated sebaceous carcinoma may be difficult to distinguish from sebaceous adenoma. This possibility has caused some investigators to assume that all sebaceous adenomas are well-differentiated sebaceous carcinomas.[54] To avoid any confusion, histopathologists should agree that the diagnosis of a sebaceous adenoma implies a benign tumor that does not metastasize. Sebaceous adenoma is a tumor usually located in the superficial dermis. A well-differentiated sebaceous tumor extending in the deep dermis showing a high mitotic activity and mild cytologic atypia is suspicious for well-differentiated sebaceous carcinoma. Sebaceous carcinoma occurring on extraocular body sites has a good prognosis if excised totally. More care is recommended concerning periocular sebaceous tumors (independent of their grade of differentiation), which are associated with higher rates of recurrence and worse prognosis.[7] If in doubt, any sebaceous tumor should be excised completely. Shave excisions or curettage material is not sufficient for judging sebaceous tumors. Sebaceous adenoma, especially the cystic variant, is a marker of MTS and needs to be stained for MMR proteins.[5]

## SEBACEOMA

Sebaceoma is a benign, well-circumscribed tumor with a plump silhouette and smooth borders that may extend in the middle and deep dermis, even in the subcutis. The size is variable from very small lesions up to 20 mm. Clinically, the tumor presents as a solitary flesh-colored or erythematous nodus or plaque, sometimes crusted or erosive in the head and neck area, rarely on other body sites. It is usually mistaken for a basal cell carcinoma, dermatofibroma, or other more common skin tumors. It may manifest with organoid growth patterns composed of multiple tumor lobules. The tumor is composed mainly of immature, monomorphic sebocytes (meaning >50% of tumor cells are basaloid cells)[19,29] (**Fig. 8**). The so-called 50% rule may serve as a rough guideline and should not be a dogmatic approach to the diagnosis, because the literature does not provide any advice concerning the number of cutting sections that are needed to estimate the percentage of immature cells within an individual tumor. The basaloid cells in sebaceoma can form distinct growth patterns (rippled, labyrinthine/sinusoidal, carcinoidlike, infundibulocystic structures, and squamous metaplasia), as mentioned earlier, that serve as clues for sebaceous differentiation[24–29] (see **Figs. 2–4**). Apart from small basaloid cells showing no lipid vacuoles, usually more mature sebocytes with a different morphology are found, such as sebocytes with just 1 or very few lipid vacuoles and a peripheral nucleus without indentations. However, the tumor may also show a considerable amount of very well-differentiated sebocytes. The mitotic activity in sebaceoma varies and can be striking in some tumor lobules but cytologic atypia is usually mild[57] (**Fig. 9**). However, the grading of cytologic atypia is a subjective criterion and the interobserver variability concerning sebaceous tumors has been well documented in a study by Harvey and colleagues.[58] Tumor necrosis does not occur in sebaceoma but is an indicator of

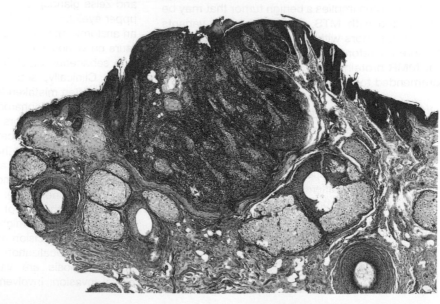

**Fig. 8.** Sebaceoma: well-circumscribed tumor with smooth borders mainly composed of monomorphic basaloid (immature) sebocytes (>50%). Mitoses can be very frequent, but cytologic atypia is still mild or moderate (H&E, original magnification ×2).

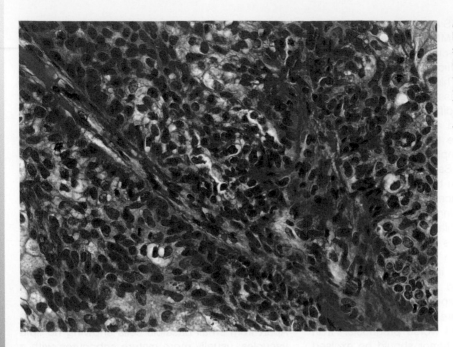

*Fig. 9.* Sebaceoma: the higher magnification shows numerous mitoses, but no gross cytologic atypia and no necroses are found (unacceptable for a benign tumor) (H&E, original magnification ×20).

malignancy. The development of sebaceous carcinoma within sebaceoma (sebaceous carcinoma ex sebaceoma) has also been described.[59] The question is whether such a lesion should be subclassified as sebaceous carcinoma.

It is difficult to decide between benign and malignant in individual tumors that do not show clearly invasive borders but cytologic atypia; all these tumors usually have an excellent prognosis if excised totally, so the debate is probably more academic than practical.

Sebaceoma implies a benign tumor that may be associated with MTS, especially cystic variants (**Fig. 10**); tumors with keratoacanthomalike architecture (therefore needing to be stained routinely for MMR proteins); and that total excision is recommended to avoid recurrence.[50]

## Differential Diagnoses

Apart from sebaceous carcinoma (discussed earlier) the most important differential diagnoses are basal cell carcinoma; trichoblastoma; and other basaloid tumors, especially adnexal neoplasms with multilineage differentiation, such as apocrine poroma (with sebaceous differentiation) and panfolliculoma. Basal cell carcinoma and trichoblastoma are usually BerEp4 positive, in contrast with sebaceoma. In the literature, BerEp4-positive sebaceomas have been described, but the author cannot support this fact by personal experience.

## PERIOCULAR SEBACEOUS CARCINOMA

Sebaceous carcinoma of the eyelid is a rare aggressive tumor that represents 1% to 2% of periorbital malignancies in the Western world. Periocular sebaceous carcinoma seems to be more common in China and India, accounting for up to 40% to 60% of malignant eyelid tumors in these countries.[60,61] The tumor usually arises in elderly people (aged >60 years) in association with the tarsal sebaceous glands (meibomian and Zeiss glands). The most common site is the upper eyelid.[62,63] The term periocular describes an anatomic site beyond the eyelids but the literature on periocular sebaceous carcinoma deals with sebaceous carcinoma of the eyelid exclusively. Clinically, sebaceous carcinoma of the eyelid is often mistaken for an inflammatory condition, such as blepharoconjunctivitis, chalazion, or more common tumors such as basal cell carcinoma and squamous cell carcinoma. Periocular sebaceous carcinoma has an estimated recurrence rate of up to 40% and a 25% risk of metastasis to regional lymph nodes and distant organs (lung, liver, bone, brain).[7] Complete radical excision reduces the risk of mortality. The high rate of local recurrence might be caused by narrow or incomplete excision of the primary caused by the difficult localization. Features predictive of poor prognosis are vascular, lymphatic, and orbital invasion; involvement of both upper and

*Fig.    10.* Sebaceoma, cystic variant: cystic sebaceous tumors are typical in patients with MTS (H&E, original magnification ×4).

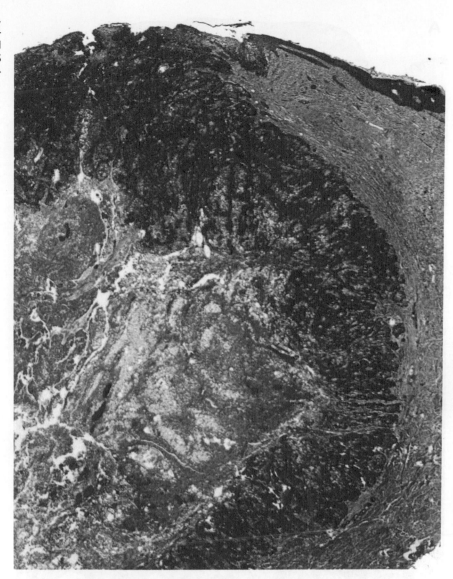

lower eyelids; poor differentiation; multicentric origin and pagetoid invasion of the overlying epithelia of the eyelids; duration of symptoms longer than 6 months; and tumor diameter exceeding 10 mm.[7,64–66] The patients require long-term follow-up.

On histology, sebaceous carcinoma of the eyelid is usually connected to the surface epithelium and may be well differentiated (low grade) showing a multilobular architecture and a clear circumscription (**Fig. 11**) or it can manifest as a mainly basaloid tumor with infiltrative borders and striking cytologic atypia (high grade) and numerous mitoses (**Figs. 12–14**). It

may show a prominent pagetoid spread of tumor cells intraepidermally (**Fig. 15**). This feature is supposed to be an important factor of the high recurrence rates of periocular sebaceous carcinoma. The neoplastic tumor cells may be small, basaloid, and difficult to identify as neoplastic sebocytes. Usually, vacuolated cells and cells with a larger foamy (gray or white) cytoplasm can be found in some of the tumor masses, and these are positive for lipid stains. Nuclear atypia can be striking. Periocular sebaceous carcinoma is rarely associated with MTS, but should be considered for MMR staining routinely.[7]

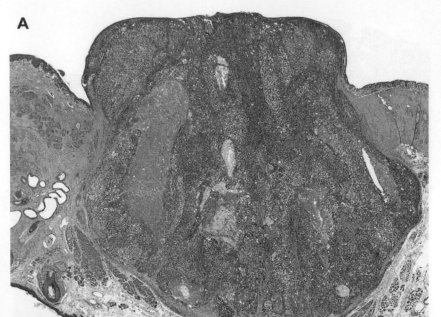

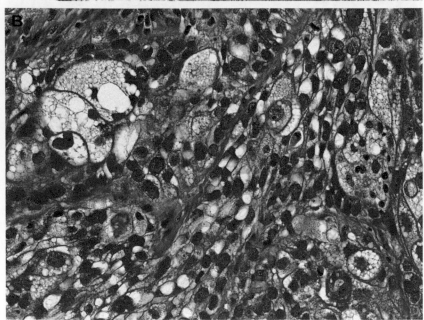

*Fig. 11.* (*A, B*) Sebaceous carcinoma: the silhouette of the tumor of this case is plump and well circumcribed resembling sebaceoma, it lacks clear infiltrative borders, but there is marked atypia, unaceeptable for a benign tumor; mitoses are frequent, also showing atypical forms. (H&E, original magnification [*a*] ×2; [*b*] ×20)

## Differential Diagnoses

It can be difficult to distinguish sebaceous carcinoma from basaloid squamous carcinoma. Both tumors show a pagetoid intraepidermal spread of tumor cells. IHC does not help reliably, because EMA and cytokeratin 7 may also be expressed by squamous cell carcinomas.[20] The markers p16 and p53 are strongly expressed by squamous cell carcinomas, squamous cell carcinoma in situ, as well as conjunctival carcinomas, but may also stain sebaceous carcinomas.[67,68] If no definitive sebaceous differentiation is found that may be additionally highlighted by lipid stains it may be impossible to rule out sebaceous carcinoma. Melanoma of the eyelid may also manifest with clear/foam cell change showing pagetoid spread, mimicking sebaceous differentiation. Periocular melanoma is usually pigmented and can easily be excluded immunohistochemically (ie, S100, MelanA, HMB45, SOX10). The most common tumor of the

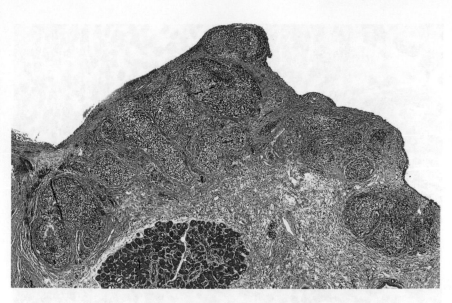

**Fig. 12.** Sebaceous carcinoma of the eyelid: a basaloid multicentric tumor with infiltrative borders. Multicentricity (and pagetoid spread of tumor cells) is held responsible for high recurrence rates of periocular sebaceous carcinoma (H&E, original magnification ×2).

eyelid (in white people) is basal cell carcinoma. In contrast with sebaceous carcinoma, basal cell carcinoma shows palisading of peripheral tumor cells and is usually BerEp4 positive. In the literature, BerEp4-positive sebaceomas have been described, but the author has not experienced such cases so far. Other tumors mimicking sebaceous carcinoma include Merkel cell carcinoma (cytokeratin 20 positive in contrast with sebaceous carcinoma), endocrine mucin-producing sweat gland carcinoma (expressing neuroendocrine markers and showing mucin and no lipids within the tumor cells), metastases of clear cell renal cell carcinoma and prostate carcinoma (being rare on the eyelids), Paget disease and clear cell hidradenocarcinoma.

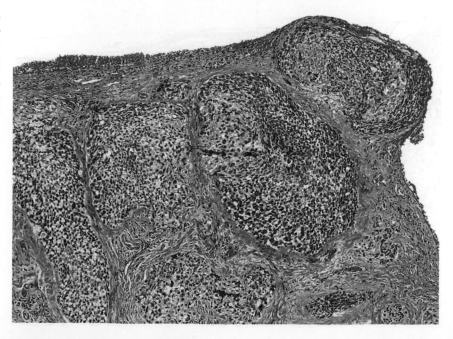

**Fig. 13.** Atypical neoplastic sebocytes in periocular sebaceous carcinoma. The basaloid cells contain different numbers of lipid droplets, and the cytoplasm varies in its size and color (H&E, original magnification ×10).

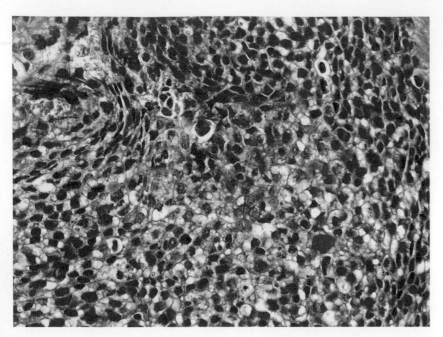

*Fig. 14.* Areas of necroses in periocular sebaceous carcinoma (H&E, original magnification ×20).

## EXTRAOCULAR SEBACEOUS CARCINOMA

Like any sebaceous tumor, extraocular sebaceous carcinoma is most often found in the head and neck area. Sebaceous carcinoma on other body sites is rare, even in MTS. Unusual sites include the salivary glands, the uterus, and the genital areas. The tumor has been described rarely in association with sebaceous nevus of Jadassohn and dermoid cysts. The prognosis of extraocular sebaceous carcinoma on the head and neck is supposed to be similar to periocular sebaceous carcinoma, but sebaceous carcinoma on any other body regions seems to have a much better prognosis.[69] However, aggressive sebaceous carcinoma on the trunk with locoregional metastases has been described, especially in patients with MTS or under immunosuppression (transplant

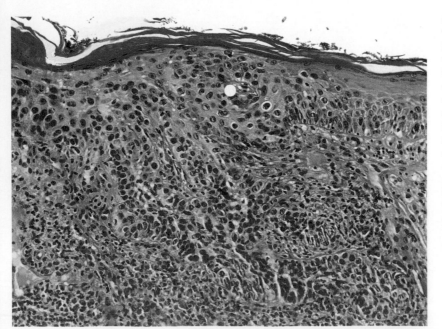

*Fig. 15.* Prominent pagetoid spread of tumor cells intraepidermally. A differentiation from (basaloid) squamous cell carcinoma by shave biopsy is impossible. IHC does not solve the problem: squamous cell carcinoma may also express cytokeratin 7, EMA, p63, and p53, and neoplastic, poorly differentiated sebocytes are usually negative for adipophilin, perilipin or other lipid markers (H&E, original magnification ×20).

recipients). Patients with extraocular carcinoma require long-term follow-up periods.

Clinically, extraocular sebaceous carcinoma presents as a solitary, circumscribed, erythematous, often crusted or erosive nodule. On histology, it may show the same spectrum as periocular sebaceous carcinoma, as described earlier. The tumors may grow in a lobular; circumscribed; or multicentric, clearly invasive fashion (the multicentric type being more common in periocular sebaceous carcinomas). Extraocular sebaceous carcinoma on other sites than the head usually shows no or little intraepidermal pagetoid spread of tumor cells. The tumor cells can be mainly basaloid and small or still show a resemblance to more mature sebocytes with indented nuclei and a large foamy cytoplasm. The cytoplasm may appear more eosinophilic than in normal sebocytes. Usually, areas with striking cytologic atypia and numerous mitoses, including atypical forms, can be identified (Fig. 16). Areas of necrosis are a strong indicator for malignancy (see Fig. 16B). Well-differentiated (low-grade) sebaceous carcinomas may be a challenge to

*Fig. 16. (A, B)* Extraocular sebaceous carcinoma: this tumor is ulcerated, well circumscribed, but shows marked cellular atypia and numerous atypical mitoses as well as focal areas of necrosis. The neoplastic sebocytes are basaloid or have a very eosinophilic cytoplasm and show polymorphic nuclei.

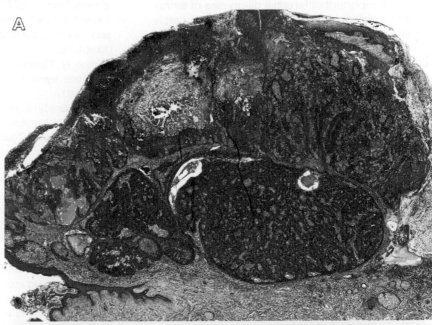

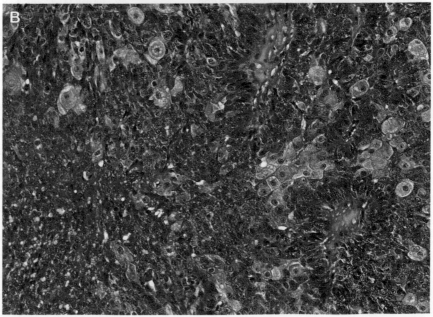

recognize[70–73] and may be mistaken for sebaceomas or even sebaceous adenoma (and vice versa). Given that there is considerable overlap of histologic features of sebaceoma and low-grade sebaceous carcinoma and a striking interobserver variability among histopathologists, the incidence of extraocular sebaceous carcinoma and its prognosis remain uncertain and all available data need to be interpreted carefully until the histologic criteria are more clear-cut.

### Differential Diagnoses

Apart from sebaceous adenoma and sebaceoma, the most important differential diagnoses of extraocular sebaceous carcinoma are basal cell carcinoma and basaloid squamous carcinoma. Merkel cell carcinoma as well as metastases of clear cell renal cell carcinoma and prostate carcinoma may also mimic sebaceous carcinoma, but can easily be excluded by IHC. Other differential diagnoses are adnexal neoplasms (often with mainly basaloid morphology; ie, microcystic adnexal carcinoma with or without sebaceous differentiation), spiradenocarcinoma, endocrine mucin-producing sweat-gland carcinoma (which has been decribed on the cheek and eylids only so far), clear cell hidradenocarcinoma, and apocrine poroma.[41–43,74]

### SUMMARY

The recognition of tumors with sebaceous differentiation is important, because all sebaceous tumors are potential markers of MTS and require screening for this syndrome. IHC is of limited use to identify sebaceous differentiation in tumors mainly composed of immature sebocytes.

The histologic distinction between sebaceous adenoma and sebaceous hyperplasia can be difficult, which is a dilemma because sebaceous hyperplasia is not associated with MTS, whereas sebaceous adenoma is the most common sebaceous tumor in MTS.

The understanding of the nature and the biological behavior of sebaceous tumors, especially sebaceomas, needs to be evaluated by further studies, including genetic approaches, combined with morphologic criteria and long-term follow-up of the patients in order to redefine and improve the morphologic criteria of sebaceous tumors. Therefore, as long as the criteria are not clear-cut, all sebaceous tumors need to be excised totally.

There is a considerable overlap of histologic criteria for sebaceous adenoma, sebaceoma, and sebaceous carcinoma and the tumors might represent different ends of 1 spectrum of sebaceous neoplasms.

## REFERENCES

1. LeBoit PE, Burg G, Weedon D, et al. World Health Organization classification of tumours. Pathology and genetics of skin tumours. Lyon (France): IARC Press; 2006.
2. Zaballos P, Ara M, Puig S, et al. Dermoscopy of sebaceous hyperplasia. Arch Dermatol 2005;141:808.
3. Kumar P, Marks R. Sebaceous gland hyperplasia and senile comedones: a prevalence study in elderly hospitalized patients. Br J Dermatol 1987;117:231–6.
4. Rulon DB, Helwig EB. Cutaneous sebaceous neoplasms. Cancer 1974;33:82–102.
5. Lazar AJF, Lyle S, Calonje E. Sebaceous neoplasia and Torre-Muir syndrome. Curr Diagn Pathol 2007;13:301–19.
6. Misago N, Narisawa Y. Sebaceous neoplasms in Muir-Torre syndrome. Am J Dermatopathol 2000;22:155–61.
7. Kyllo RL, Brady KL, Hurst EA. Sebaceous carcinoma: review of the literature. Dermatol Surg 2015;41:1–15.
8. Takeda H, Lyle S, Zouboulis CC, et al. Human sebaceous tumours harbor inactivating mutations in LEF1. Nat Med 2006;12:395–7.
9. Chan EF, Gat U, McNiff JM, et al. A common human skin tumour is caused by activating mutations in beta-catenin. Nat Genet 1999;21:395–7.
10. Papadopoulos N, Lindblom A. Molecular basis of HNPCC: mutations of MMR genes. Hum Mutat 1997;10:89–99.
11. Tetzlaff MT, Singh RR, Seviour EG, et al. Next-generation sequencing identifies high frequency of mutations in potentially clinically actionable genes in sebaceous carcinoma. J Pathol 2016;240:84–95.
12. Tetzlaff MT, Curry JL, Yin V, et al. Distinct pathways in the pathogenesis of sebaceous carcinomas implicated by differentially expressed microRNAs. JAMA Ophthalmol 2015;133:1109–16.
13. Lee MJ, Kim N, Choung HK, et al. Increased gene copy number of HER2 and concordant protein overexpression found in a subset of eyelid sebaceous gland carcinoma indicate HER2 as a potential therapeutic target. J Cancer Res Oncol 2016;142:125–33.
14. Lin SY, Liao SL, Hong JB, et al. TERT promotor mutations in periocular carcinomas: implications of ultraviolet light in pathogenesis. Br J Ophthalmol 2016;100:274–7.
15. Aslam A, Salam A, Griffiths CE, et al. Nevus sebaceus: a mosaic RASopathy. Clin Exp Dermatol 2014;39:1–6.
16. Kazakov DV, Calonje E, Zelger B, et al. Sebaceous carcinoma arising in nevus sebaceus of Jadassohn: a clinicopathological study of five cases. Am J Dermatopathol 2007;29:242–8.
17. Harvey NT, Tabone T, Erber W, et al. Circumscribed sebaceous neoplasms: a morphological,

immunohistochemical and molecular analysis. Pathology 2016;48:454–62.

18. Plaza JA, Mackinnon A, Camillo L, et al. Role of immunohistochemistry in the diagnosis of sebaceous carcinoma: a clinicopathologic and immunohistochemical study. Am J Dermatopathol 2015;37:809–21.

19. Bourlond F, Velter C, Cribier B. Clinicopathological study of 47 cases of sebaceoma. Ann Dermatol Venereol 2016;143:814–24.

20. Jakobiec FA, Mendoza PR. Eyelid sebaceous carcinoma: clinicopathologic and multiparametric immunohistochemical analysis that includes adipophilin. Am J Ophthalmol 2014;157:186–208.

21. Uhlenhake EE, Clark LN, Smoller BR, et al. Nuclear factor XIIIa staining (clone AC-1A1 mouse monoclonal) is a sensitive and specific marker to discriminate sebaceous proliferations from other cutaneous clear cell neoplasms. J Cutan Pathol 2016;43:649–56.

22. Lark LN, Elwood EE, Uhlenhake BR, et al. Nuclear factor XIIIa staining (clone AC-1A1 mouse monoclonal) is a highly sensitive marker of sebaceous differentiation in normal and neoplastic sebocytes. J Cutan Pathol 2016;43:657–62.

23. Chen WS, Chen PL, Li J, et al. Lipid synthesis and processing proteins ABHD5, PGRMC1 and squalene synthase can serve as novel immunohistochemical markers for sebaceous neoplasms and differentiate sebaceous carcinoma from sebaceoma and basal cell carcinoma with clear cell features. J Cutan Pathol 2013;40:631–8.

24. Ohata C, Ackerman AB. "Ripple pattern" in a neoplasm signifies sebaceous differentiation [sebaceoma (not trichoblastoma or trichomatricoma) if benign and sebaceous carcinoma if malignant]. Dermatopathol: Prac & Conc 2001;7:355–62.

25. Nielsen TA, Maia-Cohen S, Hessel AB, et al. Sebaceous neoplasm with reticulated and cribriform features: a rare variant of sebaceoma. J Cutan Pathol 1998;25:233–5.

26. Kazakov DV, Spagnolo DV, Kacerovska D, et al. Unusual patterns of cutaneous sebaceous neoplasms. Diagn Histopathol 2010;16:425–31.

27. Ansai S, Kimura T. Rippled-pattern sebaceoma: a clinicopathological study. Am J Dermatopathol 2009;31:364–6.

28. Kiyohara T, Kumakiri M, Kuwahara H, et al. Rippled-pattern sebaceoma: a report of a lesion on the back with a review of the literature. Am J Dermatopathol 2006;28:446–8.

29. Misago N, Mihara I, Ansai S, et al. Sebaceoma and related neoplasms with sebaceous differentiation: a clinicopathologic study of 30 cases. Am J Dermatopathol 2002;24:294–304.

30. Akasaka T, Imamura Y, Mori Y, et al. Trichoblastoma with rippled-pattern. J Dermatol 1997;24:174–8.

31. Graham BS, Barr RJ. Rippled-pattern sebaceous trichoblastoma. J Cutan Pathol 2000;27:455–9.

32. Kawakami Y, Ansai S, Nakamura-Wakatsuki T, et al. Case of rippled-pattern sebaceoma with clinically yellowish surface and histopathological paucity of lipid-containing neoplastic cells. J Dermatol 2012;39:644–6.

33. Yamamoto O, Hisaoka M, Yasuda H, et al. A rippled-pattern trichoblastoma: an immunohistochemical study. J Cutan Pathol 2000;27:460–5.

34. Kurokawa I, Nishimura K, Hakamada A, et al. Rippled-pattern sebaceoma with an immunohistochemical study of cytokeratins. J Eur Acad Dermatol Venereol 2007;21:133–4.

35. Misago N, Toda S. Sebaceous carcinoma within rippled/carcinoid pattern sebaceoma. J Cutan Pathol 2016;43:64–70.

36. Kazakov DV, Kutzner H, Rutten A, et al. Carcinoid-like pattern in sebaceous neoplasms: another distinctive, previously unrecognized pattern in extraocular sebaceous carcinoma and sebaceoma. Am J Dermatopathol 2005;27:195–203.

37. Kazakov DV, Calonje E, Rutten A, et al. Cutaneous sebaceous neoplasms with a focal glandular pattern (seboapocrine lesions): a clinicopathological study of three cases. Am J Dermatopathol 2007;29:359–64.

38. Flux K, Kutzner H, Rutten A, et al. Infundibulocystic structures and prominent squamous metaplasia in sebaceoma-a rare feature. a clinicopathologic study of 10 cases. Am J Dermatopathol 2016;38:678–82.

39. Swick BL, Baum CL, Walling HW. Rippled-pattern trichoblastoma with apocrine differentiation arising in a nevus sebaceus: report of a case and review of the literature. J Cutan Pathol 2009;36:1200–5.

40. Misago N, Narisawa Y. Sebaceous carcinoma with apocrine differentiation. Am J Dermatopathol 2001;23:50–7.

41. Nakhleh RE, Swanson PE, Wick MR. Cutaneous adnexal carcinomas with divergent differentiation. Am J Dermatopathol 1990;12:325–34.

42. Kazakov DV, Kutzner H, Spagnolo DV, et al. Sebaceous differentiation in poroid neoplasms: report of 11 cases, including a case of metaplastic carcinoma associated with apocrine poroma (sarcomatoid apocrine porocarcinoma). Am J Dermatopathol 2008;30:21–6.

43. Gianotti R, Coggi A, Alessi E. Poral neoplasm with combined sebaceous and apocrine differentiation. Am J Dermatopathol 1998;20:491–4.

44. Sanchez Yus E, Requena L, Simon P, et al. Complex adnexal tumor of the primary epithelial germ with distinct patterns of superficial epithelioma with sebaceous differentiation, immature trichoepithelioma, and apocrine adenocarcinoma. Am J Dermatopathol 1992;14:245–52.

45. Wong TY, Suster S, Cheek RF, et al. Benign cutaneous adnexal tumors with combined folliculosebaceous, apocrine, and eccrine differentiation. Clinicopathologic and immunohistochemical study of eight cases. Am J Dermatopathol 1996;18:124–36.

46. Muir EC, Beli AJ, Barlow KA. Multiple primary carcinomata of the colon, duodenum and larynx associated with kerato-acanthoma of the face. Br J Surg 1967;54:191–5.

47. Torre D. Multiple sebaceous tumors. Arch Dermatol 1968;98:549–51.

48. Abbas O, Mahalingam M. Cutaneous sebaceous neoplasms as markers of Muir-Torre syndrome: a diagnostic algorithm. J Cutan Pathol 2009;36:613–9.

49. Orta L, Klimstra DS, Qin J, et al. Towards identification of hereditary DNA mismatch repair deficiency: sebaceous neoplasm warrants routine immunohistochemistry screening regardless of patient's age or other clinical characteristics. Am J Surg Pathol 2009;33:934–44.

50. Plocharczyk EF, Frankel WL, Hampel H, et al. Mismatch repair protein deficiency is common in sebaceous neoplasms and suggests the importance of screening for Lynch syndrome. Am J Dermatopathol 2013;35:191–5.

51. Chhibber V, Dresser M, Mahalingam M. MSH-6: extending the reliability of immunohistochemistry as a screening tool in Muir-Torre syndrome. Mod Pathol 2008;21:159–64.

52. Boennelycke M, Thomsen BM, Holck S. Sebaceous neoplasms and the immunoprofile of mismatch-repair proteins as a screening target for syndromic cases. Pathol Res Pract 2015;211:78–82.

53. John AM, Schwartz RA. Muir-Torre syndrome (MTS): an update and approach to diagnosis and management. J Am Acad Dermatol 2016;74:558–66.

54. Böer-Auer A. Differential diagnostics of sebaceous tumors. Pathologe 2014;35:443–55.

55. Yoneda K, Demitsu T, Matsuda Y, et al. Possible molecular pathogenesis for plate-like sebaceous hyperplasia overlying dermatofibroma. Br J Dermatol 2008;158:840–2.

56. Davis TT, Calilao G, Fretzin D. Sebaceous hyperplasia overlying dermatofibroma. Am J Dermatopathol 2006;28:155–7.

57. Kazakov DV, Kutzner H, Spagnolo DV, et al. Discordant architectural and cytological features in cutaneous sebaceous neoplasms–a classification dilemma: report of 5 cases. Am J Dermatopathol 2009;31:31–6.

58. Harvey NT, Budgeon CA, Leecy T, et al. Interobserver variability in the diagnosis of circumscribed sebaceous neoplasms of the skin. Pathology 2013;45:581–6.

59. Wang E, Lee JS, Kazakov DV. A rare combination of sebaceoma with carcinomatous change (sebaceous carcinoma), trichoblastoma, and poroma arising from a nevus sebaceus. J Cutan Pathol 2013 Jul;40(7):676–82.

60. Kaliki S, Ayyar A, Dave TV, et al. Sebaceous gland carcinoma of the eyelid: clinicopathological features and outcome in Asian Indians. Eye 2015;29:958–63.

61. Izumi M, Mukai K, Nagai T, et al. Sebaceous carcinoma of the eyelids: thirty cases from Japan. Pathol Int 2008;58:483–8.

62. Khan JA, Doane JF, Grove AS, et al. Sebaceous and meibomian carcinomas of the eyelid. Recognition, diagnosis, and management. Ophthal Plast Reconstr Surg 1991;7:61–6.

63. Nelson BR, Hamlet KR, Gillard M, et al. Sebaceous carcinoma. J Am Acad Dermatol 1995;33:1–15.

64. Shields JA, Demirci H, Marr BP, et al. Sebaceous carcinoma of the eyelids: personal experience with 60 cases. Ophthalmology 2004;111:2151–7.

65. Rao NA, Hidayat AA, McLean IW, et al. Sebaceous carcinoma of the ocular adnexa: a clinicopathologic study of 104 cases, with five-year follow-up data. Hum Pathol 1982;13:113–22.

66. Muqit MM, Roberts F, Lee WR, et al. Improved survival rates in sebaceous carcinoma of the eyelid. Eye 2004;18:49–53.

67. Shain S, Sakharpe A, Lyle S, et al. P53 staining correlates with tumor type and location in sebaceous neoplasms. Am J Dermatopathol 2012;34:129–38.

68. Bell WR, Singh K, Rajan A, et al. Expression of p16 and p53 in intraepithelial periocular sebaceous carcinoma. Ocul Oncol Pathol 2015;2:71–5.

69. Candelario NM, Sanchez JE, Sanchez JL, et al. Extraocular sebaceous carcinoma - a clinicopathologic reassessment. Am J Dermatopathol 2016;38:809–12.

70. Bongu A, Lee ES, Peters SR, et al. Locally aggressive and multicentric recurrent extraocular sebaceous carcinoma: case report and literature review. Eplasty 2013;13:e44.

71. Seo FB, Jung HW, Choi IK, et al. Sebaceous carcinoma of the suprapubic area in a liver transplant recipient. Ann Dermatol 2014;26:395–8.

72. Moreno C, Jacyk WK, Judd MJ, et al. Highly aggressive extraocular sebaceous carcinoma. Am J Dermatopathol 2001;23:450–5.

73. Jensen ML. Extraocular sebaceous carcinoma of the skin with visceral metastases: case report. J Cutan Pathol 1990;17:117–21.

74. Pujol RM, LeBoit PE, Su WP. Microcystic adnexal carcinoma with extensive sebaceous differentiation. Am J Dermatopathol 1997;19:358–62.

# Update on Malignant Sweat Gland Tumors

Michiel P.J. van der Horst, MD[a], Thomas Brenn, MD, PhD, FRCPath[b],*

## KEYWORDS

- Sweat gland tumors • Malignant • Aggressive digital papillary adenocarcinoma
- Microcystic adnexal carcinoma • Spiradenocarcinoma • Squamoid eccrine ductal carcinoma

---

### Key Points

- Sweat gland tumors show a wide morphologic spectrum but malignant change is rare.

- Malignant sweat gland tumors are classified according to their behavior into low- and high-grade tumors. Low-grade malignant tumors are characterized by risk for locally destructive growth and local recurrence and but only rare distant metastasis, whereas high-grade tumors have significant metastatic potential and disease-related mortality.

- Precise classification and accurate diagnosis is necessary to predict behavior of these tumors.

- Immunohistochemistry and, at least as yet, molecular genetics play only a minor role in the diagnosis of sweat gland tumors.

- Cutaneous metastases from visceral primary adenocarcinomas are important considerations in the differential diagnosis of sweat gland carcinomas, and reliable separation may be impossible on morphologic and immunohistochemical grounds.

---

## ABSTRACT

Malignant sweat gland tumors are rare cutaneous neoplasms, traditionally separated according to their behavior into low- and high-grade malignant. There is significant morphologic overlap, and outright malignant tumors may show relatively bland histologic features. They may, therefore, be mistaken easily for benign neoplasms. Recognition of these tumors and accurate diagnosis is important for early treatment to prevent aggressive behavior and adverse outcome. This article provides an overview of 4 important entities with emphasis on diagnostic pitfalls, differential diagnosis and recent developments. Microcystic adnexal carcinoma, squamoid eccrine ductal carcinoma, aggressive digital papillary adenocarcinoma, and spiradenocarcinoma are discussed in detail.

## OVERVIEW

The range of skin adnexal neoplasms is broad and includes differentiation toward the hair follicle, the sebaceous gland, and the sweat gland and duct. The tumors span the spectrum from the entirely benign to high-grade malignant neoplasms with aggressive behavior and mortality. The recognition of tumors with potential for aggressive behavior is important. It poses a significant challenge for a large number of reasons. Particular problems are the rarity of skin adnexal carcinomas and the only poorly defined and often entity-specific criteria for malignancy. Furthermore, even tumors with the potential for outright aggressive disease course may show bland and innocuous histologic appearances, readily mistaken for benign neoplasms. Another important diagnostic pitfall is the separation of primary skin adnexal carcinoma

---

Disclosure Statement: The authors have nothing to disclose.
[a] Department of Pathology, Groene Hart Ziekenhuis, Bleulandweg 3, Gouda 2803 HG, The Netherlands;
[b] Department of Pathology, Western General Hospital, Alexander Donald Building, 1st Floor, Crewe Road, Edinburgh EH4 2XU, UK
* Corresponding author.
E-mail address: t_brenn@yahoo.com

Surgical Pathology 10 (2017) 383–397
http://dx.doi.org/10.1016/j.path.2017.01.010
1875-9181/17/

from cutaneous metastases of visceral primary adenocarcinomas and reliable distinction may be impossible on morphology and immunohistochemistry. According to their behavior, skin adnexal carcinomas have been traditionally separated into low- and high-grade malignant neoplasms. Low-grade malignant tumors rarely metastasize, but may cause significant morbidity owing to their locally destructive growth and risk for local recurrence. High-grade malignant tumors show significant potential for distant metastasis and disease-related mortality. This separation is, however, artificial; in reality, the boundaries are somewhat blurred. This article gives an overview and update of the recent developments of a selected group of malignant sweat gland tumors. The discussion includes examples of 2 low-grade malignant tumors, namely, microcystic adnexal carcinoma and squamoid eccrine ductal carcinoma, and 2 high-grade tumors, namely, aggressive digital papillary adenocarcinoma and spiradenocarcinoma.

## MICROCYSTIC ADNEXAL CARCINOMA

Microcystic adnexal carcinoma was first described by Goldstein in 1982.[1–9] It belongs to the group of low-grade malignant sweat duct tumors and is characterized by both sweat duct and follicular differentiation. It shows morphologic overlap with syringoid eccrine carcinoma, and the tumors are often regarded together.

### CLINICAL PRESENTATION

Microcystic adnexal carcinoma typically presents as slowly growing plaques, and paresthesia may be an accompanying symptom. The tumors are ill-defined and extend beyond the clinically visible. They have a predilection for the central face, especially the perioral area and the nasolabial folds. There is no strong gender predilection.

### MICROSCOPIC FEATURES

The tumors are based within dermis and they are characterized by a diffusely infiltrative growth with invasion of subcutis and deeper structures (Fig. 1A). They grow in cords and strands in a desmoplastic stroma (see Fig. 1B). Superficially, keratocysts and dystrophic calcifications are often seen (see Fig. 1C). Duct differentiation is an additional feature and is present in varying amounts. Although some tumors show prominent duct differentiation as seen in syringoid eccrine carcinoma (see Fig. 1D), others show almost exclusively follicular differentiation (see Fig. 1E). Cytologic atypia is mild and clear cell change may be prominent (see Fig. 1F). Mitoses are typically inconspicuous. Perineural invasion is almost invariably present. Immunohistochemistry plays no major role in the diagnosis of microscystic adnexal carcinoma. The tumors express cytokeratins and are positive for CK7 and negative for CK20. EMA and CEA staining is helpful to highlight duct differentiation and S100 and EMA are useful in identifying perineural infiltration.

## BEHAVIOR AND TREATMENT

Microcystic adnexal carcinoma is characterized by locally destructive growth and high local recurrence rates, especially if complete excision cannot be achieved. Distant metastases are, however, exceptionally rare. The treatment of choice is wide local excision with tumor-free margins. Mohs micrographic surgery is an excellent alternative. Early diagnosis and adequate surgery are necessary for local disease control.

## DIFFERENTIAL DIAGNOSIS

Owing to the bland histologic features, the diagnosis of microcystic adnexal carcinoma is extremely challenging, especially on superficial and partial biopsies. The differential diagnosis is summarized in Table 1. Microcystic adnexal carcinoma closely resembles benign skin adnexal tumors, including desmoplastic trichoepithelioma, trichoadenoma, and syringoma. Recognition of the infiltrative tumor growth is the most important differentiating feature. If the initial diagnostic biopsy does not include deeper dermis and subcutis, it is important to ask for a deeper and adequate tissue sample.

Morpheaform basal cell carcinoma and desmoplastic squamous cell carcinoma also enter the differential diagnosis. They share the infiltrative growth in a desmoplastic stroma but display more pronounced cytologic atypia and they lack the ductal differentiation. Owing to the similar behavior and treatment reliable separation on diagnostic biopsies is less important. Tumors showing predominantly duct differentiation (syringoid eccrine carcinoma) may mimic metastatic adenocarcinoma, especially of invasive ductal breast carcinoma. They are morphologically and immunohistochemically inseparable, and the diagnosis requires careful clinical correlation and screening.

## SQUAMOID ECCRINE DUCTAL CARCINOMA

Squamoid eccrine ductal carcinoma is a poorly documented and likely underreported low-grade malignant sweat duct tumor first described in

*Fig. 1.* Microcystic adnexal carcinomas are diffusely infiltrative tumors (*A*). They are characterized by a growth of cords and strands within a desmoplastic stroma (*B*). Keratocyst formation is typically seen in the more superficial aspects (*C*).

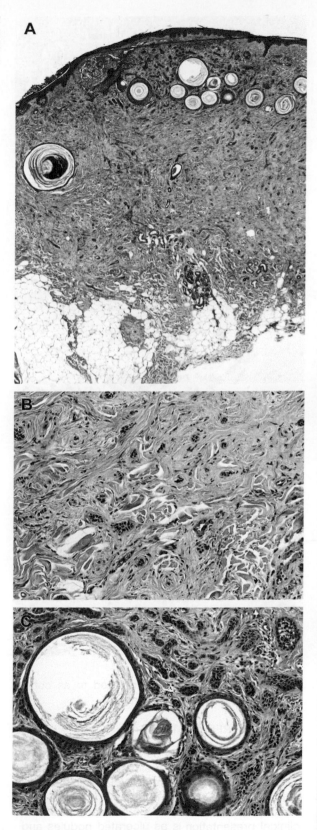

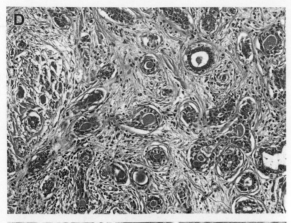

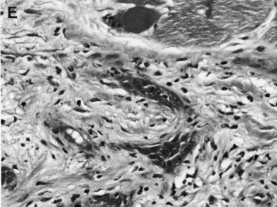

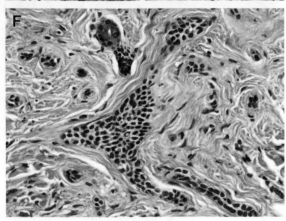

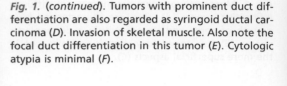

*Fig. 1.* (*continued*). Tumors with prominent duct differentiation are also regarded as syringoid ductal carcinoma (*D*). Invasion of skeletal muscle. Also note the focal duct differentiation in this tumor (*E*). Cytologic atypia is minimal (*F*).

1997.[10–13] It has also been referred to as cutaneous adenosquamous carcinoma.

## CLINICAL PRESENTATION

The tumors mainly affect dun-damaged skin of the head and neck of elderly males, and the face is the single most frequently affected anatomic location. The extremities are less commonly involved, and manifestation on the trunk is distinctly rare. The clinical presentation is as ulcerated nodules and plaques, measuring a few centimeters.

## MICROSCOPIC FEATURES

Squamoid eccrine ductal carcinomas are poorly marginated and asymmetrical tumors with a diffusely infiltrative growth pattern (**Fig. 2**A). They are based within the dermis and frequently invade subcutaneous tissues. The tumors are often ulcerated and show a multifocal connection with the epidermis. In the superficial aspects, there is overt squamous differentiation and they are indistinguishable from well-differentiated squamous cell carcinoma (see **Fig. 2**B, C). In the deeper reaches,

**Table 1**
Differential diagnosis of MAC

| MAC vs | Helpful Distinguishing Features |
|--------|-------------------------------|
| Desmoplastic trichoepithelioma | • Confined to superficial and mid dermis<br>• Lack of infiltrative growth<br>• Lack of cytologic atypia<br>• Lack of ductal differentiation |
| Trichoadenoma | • No deep and infiltrative growth<br>• Lack of ductal differentiation<br>• No perineural invasion |
| Syringoma | • Lack of cytologic atypia<br>• Lack of infiltrative growth<br>• No perineural invasion<br>• Lack of keratocysts |
| Morpheaform basal cell carcinoma | • Marked cytologic atypia<br>• Lack of ductal differentiation |
| Desmoplastic squamous cell carcinoma | • Marked cytologic atypia<br>• Lack of ductal differentiation |
| Metastatic ductal carcinoma of the breast | • Longstanding history of slowly growing plaque not typical<br>• Identification of a breast primary tumor |

*Abbreviation:* MAC, microcystic adnexal carcinoma.

the tumors are arranged in smaller nests, cords, and strands in a desmoplastic stroma. The tumor cells are large and polygonal, with moderate to severe cytologic atypia (see **Fig. 2**D). Duct differentiation is present to varying degrees. There is increased mitotic activity with occasional atypical mitotic figures. Additional findings include tumor necrosis and perineural infiltration, but lymphovascular invasion is rarely identified.

## BEHAVIOR AND TREATMENT

Squamoid eccrine ductal carcinoma is associated with a high local recurrence rate, independent of completeness of excision. This is likely owing to the deep and diffusely infiltrative growth of the tumor and the frequent presence of perineural infiltration. Importantly, the disease also shows significant potential for metastatic spread (up to 13%). Metastases are mainly to lymph nodes, but widespread metastatic disease with disease-related mortality may also be seen. Treatment recommendations include wide local excision or Mohs micrographic surgery as well as clinical screening and careful follow-up.

## DIFFERENTIAL DIAGNOSIS

Awareness of this distinctive entity is necessary to differentiate it from squamous cell carcinoma, eccrine porocarcinoma, eccrine ductal carcinoma, syringoid eccrine carcinoma, and microcystic

adnexal carcinoma. The differential diagnosis is summarized in **Table 2**.

Differentiation from squamous cell carcinoma is particularly challenging and may be impossible on superficial shave and curette biopsies. This difficulty may account for the rare reports of squamoid eccrine ductal carcinoma in the literature. Identification of the additional ductal differentiation in the deeper reaches of the tumor is necessary for the correct diagnosis.

Eccrine porocarcinoma may show squamous differentiation and differentiation from squamoid eccrine ductal carcinoma may be difficult. It is, however, of little clinical relevance because the clinical behaviors are similar. Findings in favor of eccrine porocarcinoma are the characteristic polygonal tumor cells and the identification of a benign poroma. Furthermore, the squamous and ductal areas are clearly separated in squamoid eccrine ductal carcinoma.

Eccrine ductal carcinoma lacks the squamous component. Microcystic adnexal carcinoma and syringoid eccrine carcinoma could also be considered in the differential diagnosis. Both the ductal and squamoid areas lack the degree of cytologic atypia seen in squamoid eccrine ductal carcinoma.

## "AGGRESSIVE" DIGITAL PAPILLARY ADENOCARCINOMA

Aggressive digital papillary adenocarcinoma is a distinctive high-grade malignant sweat gland

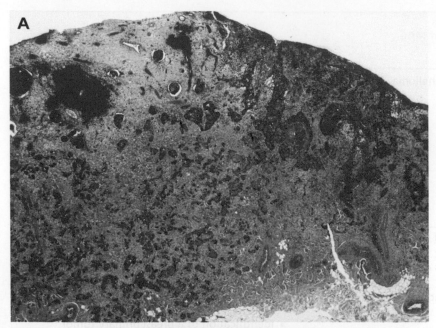

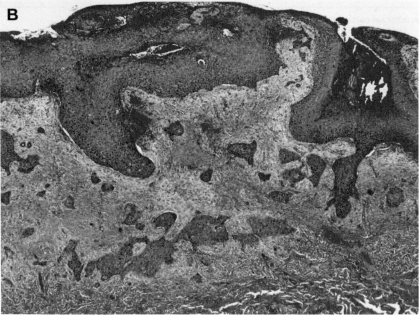

*Fig. 2.* Syringoid eccrine ductal carcinoma is a diffusely infiltrative neoplasm, often showing epidermal ulceration (*A*). In the superficial aspects, the tumor shows squamous differentiation and mimics squamous cell carcinoma. A multifocal epidermal connection is frequently present (*B, C*). In the deeper reaches the tumor is composed of pleomorphic epithelioid cells showing duct differentiation. The tumor cells are arranged in small nests and strands in a desmoplastic stroma (*D*).

tumor with a narrow clinical presentation.[14–17] Its morphologic spectrum is, however, wide ranging from tumors with bland histologic features to those with severe cytologic atypia, brisk mitotic activity, and necrosis. According to the morphologic appearances, the tumors were separated initially into adenoma and adenocarcinoma. With longer term follow-up, it has become apparent that the behavior of these tumors is independent of the morphologic findings and all tumors are currently regarded as adenocarcinoma. More recently, these tumors have also been referred to as cutaneous digital papillary adenocarcinoma because the term aggressive seems to be redundant.

## CLINICAL PRESENTATION

The tumors present as solitary nodules or cysts on the distal extremities with a marked predilection for the fingers and toes, especially around the

*Fig. 2.* (*continued*).

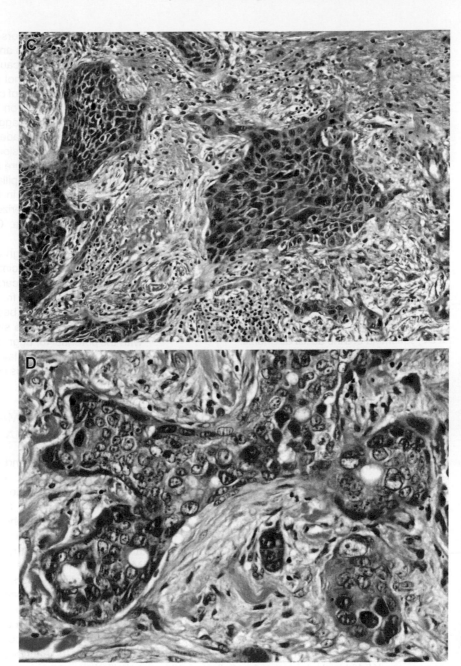

nails. Middle-aged adults are most commonly affected with a strong male predominance. The age spectrum is, however, wide and presentation in childhood and adolescence may also be observed.

## MICROSCOPIC FEATURES

Histologically aggressive digital papillary adeno-carcinomas are well-circumscribed multinodular tumors within dermis and superficial subcutis (**Fig.** 3A). They have a solid and cystic growth pattern and occasionally show infiltrative margins (see **Fig.** 3B). Papillary projections into the cyst lumen are a typical feature but may be present only focally (see **Fig.** 3C). A tubular growth may be an additional feature (see **Fig.** 3D). The tumor cells are basaloid epithelial cells and with mild to moderate cytologic atypia in the majority of cases (see **Fig.** 3E). Severe cytologic atypia and tumor

**Table 2**
**Differential diagnosis of SEDC**

| SEDC vs | Helpful Distinguishing Features |
|---|---|
| Cutaneous squamous cell carcinoma | • No duct differentiation in deeper reaches |
| Eccrine porocarcinoma with squamous differentiation | • Uniform polygonal tumor cells with poroid characteristics<br>• Lack the zonation<br>• Background of a preexisting poroma<br>• Strong predilection for the distal extremities |
| MAC | • Presence of keratocysts<br>• Lack of significant cytologic atypia |

*Abbreviations:* MAC, microcystic adnexal carcinoma; SEDC, squamoid eccrine ductal carcinoma.

necrosis is noted in a small subset of tumors. Similarly, mitoses may be inconspicuous or frequent, depending on the tumor. Spindle cell morphology, squamoid differentiation, and clear cell changes may also be encountered (see **Fig. 3**F). A second myoepithelial cell layer is present and can be highlighted by immunohistochemistry for S100, p63, SMA, and calponin (see **Fig. 3**G). By immunohistochemistry, tumor cells express cytokeratins. EMA and CEA staining highlights ductal differentiation.

## BEHAVIOR AND TREATMENT

All tumors have the potential for outright malignant behavior independent of the morphologic features. They have significant potential for local recurrence and metastasis, especially to lymph nodes and lung. The overall disease-related mortality seems to be lower. The disease course is, however, often protracted and long-term monitoring of patients is necessary. Wide local excision or (partial) amputation is the treatment of choice. It appears to result in lower recurrence and metastatic rates.

## DIFFERENTIAL DIAGNOSIS

Aggressive digital papillary adenocarcinoma has a broad differential diagnosis, which is summarized in **Table 3**. Tumors with bland cytologic features pose a particular diagnostic problem, because they may be mistaken readily for benign skin adnexal tumors or cyst.

The biggest diagnostic pitfall is with apocrine hidrocystoma or apocrine cystadenoma.

Importantly, these tumors are exceptionally rare on the distal extremities and this diagnosis should be made with extreme caution. The presence of a dual cell population is not a helpful distinguishing feature, but any degree of cytologic atypia in cystic and papillary tumors on the distal extremities should be regarded as aggressive digital papillary adenocarcinoma. Hidradenoma may affect the distal extremities occasionally. The most important distinguishing feature is lack of cytologic atypia in hidradenoma. Papillary eccrine adenoma is not seen uncommonly in then distal extremities. It is, however, characterized by a tubular growth with intervening stroma. Cytologic atypia is not present.

Morphologically high-grade tumors may resemble hidradenocarcinoma or cutaneous metastases from papillary carcinomas of visceral primary sites. Separation from hidradenocarcinoma is largely academic because they are both regarded as high-grade sweat gland carcinomas with the potential for aggressive behavior. Demonstration of a dual cell layer on morphology and immunohistochemistry is useful to exclude a cutaneous metastasis.

## SPIRADENOCARCINOMA AND CYLINDROCARCINOMA

Spiradenocarcinoma and cylindrocarcinoma are rare malignant sweat gland carcinomas.[18-22] They have been traditionally classified as high-grade malignant. More recently it has, however, been shown that morphologic features correlate well with outcome and aggressive behavior is associated with high-grade morphology only. Morphologically low-grade tumors seem to pursue an indolent clinical course. The diagnosis of these tumors is entirely dependent on sampling and recognition of a benign preexisting spiradenoma or cylindroma. This is a prerequisite for the diagnosis as the malignant component shows features of carcinoma or adenocarcinoma, not otherwise specified.

## CLINICAL PRESENTATION

The tumors present as solitary nodules, measuring up to multiple centimeters in diameter. The anatomic distribution is wide with a predilection for the head and neck area. Elderly adults in the fifth to eighth decades are typically affected and there is no gender predilection. Often there is a longstanding history with recent enlargement. Although the majority of tumors is sporadic, they may also be seen in patients with the Brooke-Spiegler syndrome.

**Fig. 3.** Aggressive digital papillary adeno-carcinoma. The tumors are solid and cystic and based within deep dermis and superficial subcutis (*A*). They are well-circumscribed and nodular. Papillary projections are a hallmark feature (*B*). The characteristic micropapillae project into the cystic spaces. Also note the second myoepithelial cell layer (*C*).

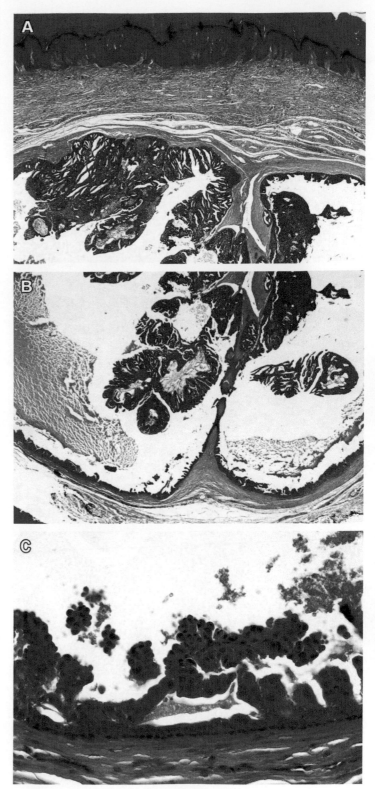

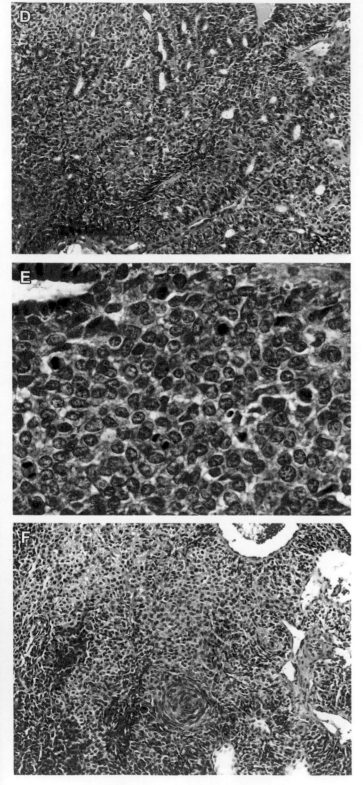

Fig. 3. (continued). Tubular differentiation is another common findings (D). Cytologic atypia is mild to moderate. Mitotic activity is increased (E). In the solid areas, squamoid whorls may be seen (F). P63 staining highlights the myoepithelial second cell layer (G).

*Fig. 3.* (*continued*).

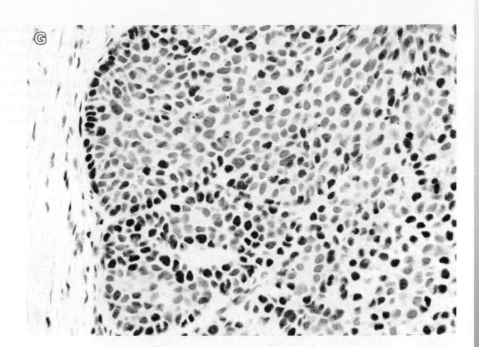

## MICROSCOPIC FEATURES

By definition, the identification of a preexisting benign spiradenoma or cylindroma is necessary for the diagnosis. These neoplasms may be focal and they are often compressed to the side (**Fig. 4**A). Careful sampling is therefore necessary. High-grade tumors are characterized by an expansile unilobular or multilobular tumor mass composed of severely atypical epithelial cells with marked nuclear pleomorphism (see **Fig. 4**B). The tumors show an infiltrative growth and may invade deeply. Gland and/or duct differentiation may be present in varying amounts (see **Fig. 4**C). The mitotic count is high and atypical mitoses may be found. Tumor necrosis may be an additional feature. The findings resemble carcinoma or adenocarcinoma, not otherwise specified.

Low-grade tumors show similar low-power architectural features to spiradenoma, for which they are readily mistaken (**Fig. 5**A). On closer examination, it becomes apparent that there is loss of the dual cell population characteristic of spiradenoma (see **Fig. 5**B). In addition, there is mild to moderate cytologic atypia and increased mitotic activity (see **Fig. 5**C). Additional features include clear cell change, keratocyst formation, and squamoid differentiation (see **Fig. 5**D). Tumor necrosis and perineural infiltration may be present. The key features of low-grade spiradenocarcinoma are listed in **Box 1**. Metaplastic change is seen in a rare subset of tumors. By immunohistochemistry, MYB expression, seen in spiradenoma and cylindroma, is lost in spiradenocarcinoma and cylindrocarcinoma. It is an additional helpful diagnostic marker in challenging cases.

## BEHAVIOR AND TREATMENT

Although the tumors have been traditionally regarded as high-grade malignancies, recent

| Table 3 | |
|---|---|
| **Differential diagnosis of ADPACa** | |
| **ADPACa vs** | **Helpful Distinguishing Features** |
| Hidradenoma | • Few, if any, papillary projections<br>• No cytologic atypia |
| Papillary eccrine adenoma | • Tubular growth with intervening stroma<br>• No solid component<br>• No cytologic atypia |
| Apocrine hidrocystoma/cystadenoma | • No solid growth component<br>• No cytologic atypia<br>• Not located on the digits |
| Metastatic papillary adenocarcinoma | • Lack of myoepithelial dual cell layer |

*Abbreviation:* ADPACa, aggressive digital papillary adenocarcinoma.

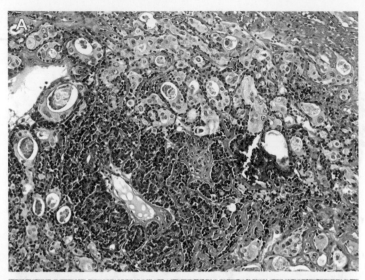

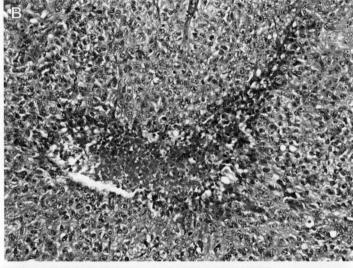

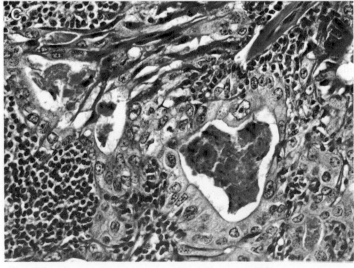

*Fig. 4.* Spiradenocarcinoma, high-grade. A preexisting benign spiradenoma is necessary for the diagnosis (*A*). The malignant component is characterized by sheets of pleomorphic cells. Brisk mitotic activity and tumor necrosis are also seen (*B*). Duct differentiation may be prominent (*C*).

*Fig. 5.* Spiradenocarcinoma, low-grade. This large tumor shows a background of a pre-existing spiradenoma in the lower parts and malignant transformation with expansile growth in the upper aspect of the image (*A*). Although the architecture of a spiradenoma is retained, there is loss of the dual cell population (*B*).

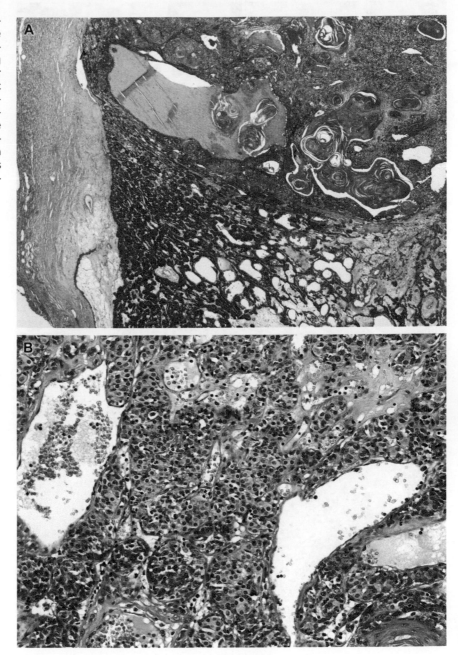

studies have demonstrated that morphology is a good predictor of outcome. Morphologically high-grade tumors are associated with an aggressive disease course with high rates of local recurrence, distant metastases to lymph nodes and lung, and mortality. In contrast, low-grade and metaplastic tumors seem to be indolent. Although they may recur locally, distant metastasis and disease-related mortality are exceptionally rare.

## DIFFERENTIAL DIAGNOSIS

Morphologically low-grade tumors resemble spiradenoma, for which they are readily mistaken. Careful examination with recognition of loss of the dual cell layer, the presence of cytologic atypia and increased mitotic activity is helpful. In view of the indolent behavior of low-grade tumors it is, however, of little clinical relevance. High-grade

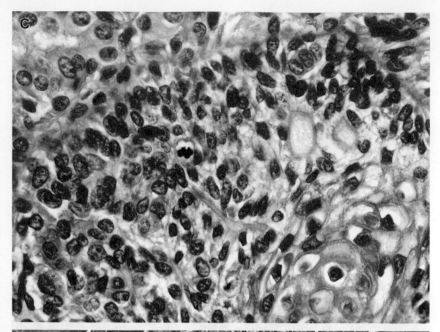

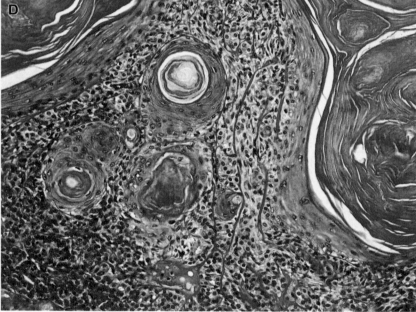

*Fig. 5. (continued).* Cytologic atypia is mild but increased mitotic activity is present (*C*). Clear cell change and keratocyst formation are additional features (*D*).

---

**Box 1**
**Key features: low-grade malignant component in spiradenocarcinoma**

*Architecturally reminiscent of benign spiradenoma, but*

1. Expansile growth in a background of a pre-existing benign spiradenoma

2. Loss of dual cell population

3. Diffuse growth of monotonous cells

4. Mild to moderate cytologic atypia

5. Mitotic activity

6. Loss of MYB expression by immunohistochemistry

tumors are easily mistaken for cutaneous metastasis from visceral adenocarcinomas. Sampling and recognition of the preexisting benign spiradenoma or cylindroma is necessary.

## REFERENCES

1. Goldstein DJ, Barr RJ, Santa Cruz DJ. Microcystic adnexal carcinoma: a distinct clinicopathologic entity. Cancer 1982;50(3):566–72.

2. Cooper PH. Sclerosing carcinomas of sweat ducts (microcystic adnexal carcinoma). Arch Dermatol 1986;122(3):261–4.

3. Friedman PM, Friedman RH, Jiang SB, et al. Microcystic adnexal carcinoma: collaborative series review and update. J Am Acad Dermatol 1999;41(2 Pt 1):225–31.

4. Chiller K, Passaro D, Scheuller M, et al. Microcystic adnexal carcinoma: forty-eight cases, their treatment, and their outcome. Arch Dermatol 2000; 136(11):1355–9.

5. Snow S, Madjar DD, Hardy S, et al. Microcystic adnexal carcinoma: report of 13 cases and review of the literature. Dermatol Surg 2001;27(4):401–8.

6. Ohta M, Hiramoto M, Ohtsuka H. Metastatic microcystic adnexal carcinoma: an autopsy case. Dermatol Surg 2004;30(6):957–60.

7. Leibovitch I, Huilgol SC, Selva D, et al. Microcystic adnexal carcinoma: treatment with Mohs micrographic surgery. J Am Acad Dermatol 2005;52(2): 295–300.

8. Gabillot-Carre M, Weill F, Mamelle G, et al. Microcystic adnexal carcinoma: report of seven cases including one with lung metastasis. Dermatology 2006;212(3):221–8.

9. Sidiropoulos M, Sade S, Al-Habeeb A, et al. Syringoid eccrine carcinoma: a clinicopathological and immunohistochemical study of four cases. J Clin Pathol 2011;64(9):788–92.

10. Fu JM, McCalmont T, Yu SS. Adenosquamous carcinoma of the skin: a case series. Arch Dermatol 2009; 145(10):1152–8.

11. Ko CJ, Leffell DJ, McNiff JM. Adenosquamous carcinoma: a report of nine cases with p63 and cytokeratin 5/6 staining. J Cutan Pathol 2009;36(4): 448–52.

12. van der Horst MP, Garcia-Herrera A, Markiewicz D, et al. Squamoid eccrine ductal carcinoma: a clinicopathologic study of 30 cases. Am J Surg Pathol 2016;40(6):755–60.

13. Wong TY, Suster S, Mihm MC. Squamoid eccrine ductal carcinoma. Histopathology 1997;30(3):288–93.

14. Duke WH, Sherrod TT, Lupton GP. Aggressive digital papillary adenocarcinoma (aggressive digital papillary adenoma and adenocarcinoma revisited). Am J Surg Pathol 2000;24(6):775–84.

15. Kao GF, Helwig EB, Graham JH. Aggressive digital papillary adenoma and adenocarcinoma. A clinicopathological study of 57 patients, with histochemical, immunopathological, and ultrastructural observations. J Cutan Pathol 1987;14(3):129–46.

16. Molina-Ruiz AM, Llamas-Velasco M, Rutten A, et al. "Apocrine hidrocystoma and cystadenoma"-like tumor of the digits or toes: a potential diagnostic pitfall of digital papillary adenocarcinoma. Am J Surg Pathol 2016;40(3):410–8.

17. Suchak R, Wang WL, Prieto VG, et al. Cutaneous digital papillary adenocarcinoma: a clinicopathologic study of 31 cases of a rare neoplasm with new observations. Am J Surg Pathol 2012;36(12):1883–91.

18. Dai B, Kong YY, Cai X, et al. Spiradenocarcinoma, cylindrocarcinoma and spiradenocylindrocarcinoma: a clinicopathological study of nine cases. Histopathology 2014;65(5):658–66.

19. Granter SR, Seeger K, Calonje E, et al. Malignant eccrine spiradenoma (spiradenocarcinoma): a clinicopathologic study of 12 cases. Am J Dermatopathol 2000;22(2):97–103.

20. Kazakov DV, Zelger B, Rutten A, et al. Morphologic diversity of malignant neoplasms arising in preexisting spiradenoma, cylindroma, and spiradenocylindroma based on the study of 24 cases, sporadic or occurring in the setting of Brooke-Spiegler syndrome. Am J Surg Pathol 2009;33(5):705–19.

21. Leonard N, Smith D, McNamara P. Low-grade malignant eccrine spiradenoma with systemic metastases. Am J Dermatopathol 2003;25(3):253–5.

22. van der Horst MP, Marusic Z, Hornick JL, et al. Morphologically low-grade spiradenocarcinoma: a clinicopathologic study of 19 cases with emphasis on outcome and MYB expression. Mod Pathol 2015;28(7):944–53.

# Merkel Cell Carcinoma

Melissa Pulitzer, MD

## KEYWORDS

• Neuroendocrine • Merkel cell • Polyomavirus • UV

## Key Points

- Merkel cell carcinoma (MCC) is an aggressive neoplasm with a high risk of metastasis, relapse, and disease-related mortality.
- The presence of lymphovascular invasion and the pattern of involvement of MCC in lymph nodes may have bearing on prognosis.
- An evolving paradigm suggests 2 distinct types of MCC, most easily stratified by Merkel cell polyomavirus (MCV) presence but also exhibited by morphologic, immunophenotypic, molecular, and clinical features.

## ABSTRACT

Merkel cell carcinoma (MCC) encompasses neuroendocrine carcinomas primary to skin and occurs most commonly in association with clonally integrated Merkel cell polyomavirus with related retinoblastoma protein sequestration or in association with UV radiation–induced alterations involving the TP53 gene and mutations, heterozygous deletion, and hypermethylation of the *Retinoblastoma* gene. Molecular genetic signatures may provide therapeutic guidance. Morphologic features, although patterned, are associated with predictable diagnostic pitfalls, usually resolvable by immunohistochemistry. Therapeutic options for MCC, traditionally limited to surgical intervention and later chemotherapy and radiation, are growing, given promising early results of immunotherapeutic regimens.

## OVERVIEW

Diagnosis of stage IV MCC is associated with an approximate 11% survival and a median survival of 6 months. Overall, the 5-year disease-specific survival (DSS) rate for MCC is estimated to be between 30% and 64%,[1] with a DSS rate greater than 90% for those with local disease.[2] It is thus clear that the timely and accurate diagnosis of this aggressive primary cutaneous neuroendocrine carcinoma (NEC) is critical, yet as many

as 56% of MCCs are thought to be clinically benign at biopsy.[3] The thoughtful evaluation of poorly differentiated/basaloid infiltrates in the skin, subcutaneous tissues, salivary glands, and lymph nodes can allow for earlier recognition, correct diagnosis, and clinically useful pathologic characterization of MCC. Pathologic pitfalls in the diagnosis of MCC derive from lack of exposure to these rare tumors, lack of adequate sectioning of nondiagnostic tissue, hasty interpretation of small round blue cell tumors in the skin, inadequate provision of clinical history, and underutilization of immunohistochemistry in the diagnostic work-up. A basic understanding of the lymphovascular nature of tumor spread as well as the two major and apparently distinct pathways of MCC pathogenesis can serve as a reminder of the most salient reportable features of these tumors to enable the best prognostic and therapeutic algorithms for individual patients with this disease.

## GROSS FEATURES

MCC most often presents in an older white population with a male predominance. The median age of presentation falls within the late seventh decade, despite a broad age range (fourth to tenth decades). Sun-exposed sites, including the head/neck and limbs, are the most common sites of presentation. There seem to be 2 patterns of clinical presentation that align with either MCV-positive,

Sources of Support: This research was funded in part through the NIH/NCI Cancer Center Support Grant P30CA008748.

Department of Pathology, Memorial Sloan Kettering Cancer Center, 1275 York Avenue, New York, NY 10021, USA

E-mail address: pulitzem@mskcc.org

Surgical Pathology 10 (2017) 399–408
http://dx.doi.org/10.1016/j.path.2017.01.013

surgpath.theclinics.com

morphologically monophenotypic, and/or cytokeratin 20 (CK20)-positive tumors versus MCV-negative, often morphologically heterogeneous, tumors. The first, more prevalent group (80% of cases) arises in a slightly younger population and is equally present on the limbs and head/neck, sometimes found on the buttock or other non–sun-exposed sites. These tumors are often (>45%) indeterminate to clinically benign flesh-colored to violaceous dome-shaped nodules with chief differential diagnoses of cysts, pimples, dermatofibromas, lipomas, and lymphomas; 10% are suspected to be nonmelanoma skin cancer. The second group of patients more commonly presents with tumors in sun-damaged skin of the head and neck, in a background of other nonmelanoma skin cancers, and are clinically more likely to be diagnosed as a new nonmelanoma skin cancer (58%), with only 15% suspected to be benign.[4] Clinical features, such as overlying scale and nearby actinic keratoses, solar lentigines, and telangiectasia, are common. A third, smaller group of patients presents with nodal adenopathy, eventuating in a biopsy-diagnosis of apparently metastatic MCC of unknown primary skin site.[5]

## MICROSCOPIC FEATURES

The quintessential small round blue cell tumor with salt-and-pepper chromatin, MCC practically defines pattern recognition. Most often, the tumor cells are uniform, with round to oval nuclei, finely dispersed chromatin, inconspicuous nucleoli, distinct nuclear membranes, scant cytoplasm, and numerous mitoses with nuclear fragmentation (Fig 1A). Small cell variants also show nuclear molding and crush artifact. Morphologic subtypes have been suggested evaluating the presence/absence of second tumor-types (eg, squamous cell carcinoma [SCC], in up to 15% of cases [see Fig 1B], or basal cell carcinoma [BCC]),[6] epithelial involvement (within epidermis [see Fig 1C] or adnexal epithelium [see Fig 1D]),[7,8] architectural arrangement (infiltrative periphery vs smooth nodular borders [see Fig 1E]),[9] cell size (small, medium, or large), and cell shape.[10] Regardless of pattern, tumors localize predominantly to the dermis as 1 or multiple nodules and may invade deeply into the subcutis. Tumor microemboli are frequently found within peritumoral lymphatic spaces (see Fig 1F).

A majority of MCC express cytokeratins, most characteristically CK20 in 95% of cases (Fig 2A) or Cam5.2 in a paranuclear dot-like and/or cytoplasmic pattern, neuroendocrine markers (most commonly synaptophysin, chromogranin, and CD56), and neurofilament (NF). Thyroid transcription factor-1 (TTF-1) and CDX-2 are negative. P63

is reported present in 60% of MCC and may be associated with a poorer overall and disease specific survival rates.[11–13] CK7 is generally negative, but occasional reported cases are positive.[14,15]

MCV is present in 55% to 90% of MCC by immunohistochemistry (see Fig 2B). NF is more frequently negative in MCV-negative cases with combined morphology.[16] These cases are more highly represented among the CK20-negative MCC population and have been shown to uniquely express follicular stem cell markers[17] and higher labeling with p53.[16,18]

## DIFFERENTIAL DIAGNOSIS

### BASAL CELL CARCINOMA

Distinguishing MCC from BCC requires attention to cytologic and stromal detail. Specifically, MCC lacks palisading peripheral cells and displays characteristic neuroendocrine cytology. MCC may be seen within the epidermis/adnexal epithelium, but does not bud from the base of the epidermis. Other confounders in MCC include mucinous stroma, stroma-tumor clefts, mucinous intratumoral glandular spaces (see Fig 3A), and focal peripheral palisading,[15] but these are limited. Ber-EP4 and epithelial membrane antigen (EMA) may be positive in MCC.[19] BCC can show neuroendocrine-type chromatin and immunolabeling, for example, with chromogranin.[20] Cam5.2 can be seen in BCC.[15] Strong dot-like labeling by CK20 strongly favors MCC,[21] and MCV is negative in BCC.

### MELANOMA

Small cell melanoma occasionally enters the differential diagnosis of MCC. Both tumors may exhibit irregular nesting at the dermoepidermal junction,[15] and pagetoid/bowenoid extension in the epidermis (see Fig 3B).[22] Large irregular nuclei and prominent cherry-red nucleoli are unusual in MCC and favor melanoma, although in one study 20% of MCCs showed intranuclear inclusions.[15] Pigment granules favor melanoma, although melanophages may be noted in MCC. Immunohistochemistry resolves the diagnosis in most cases. Occasional MCCs are S100 positive but HMB-45 negative and NKI/C3 negative.[23] MCV is negative in melanoma.

### METASTATIC NEUROENDOCRINE CARCINOMA

Clinical evaluation is paramount to diagnose metastatic neuroendocrine carcinoma (NEC) to skin. A few pathologic features may be helpful. Architectural and cytologic features of concern include extensive lymphovascular involvement, adenoidal patterns of growth, anisocytosis, large irregular

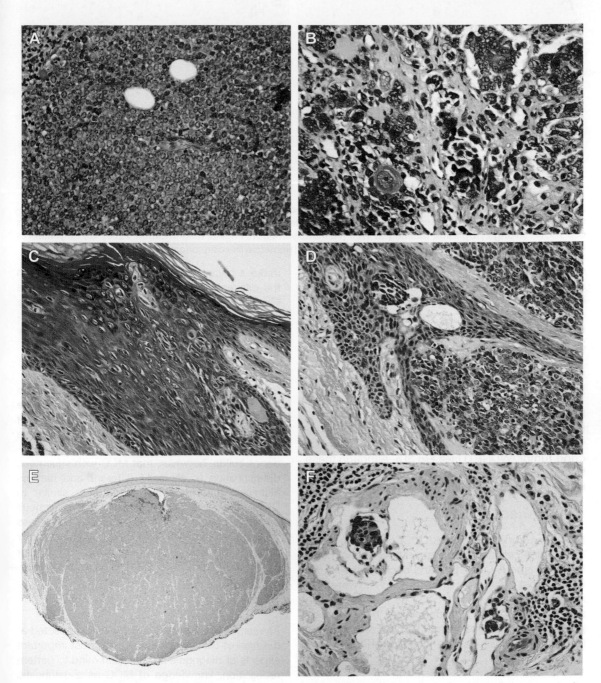

*Fig. 1.* (*A*). Cytomorphology of MCC showing round nuclei, scant cytoplasm, salt-and-pepper chromatin, indistinct nucleoli [Hematoxylin-eosin, original magnification ×200]. (*B*) Combined MCC; a small cell component demonstrates small round nuclei with crush artifact whereas a second more epitheloid population is punctuated by large keratinizing squamous cells [Hematoxylin-eosin, original magnification ×400]. (*C*) Intraepidermal pagetoid extension of MCC overlying a dermal tumor nodule (focally seen in left lower corner) [Hematoxylin-eosin, original magnification ×400]. (*D*) MCC in situ arising within severely dysplastic squamous epithelium/SCC in situ of epithelium, associated with invasive NEC in adjacent dermis [Hematoxylin-eosin, original magnification ×400]. (*E*) Low-power photomicrograph showing nodular circumscription of a dermal tumor [Hematoxylin-eosin, original magnification ×40]. (*F*) Intralymphatic tumor emboli of MCC within ectatic deep dermal lymphatics [Hematoxylin-eosin, original magnification ×400].

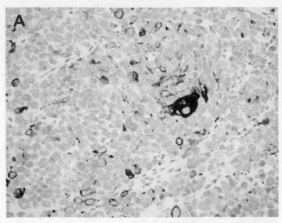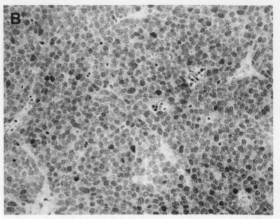

*Fig. 2.* (*A*) CK20 stain in a combined tumor shows a varied pattern of labeling, including patchy but diffuse perinuclear dots as well as areas of membranous accentuation [Hematoxylin-eosin, original magnification ×400]. Squamous cell shows strong cytoplasmic labeling as well [Hematoxylin-eosin, original magnification ×200]. (*B*) Polyomavirus immunohistochemical stain diffusely labels tumor nuclei [Hematoxylin-eosin, original magnification ×400].

nucleoli, coarse chromatin, and more abundant cytoplasm than seen in MCC (see **Fig** 3C). Immunohistochemistry favoring metastatic disease includes TTF-1 (eg, lung or thyroid [up to 85%]),[24] CK7 (73% of metastatic NEC),[14,25–27] and CDX-2.[28] MCV is negative in metastatic NEC.[29]

## METASTATIC WELL-DIFFERENTIATED NEUROENDOCRINE TUMOR

Histologic lack of high-grade neuroendocrine features can exclude metastatic NEC but may be seen in metastatic well-differentiated neuroendocrine tumor (WDNET) (see **Fig** 3D). Although these tumors are often positive for synaptophysin, chromogranin, and CD56, they are negative for CK20.

## EWING SARCOMA

Ewing sarcoma (EWS) and MCC are both small round blue cell tumors that may show strong membranous labeling for CD99 and nuclear labeling for FLI-1. Most cutaneous EWS show EWS rearrangements, for example, t (11; 22), by fluorescence in situ hybridization (FISH) or reverse transcription–polymerase chain reaction (RT-PCR). All cases are immunohistochemically negative for MCV.[30]

## LYMPHOMA

Peripheral lymphomas may mimic small cell MCC morphologically and immunohistochemically; PAX-5, Terminal deoxynucleotidyl Transferase (TdT), CD56, and CD99 may be positive in MCC.[15,19] A small panel of immunohistochemistry, including CD43 and/or CD45, CK20, and MCV, typically resolves the diagnosis.

## SEBACEOUS CARCINOMA

Rippled architecture, sebaceous mantle involvement, and pagetoid intraepidermal spread can make sebaceous carcinoma a suspect entity in the differential diagnosis of superficial MCC (see **Fig** 3E). Occasional EMA, p53, and p63 positivity in MCC confounds. A helpful feature is that sebaceous carcinoma is CK20[31] and MCV negative.

## SQUAMOUS CELL CARCINOMA

SCC with robust neuroendocrine differentiation may be impossible to tease apart from MCC (see **Fig** 3F). If CK20 is positive or there is abundant NF and/or neuroendocrine granule positivity, these tumors are traditionally categorized as MCC. Evidence builds, however, that MCC with squamous differentiation is clinically different and harbors histologic and molecular signatures, similar to CK20-negative MCC,[32] of UV-related squamous epithelial tumors.[4,16,17] Such tumors show less CK20 and NF positivity and more p53 and follicular stem cell markers[16–18] and are always negative for MCV. Well-differentiated SCC is easily diagnosed.

## DIAGNOSIS

As many as half of all MCCs are unsuspected at the time of biopsy; therefore, the most important aspects of diagnosis are an open mind to pattern recognition, knowledge of MCC as a diagnostic possibility in solitary cutaneous growths, and attention to the clinical description of a nodular lesion in the context of superficial biopsies. Although the most common diagnostic pitfall is probably misdiagnosis of MCC as BCC, a significant runner-up is the failure to diagnose MCC in a too-superficial biopsy. As with all superficial biopsies, if the histopathologic findings do not match the clinical suspicion, deeper levels and a recommendation to the clinician to perform a deeper or excisional biopsy are strongly encouraged.

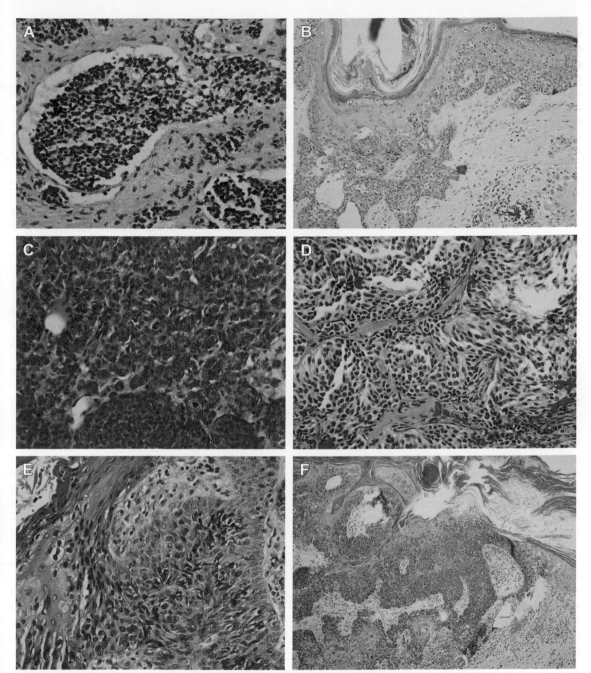

*Fig. 3.* Differential diagnostic considerations of MCC. (*A*) Islands of small round blue cells with mucinous tumor-stroma retraction in MCC mimicking BCC [Hematoxylin-eosin, original magnification ×400]. (*B*) Extensive intraepidermal and pagetoid spread in MCC mimicking melanoma in situ [Hematoxylin-eosin, original magnification ×200]. (*C*) Pleomorphism (architecturally and cytologically) characteristic of a metastatic NEC, in a tumor derived from the lung [Hematoxylin-eosin, original magnification ×400]. (*D*) WDNET/carcinoid metastatic to the skin shows organized, organoid architecture and lacks high grade nuclear features [Hematoxylin-eosin, original magnification ×400]. (*E*) In situ component of MCC; some intraepidermal tumor cells appear to have bubbly cytoplasm and an intrafollicular localization reminiscent of sebaceous carcinoma [Hematoxylin-eosin, original magnification ×400]. (*F*) Combined MCC/SCC; immunohistochemistry would be needed to distinguish from poorly differentiated SCC [Hematoxylin-eosin, original magnification ×100].

Cytomorphologic neuroendocrine features, when recognized in a skin tumor, require evaluation by CK20 for any type of staining (membranous, cytoplasmic, or Golgi, although dot-like perinuclear pattern is common) as well as limited markers of extracutaneous NEC, including TTF-1 and CDX-2.[21] CK20 labeling may require higher-power microscopic assessment to identify occasional sparse and/or faint dot-like staining. Along with CK20, assessment of at least 1 marker of neuroendocrine differentiation (eg, synaptophysin) can be helpful to confirm the neuroendocrine nature of the tumor and to prevent missed diagnoses in the occasional CK20-negative MCC. In such a case, positive evidence of neuroendocrine granules should prompt evaluation of another low-molecular-weight cytokeratin, in particular, Cam5.2, which labels many of the CK20-negative MCCs. Immunohistochemistry for MCV is specific but not sensitive and is not available in all laboratories. If a truly undifferentiated small round blue cell tumor is encountered in a routine biopsy sample, it may be reasonable to request a limited immunohistochemical panel to rule out melanoma and lymphoma (S100 or SOX10 and CD43). If there is distinct dermoepidermal junction nesting, then a second melanocytic differentiation marker, such as Melan-A, may be assessed (**Fig. 4**).

Pathologic reporting should include, at a minimum, tumor size, peripheral and deep margin status, lymphovascular invasion, and the presence/absence of bone/muscle/fascia or cartilage involvement.[33] The authors encourage the reporting of second tumor phenotypes, for example, SCC or BCC. Additional reporting considerations include thickness, mitotic rate, growth pattern,[9] tumor infiltrating lymphocytes,[34] and MCV immunohistochemistry.

Sentinel lymph node evaluation is commonly requested. For tumors that do not show diffuse involvement or large clusters of metastatic tumor, immunohistochemistry may be needed to identify scattered intranodal tumor cells. Most commonly, if the nodal tumor volume is low, cells present in a peripheral intraparenchymal pattern of single cells, most easily found with CK20 (and/or Cam5.2 as appropriate).[35] The American Joint Committee on Cancer recommendation for lymph node reporting includes tumor burden, size, and the presence/absence of extracapsular invasion.[5]

## PROGNOSIS

DSS in MCC is difficult to measure, given the overwhelming occurrence of this disease in an older population.[36] Between 50% and 76% of MCCs present as localized skin disease.[2,36,37] Most people with a diagnosis of local, cutaneous-only disease have the same life expectancy as those without

the disease,[38] keeping in mind that MCC presents predominantly in the seventh to eighth decades. Recurrences of all MCCs are common and only partly related to the adequacy of excision, with recurrence occurring even in patients with greater than 2.5-cm surgical margins.[39–41] Nodal metastases to local regional lymph nodes occur early, and patients may have disease progression to distant sites, such as liver, bones, lung, brain, and distant lymph nodes. When the disease involves noncutaneous sites, more than half of MCC patients seem to succumb.[38] MCC survival analyses that control for the impact of deaths due to other causes are drawn from small groups but confirm a significant impact of the disease at all stages, with a reported 5-year relative percent survival of 69 in stage I disease and 64 in all local disease, 39 in regional nodal disease, and 18 in patients with distant metastases, indicating a broad and highly stage-dependent prognostic range for a diagnosis with this cancer.[36] Recent analyses failed to control for the effect of death due to other causes in this population[33] but have higher statistical power due to greater numbers of patients in tumor registries. In these studies, pathologically node-negative skin-limited disease (without involvement of deep structures) is associated with a 5-year overall survival rate of 54% to 63.8%, whereas involvement of deep cutaneous structures (fascia, muscle, cartilage, or bone) and/or lymph node positivity by either clinical or sentinel lymph node evaluation correlates with decreased overall survival rates of 26% to 40.3%.[33] Primary tumor size cutoff of 2 cm is still considered a significant break point in prognosis.[37] Microscopic lymph node analysis allows for a more clear-cut prognostic stratification of 5-year overall survival rates in stage I (<2 cm) and stage II or above,[5] Nodal tumors of unknown primary skin site seem to have a better prognosis and are considered separately.[5]

Additional features that may affect prognosis of patients with MCC include other disease states that associate with MCC, including immunodeficiencies, such as chronic lymphocytic leukemia/lymphoma, HIV, and post-transplant–related immunosuppression. In future algorithms, the impact of immunosuppression, polyomavirus positivity, and molecular/morphologic-based stratification may be useful.

Regarding pathologically prognostic features, on multivariate as well as univariate analysis, the presence of lymphovascular invasion has been repeatedly shown to risk-stratify patients.[42,43] Univariate analysis of pathologic features, such as tumor size,[44] cell size,[11,44] inflammatory reaction,[45] number of mitoses/high-power field,[44] and p63,[11,46] and a few other features have occasionally suggested slight associations with outcomes but require additional validation.

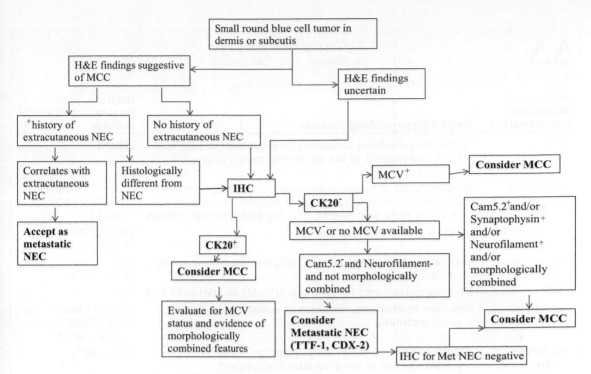

**Fig. 4.** Diagnostic algorithm for MCC. H&E, hematoxylin-eosin stain.

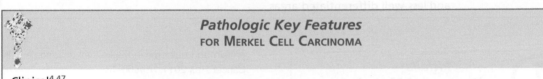

*Pathologic Key Features*
FOR MERKEL CELL CARCINOMA

Clinical[4,47]

- Nonspecific dome-shaped firm nodule or tumor
- Flesh-colored to erythematous to violaceous
- +/− overlying scale and telangiectasia (more in UV areas)

Dermoscopic[4,48,49]

- Polymorphic vascular pattern
- Milky-white structureless areas

Histologic[9,50]

- Small round blue cell tumor in dermis/subcutis ± epidermal/adnexal involvement
- +/− overlying/intermingled atypical epidermis or intratumoral squamous islands/eddies
- Circumscribed or infiltrative borders
- Sometimes extensive surrounding lymphovascular tumor emboli
- Sometimes islands of tumor necrosis
- Numerous mitotic figures
- Cell types include
  - Small: hyperchromatic nuclei, fragile chromatin, molding, crush artifact
  - Medium: cleared out nuclei, salt-and-pepper chromatin, defined nuclear borders, inconspicuous cytoplasm
  - Large: large size, pleomorphic, irregular chromatin, abundant cytoplasm, +/− nucleoli

## Differential Diagnosis
### OF MERKEL CELL CARCINOMA

| Differential Diagnostic Consideration | Helpful Distinguishing Features | Helpful Immunohistochemical Findings |
|---|---|---|
| BCC | Abundant peripheral palisading, low cuboidal to columnar cells, budding off of the epidermis, mucin, single-cell necrosis | BEREP4$^+$ MCV$^-$ |
| Melanoma | Predominance of irregular intraepidermal nests, cytologic pleomorphism, irregular nuclear borders, prominent nucleoli, melanin pigment, +/− regressive dermal changes | MelanA$^+$, HMB-45$^+$, MART-1$^+$, SOX10$^+$, NKI-C3$^+$ |
| Metastatic NEC | Large, pleomorphic cytology | TTF-1$^+$, CDX-2$^+$ CK20$^-$, MCV$^-$ |
| Metastatic WDNET | Lobulated islands/trabeculae of cells, pooling of hemorrhage, uniform cytology | TTF-1$^+$, CDX-2$^+$ CK20$^-$, MCV$^-$ |
| EWS | EWS rearrangements for example, t(11;22), by FISH or RT-PCR | MCV$^-$ |
| Lymphoma | Vesicular, cerebriform, reniform or wreath-shaped nuclei, scant cytoplasm | CD3$^+$ or CD20$^+$ CD43$^-$, CD45$^-$, CK20$^-$, MCV$^-$ |
| Sebaceous carcinoma | Crenulated nuclei, vacuolated cytoplasm, often extensive intraepidermal or intra-adnexal involvement | CK20$^-$, MCV$^-$ |
| SCC | Preponderance of squamous differentiation, in situ SCC component, clear transition between well differentiated and less well differentiated areas | CK20$^-$, MCV$^-$ |

## Pitfalls
### IN DIAGNOSIS OF MERKEL CELL CARCINOMA

! Mucin, stromal-tumor clefts, and focal palisading may lead to an erroneous diagnosis of BCC. Remember that Ber-EP4 can be positive in MCC as well as BCC.

! Superficial biopsies showing SCC with basaloid cells at the base — consider CK20!

! CK20 negativity does not exclude MCC; Cam5.2 and/or synaptophysin should allow correct diagnosis.

! Large nucleoli do not exclude MCC, although extracutaneous NEC should be considered.

## REFERENCES

1. Bichakjian CK, Lowe L, Lao CD, et al. Merkel cell carcinoma: critical review with guidelines for multidisciplinary management. Cancer 2007;110:1–12.
2. Agelli M, Clegg LX. Epidemiology of primary Merkel cell carcinoma in the United States. J Am Acad Dermatol 2003;49:832–41.
3. Sihto H, Kukko H, Koljonen V, et al. Merkel cell polyomavirus infection, large T antigen, retinoblastoma protein and outcome in Merkel cell carcinoma. Clin Cancer Res 2011;17:4806–13.
4. Suarez AL, Louis P, Kitts J, et al. Clinical and dermoscopic features of combined cutaneous squamous cell carcinoma (SCC)/neuroendocrine [Merkel cell] carcinoma (MCC). J Am Acad Dermatol 2015;73:968–75.
5. Bichakjian CK, Hghiem P, Johnson T, et al. Merkel cell carcinoma. New York: Springer; 2016.
6. Walsh NM. Primary neuroendocrine (Merkel cell) carcinoma of the skin: morphologic diversity and implications thereof. Hum Pathol 2001;32:680–9.
7. LeBoit PE, Crutcher WA, Shapiro PE. Pagetoid intraepidermal spread in Merkel cell (primary neuroendocrine) carcinoma of the skin. Am J Surg Pathol 1992;16:584–92.
8. Rocamora A, Badía N, Vives R, et al. Epidermotropic primary neuroendocrine (Merkel cell) carcinoma of the skin with Pautrier-like microabscesses. Report of three cases and review of the literature. J Am Acad Dermatol 1987;16:1163–8.
9. Andea AA, Coit DG, Amin B, et al. Merkel cell carcinoma: histologic features and prognosis. Cancer 2008;113:2549–58.
10. Kuwamoto S, Higaki H, Kanai K, et al. Association of Merkel cell polyomavirus infection with morphologic differences in Merkel cell carcinoma. Hum Pathol 2011;42:632–40.

11. Asioli S, Righi A, Volante M, et al. p63 expression as a new prognostic marker in Merkel cell carcinoma. Cancer 2007;110:640–7.

12. Fleming KE, Ly TY, Pasternak S, et al. Support for p63 expression as an adverse prognostic marker in Merkel cell carcinoma: report on a Canadian cohort. Hum Pathol 2014;45:952–60.

13. Hall BJ, Pincus LB, Yu SS, et al. Immunohistochemical prognostication of Merkel cell carcinoma: p63 expression but not polyomavirus status correlates with outcome. J Cutan Pathol 2012;39:911–7.

14. Sidiropoulos M, Hanna W, Raphael SJ, et al. Expression of TdT in Merkel cell carcinoma and small cell lung carcinoma. Am J Clin Pathol 2011;135:831–8.

15. Ball NJ, Tanhuanco-Kho G. Merkel cell carcinoma frequently shows histologic features of basal cell carcinoma: a study of 30 cases. J Cutan Pathol 2007;34:612–9.

16. Pulitzer MP, Brannon AR, Berger MF, et al. Cutaneous squamous and neuroendocrine carcinoma: genetically and immunohistochemically different from Merkel cell carcinoma. Mod Pathol 2015;28: 1023–32.

17. Narisawa Y, Koba S, Inoue T, et al. Histogenesis of pure and combined Merkel cell carcinomas: an immunohistochemical study of 14 cases. J Dermatol 2015; 42:445–52.

18. Lai JH, Fleming KE, Ly TY, et al. Pure versus combined Merkel cell carcinomas: immunohistochemical evaluation of cellular proteins (p53, Bcl-2, and c-kit) reveals significant overexpression of p53 in combined tumors. Hum Pathol 2015;46:1290–6.

19. Ferringer T. Immunohistochemistry in dermatopathology. Arch Pathol Lab Med 2015;139:83–105.

20. Visscher D, Cooper PH, Zarbo RJ, et al. Cutaneous neuroendocrine (Merkel cell) carcinoma: an immunophenotypic, clinicopathologic, and flow cytometric study. Mod Pathol 1989;2:331–8.

21. Yang DT, Holden JA, Florell SR. CD117, CK20, TTF-1, and DNA topoisomerase II-alpha antigen expression in small cell tumors. J Cutan Pathol 2004;31:254–61.

22. Gillham SL, Morrison RG, Hurt MA. Epidermotropic neuroendocrine carcinoma. Immunohistochemical differentiation from simulators, including malignant melanoma. J Cutan Pathol 1991;18:120–7.

23. Kontochristopoulos GJ, Stavropoulos PG, Krasagakis K, et al. Differentiation between merkel cell carcinoma and malignant melanoma: an immunohistochemical study. Dermatology 2000;201:123–6.

24. Bobos M, Hytiroglou P, Kostopoulos I, et al. Immunohistochemical distinction between merkel cell carcinoma and small cell carcinoma of the lung. Am J Dermatopathol 2006;28:99–104.

25. Ralston J, Chiriboga L, Nonaka D. MASH1: a useful marker in differentiating pulmonary small cell carcinoma from Merkel cell carcinoma. Mod Pathol 2008;21:1357–62.

26. Koba S, Inoue T, Okawa T, et al. Merkel cell carcinoma with cytokeratin 20-negative and thyroid transcription factor-1-positive immunostaining admixed with squamous cell carcinoma. J Dermatol Sci 2011;64:77–9.

27. Buresh CJ, Oliai BR, Miller RT. Reactivity with TdT in Merkel cell carcinoma: a potential diagnostic pitfall. Am J Clin Pathol 2008;129:894–8.

28. Erickson LA, Papouchado B, Dimashkieh H, et al. Cdx2 as a marker for neuroendocrine tumors of unknown primary sites. Endocr Pathol 2004;15:247–52.

29. Busam KJ, Jungbluth AA, Rekthman N, et al. Merkel cell polyomavirus expression in merkel cell carcinomas and its absence in combined tumors and pulmonary neuroendocrine carcinomas. Am J Surg Pathol 2009;33:1378–85.

30. Pulitzer M, Jungbluth A, Scolyer R, et al. Primary Cutaneous Ewing Sarcoma/Primitive Neuroectodermal Tumor are immunohistochemically negative for Merkel Cell Polyomavirus. in European Congress of Pathology. Florence (Italy); 2009.

31. Goto K, Anan T, Fukumoto T, et al. Carcinoid-Like/Labyrinthine Pattern in Sebaceous Neoplasms Represents a Sebaceous Mantle Phenotype: immunohistochemical Analysis of Aberrant Vimentin Expression and Cytokeratin 20-Positive Merkel Cell Distribution. Am J Dermatopathol 2016, [Epub ahead of print].

32. Wong SQ, Waldeck K, Vergara IA, et al. UV-Associated Mutations Underlie the Etiology of MCV-Negative Merkel Cell Carcinomas. Cancer Res 2015;75:5228–34.

33. Harms KL, Healy MA, Nghiem P, et al. Analysis of Prognostic Factors from 9387 Merkel Cell Carcinoma Cases Forms the Basis for the New 8th Edition AJCC Staging System. Ann Surg Oncol 2016;23:3564–71.

34. Miller NJ, Church CD, Dong L, et al. Tumor-Infiltrating Merkel Cell Polyomavirus-Specific T Cells Are Diverse and Associated with Improved Patient Survival. Cancer Immunol Res 2017;5:137–47.

35. Ko JS, Prieto VG, Elson PJ, et al. Histological pattern of Merkel cell carcinoma sentinel lymph node metastasis improves stratification of Stage III patients. Mod Pathol 2016;29:122–30.

36. Lemos BD, Storer BE, Iyer JG, et al. Pathologic nodal evaluation improves prognostic accuracy in Merkel cell carcinoma: analysis of 5823 cases as the basis of the first consensus staging system. J Am Acad Dermatol 2010;63:751–61.

37. Allen PJ, Busam K, Hill AD, et al. Immunohistochemical analysis of sentinel lymph nodes from patients with Merkel cell carcinoma. Cancer 2001;92:1650–5.

38. Lemos B, Nghiem P. Merkel cell carcinoma: more deaths but still no pathway to blame. J Invest Dermatol 2007;127:2100–3.

39. Meeuwissen JA, Bourne RG, Kearsley JH. The importance of postoperative radiation therapy in the treatment of Merkel cell carcinoma. Int J Radiat Oncol Biol Phys 1995;31:325–31.

40. O'Connor WJ, Roenigk RK, Brodland DG. Merkel cell carcinoma. Comparison of Mohs micrographic surgery and wide excision in eighty-six patients. Dermatol Surg 1997;23:929–33.

41. Boyer JD, Zitelli JA, Brodland DG, et al. Local control of primary Merkel cell carcinoma: review of 45 cases treated with Mohs micrographic surgery with and without adjuvant radiation. J Am Acad Dermatol 2002;47:885–92.

42. Fields RC, Busam KJ, Chou JF, et al. Five hundred patients with Merkel cell carcinoma evaluated at a single institution. Ann Surg 2011;254:465–73, [discussion: 473–65].

43. Fields RC, Busam KJ, Chou JF, et al. Recurrence and survival in patients undergoing sentinel lymph node biopsy for merkel cell carcinoma: analysis of 153 patients from a single institution. Ann Surg Oncol 2011;18:2529–37.

44. Skelton HG, Smith KJ, Hitchcock CL, et al. Merkel cell carcinoma: analysis of clinical, histologic, and immunohistologic features of 132 cases with relation to survival. J Am Acad Dermatol 1997;37:734–9.

45. Llombart B, Monteagudo C, López-Guerrero JA, et al. Clinicopathological and immunohistochemical analysis of 20 cases of Merkel cell carcinoma in search of prognostic markers. Histopathology 2005;46:622–34.

46. Asioli S, Righi A, de Biase D, et al. Expression of p63 is the sole independent marker of aggressiveness in localised (stage I-II) Merkel cell carcinomas. Mod Pathol 2011;24:1451–61.

47. Heath M, Jaimes N, Lemos B, et al. Clinical characteristics of Merkel cell carcinoma at diagnosis in 195 patients: the AEIOU features. J Am Acad Dermatol 2008;58:375–81.

48. Dalle S, Parmentier L, Moscarella E, et al. Dermoscopy of Merkel cell carcinoma. Dermatology 2012;224:140–4.

49. Harting MS, Ludgate MW, Fullen DR, et al. Dermatoscopic vascular patterns in cutaneous Merkel cell carcinoma. J Am Acad Dermatol 2012;66:923–7.

50. Toker C. Trabecular carcinoma of the skin. Arch Dermatol 1972;105:107–10.

# Cutaneous Lymphomas with Cytotoxic Phenotype

Adriana García-Herrera, MD, PhD[a], Eduardo Calonje, MD, DipRCPath[b],*

## KEYWORDS

- Primary cutaneous lymphoma • Cytotoxic phenotype • CD8$^+$ mycosis fungoides
- Primary acral CD8$^+$ lymphoma • Subcutaneous panniculitis-like T-cell lymphoma
- Primary cutaneous γ/δ T-cell lymphoma
- Primary cutaneous CD8$^+$ aggressive epidermotropic cytotoxic T-cell lymphoma

## Key Points

- The histologic diagnosis of PCCLs can be difficult and clinicopathologic correlation is of upmost importance to reach a correct diagnosis.

- The clinical and histologic overlap between lupus erythematosus panniculitis (LEP) and subcutaneous panniculitis-like T-cell lymphoma (SPTCL) also needs to be taken into consideration to avoid pitfalls in diagnosis.

- The presence of a γδ phenotype in cutaneous lymphoid proliferations should not be misconstrued as evidence of an aggressive cytotoxic cutaneous lymphoma.

- The work-up of all suspected cases of primary cytotoxic T cells/natural killer (NK) cells should include in situ hybridization for Epstein-Barr virus (EBV).

## ABSTRACT

Primary cutaneous cytotoxic lymphomas are T-cell or natural killer–cell lymphomas that express 1 or more cytotoxic markers. These neoplasms constitute a spectrum of diseases. In this review, an overview of clinical, morphologic, and phenotypical features of each subtype is provided. Differential diagnosis is discussed with attention to scenarios in which diagnostic difficulties are most frequently encountered.

## OVERVIEW

Primary cutaneous cytotoxic lymphomas (PCCLs) (Table 1) are T-cell or NK-cell lymphomas that present in the skin with no evidence of extracutaneous disease at the time of diagnosis and express 1 or more cytotoxic markers, such as T-cell intracellular antigen (TIA)-1, perforin, or granzyme B. Expression of TIA-1 is characteristic of cytotoxic cells regardless of their activation status, whereas expression of perforin and granzyme is highly increased in activated cytotoxic cells and correlates with the induction of cytolytic activity. Although most PCCLs are CD8$^+$, such as SPTCL, some are double negative (CD4$^{-/-}$CD8$^-$), such as primary cutaneous γ/δ T-cell lymphoma (PCGDTCL) and less often CD4$^+$, such as lymphomatoid papulosis (LyP) types A and B or primary cutaneous anaplastic large cell lymphoma.[1,2] EBV$^+$ NK/T-cell lymphoproliferative disorders (LPDs) can also involve the skin primarily and include hydroa vacciniforme-like LPD (HVLLPD) and extranodal NK/TCL (ENKTL), nasal type. In addition, a small subset of mycosis fungoides (MF) can also express cytotoxic markers, but the cases are not segregated on the basis of this phenotype, because this feature does not influence behavior. PCCLs constitute a heterogeneous group of diseases and close clinicopathologic correlation is of utmost importance to classify these

Disclosure Statement: The authors have nothing to disclose.
$^a$ Department of Pathology, Hospital Clínic de Barcelona, Villarroel, 170, Escalera 3, Planta 5, Barcelona 08036, Spain; $^b$ Dermatopathology Laboratory, St John's Institute of Dermatology, St Thomas' Hospital, South Wing, Staircase C, Westminster Bridge Road, London SE1 7EH, UK
* Corresponding author.
*E-mail address:* jaime.calonje@kcl.ac.uk

Surgical Pathology 10 (2017) 409–427
http://dx.doi.org/10.1016/j.path.2017.01.003
1875-9181/17/© 2017 Elsevier Inc. All rights reserved.

**Table 1**
Primary cutaneous cytotoxic T-cell and natural killer–cell lymphomas recognized in the updated 2016 World Health Organization classification

| Entity | Clinical Presentation | Cell Origin | Phenotype | Epstein-Barr Virus Status |
|---|---|---|---|---|
| SPTCL | Solitary or multiple nodules or deeply seated plaques, which mainly involve extremities and trunk | $\alpha\beta$ T cells | CD3$^+$, CD8$^+$, betaF1$^+$, CD56$^+$, CD30$^+$, CD5$^{+/+}$, CD7$^{+/+}$, CD2$^{+/+}$, activated cytotoxic profile, Ki-67 hotspots | Negative |
| *Primary cutaneous CD8$^+$ AECTCL* | Localized or generalized papulonodules with ulceration or hyperkeratotic patches/plaques | $\alpha\beta$ T cells | CD3$^+$, CD8$^+$, betaF1$^+$, CD56$^-$, CD30$^-$, CD2$^{-/+}$, CD5$^{-/+}$, CD7$^{+/-}$, CD45RA$^+$, activated cytotoxic profile, high Ki-67 | Negative |
| PCGDTCL | Disseminated plaques and/or ulceronecrotic plaques or nodules | $\gamma\delta$ T cells | CD4$^-$/CD8$^-$ > CD4$^-$/CD8$^+$, CD3$^+$, TCR-$\delta^+$, CD2$^+$, CD56$^{+/-}$, betaF1$^-$, CD5$^{-/+}$, CD30$^-$ | Negative |
| *Primary cutaneous acral CD8$^+$ TCL* | Slowly enlarging papulonodular lesions arising on peripheral locations (ear, nose, acral sites) | $\alpha\beta$ T cells | CD3$^+$, CD8$^+$, CD4$^-$, CD7$^{-/+}$, CD2$^{+/-}$, CD5$^{+/-}$, betaF1$^+$, CD30$^-$, CD56$^-$, TIA-1$^+$, but granzyme B$^-$, low proliferation index | Negative |
| CD8$^+$ MF | More frequently in childhood MF and is more commonly associated with hypopigmented and poikilodermatous lesions | $\alpha\beta$ T cells | CD3$^+$, CD8$^+$, CD4-, CD7$^{-/+}$, CD5$^{+/-}$, CD2$^{+/-}$, CD30$^-$, rarely CD56$^+$, TIA-1$^+$ | Negative |
| CD30$^+$ primary cutaneous LPD with cytotoxic phenotype | LyP: recurrent, and self-healing papulonecrotic or papulonodular eruption PCAL solitary nodules or tumors | $\alpha\beta$ T cells > $\gamma\delta$ T cells | Uniform CD3$^+$, CD8$^+$, CD30$^+$ (primary cutaneous with concurrent CD8 expression: LyP D and uncommon LyP B, LyP C, and PCAL) *In addition, cases CD4$^+$ with expression of cytotoxic granules | Negative |
| HVLLPD | Papulovesicular eruptions with ulceration and scarring in sun-exposed areas | $\alpha\beta$ T cells > NK cells > $\gamma\delta$ T cells | CD4$^-$, CD8$^{+/-}$, betaF1$^+$ often CD30 expression or CD4$^-$/CD8$^-$, CD56$^+$, betaF1$^-$, TCR-$\gamma^-$ or CD4$^-$/CD8$^-$, TCR-$\gamma^+$ | Positive |
| ENKTL, nasal type | Nodular lesions, cellulitis or abscess-like swellings, erythematous to purpuric patches | NK cells > $\gamma\delta$ T cells > $\alpha\beta$ T cells | Cytoplasmic CD3$^+$, CD2$^+$, CD56$^+$, CD5$^-$, CD30$^{+/-}$, activated cytotoxic profile | Positive |

Italic text denotes entities regarded as provisional.

entities accurately. PCCLs are reviewed according to the most recent updated World Health Organization (WHO) lymphoma classification and criteria.[3,4] A clinical overview and the morphologic and phenotypical features of each subtype of primary cutaneous lymphomas with cytotoxic phenotype are presented. The differential diagnosis is discussed with particular attention to situations in which diagnostic difficulties are frequently encountered. CD30[+] primary cutaneous LPD and EBV[+] NK/T-cell LPD are covered in detail in other sections of this issue.

## KEY POINTS T-CELL AND NATURAL KILLER CELL SUBSETS

Historically, the classification of lymphomas has been based on the presumed normal counterpart. Thus, some of the subtypes of primary cutaneous cytotoxic T-cell lymphomas (TCLs) reflect the putative cell of origin, for example, naive CD8[+] $\alpha\beta$ T cell versus memory CD8[+] $\alpha\beta$ T cell.

1. T-cell sublineages are divided into 2 large classes—$\alpha\beta$ and $\gamma\delta$ T cells—which relate to the expression of an $\alpha\beta$ T-cell receptor (TCR) or a $\gamma\delta$ TCR and the intrathymic progression through the double-positive stage (CD4[+]/CD8[+] $\alpha\beta$) to single-positive (CD4[+] $\alpha\beta$ or CD8[+] $\alpha\beta$) or lack thereof (CD4[-]/CD8-$\gamma\delta$ lineage).[5]
2. Unlike T cells, most of the NK cells do not require the thymus for their development, do not use recombination activating gene enzymes for rearrangement of their TCR genes and, consequently, express no TCR. NK cells are usually CD4[-] and CD8[-] and they express NK-associated antigens (CD16, CD56, CD57, and killer cell immunoglobulin-like receptor [KIR]), which are, not entirely specific.[6]
3. Functionally, the majority of $\alpha\beta$ T cells recognizing an antigen in a major histocompatibility complex–restricted fashion in the presence of an antigen-presenting cell are part of the adaptative immune system that is characterized by specificity and memory of the immunologic response. On the other hand, NK cells, a subset of the $\gamma\delta$ T cells and a minor subset of $\alpha\beta$ T cells, are part of the innate immunity that provides immune surveillance and may lead to a rapid proinflammatory response.
4. In T cells, CD45 can be expressed as one of several isoforms by alternative splicing. The largest isoform CD45RA is expressed on naive T cells. Activated and memory T lymphocytes express the shortest CD45 isoform, CD45RO.[7]

## SUBCUTANEOUS PANNICULITIS-LIKE T-CELL LYMPHOMA

### OVERVIEW

SPTCL is a rare subset of cutaneous lymphoma with an indolent course and long survival, characterized by subcutaneous infiltration of neoplastic CD8[+] CD56[-], and betaF1[+] cytotoxic T cells. In the WHO–European Organisation for Research and Treatment of Cancer (EORTC) classification of cutaneous lymphomas in 2005,[8] the term SPTCL was restricted to cases with an $\alpha\beta$ T-cell phenotype. Prior to this definition, the term SPTCL was used to include all TCLs with a panniculitic-like pattern, thus making review of the literature confusing due to the heterogeneous entities included with variable clinical outcomes.[9] SPTCL is most common in young adults (median age, 36 years old),[10] although it can occur in a wide age range, including pediatric patients.[11–14] There is a female predominance, with a male-to-female ratio of 0.5.[10]

### CLINICAL FEATURES

Patients usually present with multiple subcutaneous nodules and/or indurated, erythematous, or bruiselike plaques that are primarily seen on the limbs and trunk (Fig. 1A). Rarely, cases of solitary lesions may occur. Lesions are rarely ulcerated and may show a waxing and waning course. The most common systemic symptom is fever, occasionally accompanied by chills, malaise, and weight loss. These B symptoms are present in approximately 60% of the patients. Laboratory abnormalities, mainly anemia, leukopenia, thrombocytopenia or combined cytopenias, and elevated liver function tests, are common.[10,11,15] Approximately 20% of patients with SPTCL have been reported to have autoimmune disorders, such as lupus erythematosus, Sjögren disease, rheumatoid arthritis, and dermatomyositis.[10,11,16–18]

### MICROSCOPIC FEATURES

SPTCL displays a lobular panniculitis-like infiltrate (see Fig. 1B), with no evidence of dermal or epidermal involvement.[10,11,15] Although dermal perivascular or periadnexal lymphocytic infiltrate can be observed, these lymphocytes are not cytologically atypical and do not have an abnormal immunophenotype. Rimming of individual adipocytes by neoplastic T cells (see Fig. 1C) is a common feature although it is nonspecific, because this feature may also be seen in other primary and secondary cutaneous lymphomas as well as

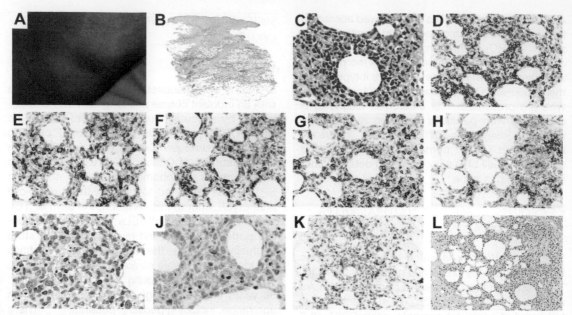

**Fig. 1.** Subcutaneous panniculitis-like TCL. Erythematous nodule on a lower limb (*A*). Lobular panniculitis-like dense infiltrate (*B*), with atypical lymphoid cells displaying rimming of adipocytes (*C*). Neoplastic cells express CD3 (*D*), with partial loss of expression of CD5 (*E*) and CD7 (*F*). They are positive for CD8 (*G*) and negative for CD4 (*H*). BetaF1 is also positive (*I*), whereas δ chain (*J*), CD56 (*K*), and EBER (*L*) are negative (H&E, original magnification, [*A*] ×20; [*B*] ×400; [*C*] ×200; [*D*] ×200; [*E*] ×200; [*F*] ×200; [*G*] ×200; [*H*] ×400; [*I*] ×400; [*J*] ×200; [*K*] ×100; [*L*] ×100).

in various lobular panniculitis.[19] Fat necrosis with a focal granulomatous reaction is present in some cases. Angioinvasion or angiodestruction is uncommon. The neoplastic infiltrate is composed of small to medium-sized lymphocytes with irregular nuclear contours. Nucleoli may be observed in some cells. Mitotic figures are easily identified. Karyorrhexis with macrophages engulfing cellular debris is present at least partially within the panniculitic infiltrates in a majority of SPTCL biopsies and often in association with patchy foci of fibrinoid or coagulative necrosis. Variable numbers of inflammatory cells, including small lymphocytes, histiocytes, plasma cells, neutrophils, or eosinophils, are also identified.

The neoplastic cells express CD3[+], CD8[+], and cytotoxic proteins (granzyme B, TIA-1, perforin), with variable loss of pan T-cell antigens. The order of frequency of loss of pan T-cell antigens is CD5 (50%) followed by CD7 (44%) and CD2 (10%). BetaF1 is positive, confirming the αβ T-cell phenotype and CD30, CD56, and EBV-encoded small RNA (EBER) are negative (see **Fig. 1**).

## PROGNOSIS

The clinical course of SPTCL depends on the presence or absence of a hemophagocytic syndrome (HPS).[10] The development of HPS in SPTCL is associated with a dramatic decrease in 5-year overall survival, from 91% in patients without HPS to 46% in patients with HPS. The reported rate of HPS in SPTCL has ranged from 6% to 50%. HPS affects children more frequently than adults (incidence of 54%)[13,14] and the extent of cutaneous lesions or systemic symptoms does not seem to influence its development.[10]

## DIFFERENTIAL DIAGNOSIS

Morphologically, SPTCL can mimic PCGDTCL. Although both entities may have a panniculitis-like picture, PCGDTCL shows involvement of the epidermis and dermis in several cases and is more commonly associated with ulceration (see **Fig. 3**A). Immunophenotypic differences include positive CD56 and often lack of expression of both CD4 and CD8 in PCGDTCL.[10] Immunohistochemical stains for TCR-betaF1, TCR-γ, and/or TCR-δ may also be valuable if available, because SPTCL has an αβ phenotype.

The main histologic differential diagnosis is with LEP,[17,20–23] an autoimmune disorder characterized by a predominantly lobular panniculitis. An additional complicating factor is that SPTCL has been associated with several autoimmune disorders, including lupus erythematosus. Recently, cases of overlapping histologic features on the same biopsy have been described, suggesting that SPTCL and LEP may represent 2 ends of a spectrum.[22–24] Histologic criteria that may be helpful in differentiating LEP from SPTCL include the following: (1) scattered to absent plasma cells favoring the diagnosis of SPTCL,[23] (2) CD123-positive plasmocytoid dendritic cell clusters that are more common in LEP than in SPTCL,[21] and (3) foci of Ki-67 hotspots prominent in cytotoxic atypical CD8[+] T cells a feature of SPTCL.[23] Other morphologic features, such as hyaline fat necrosis with lipomembranes, dermal mucin deposition, and interface vacuolar change, although more common in LEP, have also been observed in SPTCL and thus do not offer any help in the differential diagnosis.[17,20,22,23]

Molecular studies to demonstrate a monoclonal T-cell population by polymerase chain reaction are diagnostically helpful but not entirely specific. A monoclonal population of T lymphocytes has been detected in 44% to 100% of SPTCL,[10,11,23] whereas clonal expansions have been observed in 0% to 12% of cases of LEP,[20,25] thus limiting the discriminative value of the method. To improve diagnostic sensitivity when histologic findings are suspicious of focal involvement by lymphoma with a prominent inflammatory cell infiltrate in the background, some investigators recommend laser microdissection combined with either traditional polymerase chain reaction or high-throughput sequencing of the TCR gene.[23]

## PRIMARY CUTANEOUS CD8[+] AGGRESSIVE EPIDERMOTROPIC CYTOTOXIC T-CELL LYMPHOMAS

### OVERVIEW

Primary cutaneous CD8[+] aggressive epidermotropic cytotoxic TCL (AECTCL) is a rare, provisional entity characterized by a proliferation of epidermotropic CD8[+] cytotoxic T cells.[3,4] Since the first description by Berti and colleagues,[26] fewer than 100 cases of this lymphoma have been reported in the literature.[26–32] Probably some cases of CD8[+] AECTCL were categorized in the past as generalized pagetoid reticulosis (PR), Ketron-Goodman type. Patients present de novo with disseminated cutaneous lesions. Unlike classic MF, there is an absence of long-standing precursor lesions (patches or poikiloderma). The disease occurs mainly in adults, with a mean age of 54 years.[32] There is predilection for men, with a male:female ratio of approximately 2:1.

### CLINICAL FEATURES

The clinical presentation is characterized by a sudden eruption of localized or disseminated nodules and tumors, often with ulceration, hemorrhage, blistering, and necrosis, or less frequently with superficial hyperkeratotic patches and plaques (Fig. 2A).[26,30–32] Papulonodular and tumoral lesions sometimes show spontaneous central resolution. Involvement of mucosal surfaces, especially the oral mucosa, and acrally accentuated lesions on the palms and soles, are commonly seen. The disease is characterized by rapid progression with dissemination to visceral sites, including lung, testis, and central nervous system, and sparing of lymph nodes. There is usually no bone marrow involvement.

### MICROSCOPIC FEATURES

A histologic hallmark is the presence of striking epidermotropism (see Fig. 2C) of atypical lymphocytes.[26–32] Replacement of the epidermis and of the epithelium of neighboring adnexal structures in a pagetoid pattern most extensively involving the basal layer is characteristic in the absence of Pautrier microabscesses or tagging. Numerous apoptotic keratinocytes and spongiosis are common features. The epidermis may be acanthotic or atrophic, with ulceration and occasional blister formation. Extension of the infiltrate into the deeper dermis and subcutis and angiocentricity may be seen. Malignant cells are mostly medium-sized with enlarged hyperchromatic rounded nuclei, frequently with a coarse chromatin pattern.

Tumor cells are positive for CD3, CD8, betaF1, and cytotoxic granules with a high Ki-67 proliferation index. CD45RA[+] is often expressed, whereas CD30 and CD56 are typically negative (see Fig. 2). Focal or complete loss of expression of CD2 and/or CD5 is also common. There is no association with EBV.

### PROGNOSIS

The disease runs an aggressive course with a median survival of less than 32 months and a 5-year survival rate of 18%.[26,31,32]

### DIFFERENTIAL DIAGNOSIS

Distinction from other CD8[+] T-cell epidermotropic neoplasms may be challenging and correlation with clinical, histologic, and immunohistochemical features is crucial to reach a correct diagnosis. The main differential diagnoses include LyP type D[33–37] and PR.[38]

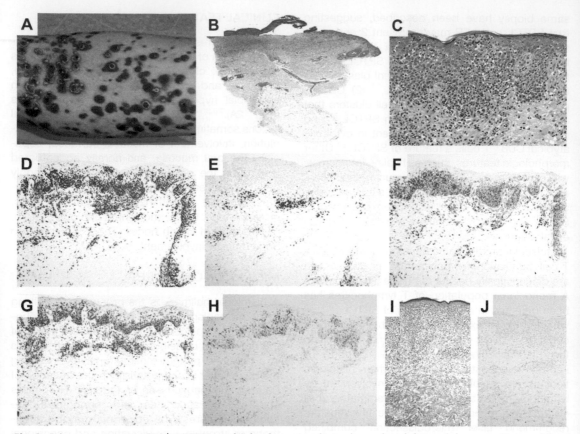

**Fig. 2.** Primary cutaneous CD8$^+$ AECTCL: multiple plaques and papules and nodules and desquamation and focal necrosis (*A*). Superficial ulceration with an underlying dense superficial and mid-dermal (*B*) and epidermotropic lymphocytic infiltrate (*C*). Neoplastic cells are diffusely positive for CD3 (*D*), with loss of expression of CD5 (*E*). Infiltrate shows adnexotropism and positivity for CD8 (*F*), betaF1 (*G*), and CD45RA (*H*). EBER (*I*) and CD56 (*J*) are negative (H&E, original magnification, [*B*] ×20; [*C*] ×100; [*D*] ×40; [*E*] ×40; [*F*] ×40; [*G*] ×40; [*H*] ×40; [*I*] ×40; [*J*] ×40).

The clinical presentation of LyP type D is typical of other types of LyP with a history of a cyclic eruption of erythematous papulonodular lesions followed by necrosis, spontaneous healing, and scar formation.[33–35] The most striking histopathologic finding observed in LyP type D is the presence of large numbers of medium-sized, pleomorphic lymphocytes, with a cytotoxic phenotype, infiltrating the epidermis with prominent pagetoid spread. This presentation is strikingly similar to that of AECTCL. In the latter, however, infiltrating cells are negative for CD30 and the infiltrate does not have a wedge-shaped distribution. LyP lesions may also be associated with pseudoepitheliomatous hyperplasia and are often associated with other reactive inflammatory cells in the background, including neutrophils and eosinophils, features not usually seen in AECTCL.[36] Additionally, CD8/CD30$^+$ LPD are frequently focally or diffusely positive for MUM-1.[37]

PR, regarded as a subtype of MF in both the WHO-EORTC[8] and WHO classifications,[4] displays prominent epidermotropism of atypical lymphoid cells and not uncommonly shows a CD8$^+$ phenotype. Histologic distinction from AECTCL may be, therefore, impossible. PR is restricted to an anatomic area, however, and has an invariable indolent clinical course.[32,38]

Pityriasis lichenoides et varioliformis (PLEVA) is another histologic differential diagnosis of AECTCL because lesions are characterized by numerous necrotic keratinocytes, prominent infiltration of the epidermis by lymphocytes, and frequent CD8 expression.[39] The clinical presentation with maculopapular scaly lesions that develop necrosis along with the lack of significant nuclear atypia in PLEVA, however, allows easy distinction between both entities.

A small percentage of cases of MF are CD8$^+$ (discussed later) and, in occasional biopsies from these patients, epidermotropism may be prominent. The clinical presentation, however, along with the absence of a mid to deep dermal infiltrate in early lesions of MF, makes distinction easy. Furthermore, whereas a naive phenotype (CD45 RA+) is characteristic of primary cutaneous CD8+ AECTCL, the CD8+ cells in MF are more often CD45 RO+.[40]

## PRIMARY CUTANEOUS γ/δ T-CELL LYMPHOMA

### OVERVIEW

In the latest WHO classification, PCGDTCL is considered a distinct entity composed of a clonal proliferation of mature, activated γ/δ T-cells with expression of CD3, CD2, and CD56 and negativity for betaF1, CD4, and usually CD8.[3,4] Historically, the diagnosis of PCGDTCL could only be established with certainty in tissue samples by flow cytometry or frozen sections by immunohistochemistry. The diagnosis based on formalin-fixed

paraffin-embedded (FFPE) material was basically a presumptive diagnosis, relying on the absence of the αβ TCR expression (using the betaF1 antibody) under appropriate circumstances. Recently, more specific antibodies that identify the γ or the δ chain of the γδ TCR heterodimer in FFPE tissue have been described.[41,42] Their use allows better recognition of lymphomas derived from γδ T cells. PCGDTCLs are heterogenous, exhibiting a wide spectrum of clinical and histologic features (discussed later).[10,43] PCGDTCL is considered a very aggressive neoplasm, although variation in clinical outcome has been described.[10,43–46]

### CLINICAL FEATURES

Most of the patients are middle-aged to elderly, with a median age at diagnosis of 61 years.[10,43,47] There is no gender predilection. Presentation is with multiple multifocal or generalized, nodules and large and deep indurated plaques often with a panniculitic appearance. Ulceration is common (**Fig. 3**A). Less frequently, localized or solitary

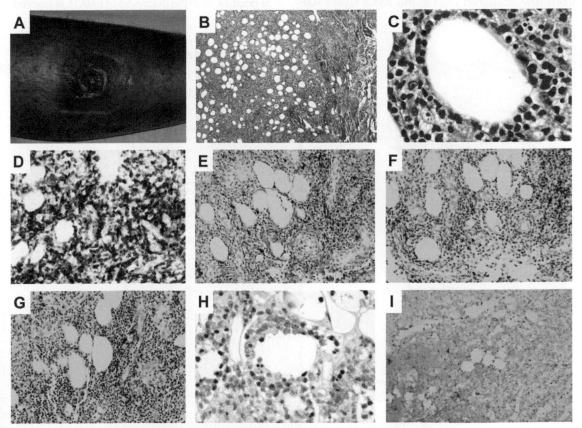

**Fig. 3.** PCGDTCL: ulcerative nodule on the lower extremity (A). On histology the subcutaneous adipose tissue is diffusely infiltrated (B) by atypical cells that surround adipocytes (C). Neoplastic cells show expression of CD3 (D), and they are double negative for CD4 (E) and CD8 (F). Beta F1 is negative (G), whereas δ chain (H) is expressed in neoplastic lymphocytes, giving support to the γδ T-cell derivation (I). In situ hybridization for EBV is negative (H&E, original magnification, [A] ×40; [B] ×600; [C] ×200; [D] ×200; [E] ×200; [F] ×200; [G] ×400; [H] ×100).

lesions have been described. Lesions may mimic conditions like cellulitis, hematoma, pyoderma, or an arthropod bite reaction. The most common site of involvement at presentation is the lower limbs, followed by the arms and trunk. Cutaneous lesions are associated with constitutional symptoms, including fever, weight loss, asthenia, or night sweats in approximately half of patients. The predominant laboratory findings are cytopenia(s), elevated lactate dehydrogenase levels, and deranged liver enzymes. Development of mucosal lesions, especially gastrointestinal tract, and dissemination to other extranodal sites are frequently observed, but involvement of the bone marrow, spleen, and lymph nodes is rare.

## MICROSCOPIC FEATURES

Histologically, 3 main patterns of infiltration can be recognized: epidermotropic, dermal, and subcutaneous.[10,20,43,47] All of these patterns can be present in the same patient and even within the same lesion (**Fig. 4**). Epidermal infiltration might range from few scattered cells in the basal layers (MF-like) to overt pagetoid spread or marked lichenoid infiltrate with extensive necrosis of keratinocytes and ulceration. Folliculotropism may be observed. Pautrier microabscesses are not often a feature. Infiltration of the subcutaneous tissue is usually associated with dermal or epidermal involvement and can show a distribution of the neoplastic cells around adipocytes with rimming, similar to that seen in SPTCL (see **Fig. 3**C). Infiltrates tend to be more monotonous and diffuse, however, and rimming is less pronounced. Neoplastic cells are usually medium-sized with coarsely clumped chromatin. Immunophenotypically, tumor cells exhibit a CD3$^+$, CD2$^+$, CD56$^+$ phenotype and are often CD4/CD8 double negative. Cytotoxic molecules (TIA-1, granzyme B, and perforin) are strongly expressed. In addition, the expression of CD7 may be found. As discussed previously, the defining criterion resides in the fact that the neoplastic cells in PCGDTCL express $\gamma\delta$ TCR (TCR-$\delta^+$ or TCR-$\gamma^+$) and lack $\alpha\beta$ TCR (betaF1) (see **Fig. 3**). As currently defined, the cells of PCGDTCL are EBV$^-$ and show clonal rearrangement of TCR genes. If EBV is positive, then the diagnosis of ENKTL is favored.[3]

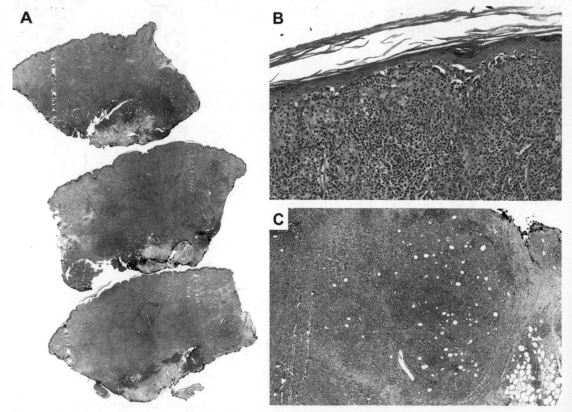

*Fig. 4.* PCGDTCL: low-power view showing dense lymphoid infiltrate with epidermal, dermal, and subcutaneous tissue involvement (*A*). The epidermotropic infiltrate is composed of small lymphocytes with conspicuous epidermotropism (*B*). Neoplastic lymphoid cells replace mainly lobular areas of the subcutaneous tissue (*C*) (H&E, original magnification, [*A*] ×20; [*B*] ×100; [*C*] ×40).

## PROGNOSIS

PCGDTCLs usually have an aggressive clinical course, with an approximately 10% 5-year overall survival.[10,48] Occasional cases have been reported, however, with indolent clinical courses, including pediatric cases.[12,44–46] Tumors with involvement restricted to superficial sites seem to have a more indolent clinical course, as do MF-like lesions with or without a panniculitis-like presentation. A characteristic feature is the presence of a long indolent evolution over years with progression into a more aggressive behavior in some cases.[49] Unlike other cutaneous lymphomas, the skin tumor burden does not seem to correlate with prognosis.[10]

## DIFFERENTIAL DIAGNOSIS

The desire to categorize lymphomas according to the precise cellular origin is attractive, but among the mature TCLs, promiscuity of phenotype is often seen. As discussed previously, some years ago it was recognized that SPTCL, with a $\gamma\delta$ phenotype compared with those expressing an $\alpha\beta$ subset, have discrepant clinical courses.[10,47,48] This led to the WHO-EORTC separating the 2 entities into SPTCL and PCGDTCL.[8] A $\gamma\delta$ phenotype, however, is not restricted to PCGDTCL, and variants of bona fide MF[50,51] or LyP[52] with an indolent clinical course and $\gamma\delta$ expression have been described. In addition, approximately 10% of HVLLPD have been reported to express the $\gamma\delta$ TCR.[53] The clinical course of the latter, however, is unlike that of PCGDTCL, and HVLLPD is consistently positive for EBER (**Fig. 5**).

Most of the PCGDTCLs are cytotoxic lymphomas with null phenotype (CD4−/CD8−), CD56+, and CD30−. An epidermotropic lymphoma with $\gamma\delta$ TCR expression and negativity for TIA-1 and granzyme B should suggest a diagnosis of MF whereas a history of recurrent and self-healing papules and nodules and positivity for CD30 are features of LyP.

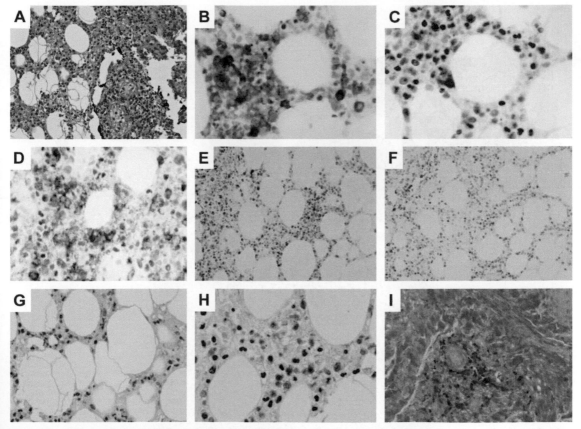

**Fig. 5.** The differential diagnosis between PCGDTCL and HVLLPD sometimes can be challenging. This case displays a diffuse atypical lymphocytic infiltrate that invades the subcutaneous fat (*A*). Atypical cells are $\gamma\delta$ T cells, with a cytotoxic activated phenotype: CD3+, CD5−, CD8+, granzyme B+, CD56−, betaF1−, $\delta$ chain+ ([*B–H*], respectively). In contrast to PCGDTCL, however, atypical cells of HVLLPD are EBER+ (*I*) (H&E, original magnification, [*A*] ×100; [*B*] ×600; [*C*] ×600; [*D*] ×400; [*E*] ×100; [*F*] ×100; [*G*] ×400; [*H*] ×600; [*I*] ×100).

Cutaneous ENKTL, nasal type, should be included in the differential diagnosis of PCGDTCL. These entities show significant phenotypic overlap; there are few described cases of cutaneous ENKTL cases derived from γδ T cells.[54–56] Even gene expression profiles may be similar in both entities.[57] An angiocentric and often angiodestructive infiltrate of atypical lymphoid cells (**Fig. 6**) and demonstration of EBV by in situ hybridization should point to a diagnosis of cutaneous ENKTL (**Fig. 7**).

## PRIMARY CUTANEOUS ACRAL CD8[+] T-CELL LYMPHOMA

### OVERVIEW

Primary cutaneous acral CD8[+] TCL has been included as a provisional entity in the recent 2016 revision of the WHO classification of lymphoid neoplasms.[3] It is defined as a clonal disorder composed of CD8[+] cells with an indolent clinical course and was described by Petrella

and colleagues in 2007.[58] Four patients with lesions restricted to the skin of the ear were described and the name, indolent CD8[+] lymphoid proliferation of the ear, was proposed. Since the original description, 47 additional cases have been reported,[59–67] and the realization that involvement is not restricted to the ear but may include other sites, including the nose, eyelids, and lower limbs, has led to the most recent proposed term to denote the entity.[60,64–67]

### CLINICAL FEATURES

Affected individuals are adults with a mean age of 56 years and there is a male predilection (male:female ratio of 1.7:1).[58,62,67] Clinically, primary cutaneous acral CD8[+] TCL usually presents as a slow-growing solitary papule on the ear. Lesions located on the nose, eyelid, and distal extremities, however, have been described as well as bilateral symmetric presentation. Multifocal cutaneous disease has only been reported in 4 cases to date and seems associated with a similarly benign

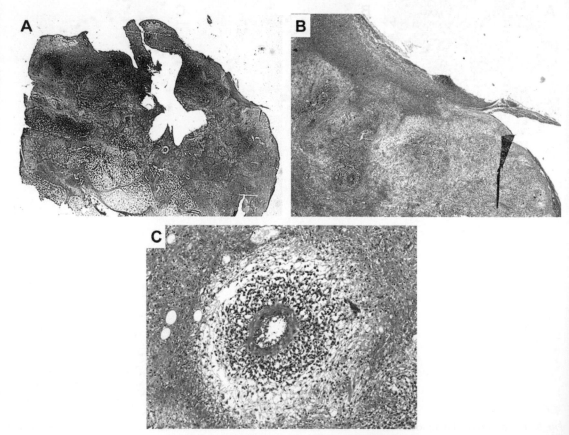

*Fig. 6.* Histopathologic features of cutaneous ENKTL: dense atypical lymphoid cell infiltration in the dermis with extension to the subcutis with a lobular panniculitis-like pattern (*A*). There is extensive epidermal ulceration (*B*) and prominent angiocentric tumoral infiltration with necrosis (*C*) (H&E, original magnification, [*A*] ×20; [*B*] ×40; [*C*] ×100).

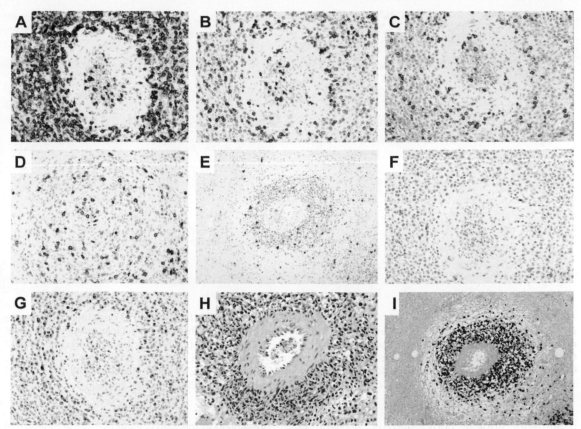

*Fig. 7.* Phenotypic features of cutaneous ENKTL: angiocentric tumoral population expressed CD2 (*A*), with loss of expression of CD3 and CD5 (*B*, *C*). Neoplastic cells are double negative CD4⁻/CD8⁻ (*D*, *E*) with no expression of CD56 (*F*). (*G*) Granzyme B is positive and (*H*) betaF1 is negative. There is a high concentration of (*I*) EBER⁺ cells around vessels (H&E, original magnification, [*A*] ×200; [*B*] ×200; [*C*] ×200; [*D*] ×100; [*E*] ×100; [*F*] ×200; [*G*] ×200; [*H*] ×200; [*I*] ×100).

clinical course. Systemic involvement is not seen. The duration of skin lesions before diagnosis ranges from 1 week to several years (median: 15.5 months).

## HISTOLOGIC FEATURES

Histology typically shows a nondestructive, dense, monomorphic, dermal lymphoid infiltrate composed of medium-sized atypical T cells (**Fig. 8**A, B).[58–67] Epidermotropism is not observed and a grenz zone is typically identified. Ulceration and necrosis have not been described. Atypical cells show a blastlike appearance with irregular nuclear margins, small nucleoli, and scant cytoplasm. Histiocytes and small B-cell lymphocytes are present and no other significant component of inflammatory cells (eosinophils, neutrophils, and plasma cells) is seen. Neoplastic cells are positive for CD8, betaF1, CD45RO, and TIA-1 but negative for granzyme B, CD30, CD56, and EBV. Perforin is expressed in half of the tested cases.

Loss of 2 of the pan T-cell antigens (CD3, CD5, CD2, or CD7) is seen in 50% of cases (see **Fig. 8**). Mitotic figures are rare, and the overall Ki-67 proliferation index is low. Molecular testing for TCR clonality is positive in approximately 90% of the tested cases.

A unique aspect of the primary cutaneous acral CD8⁺ TCL phenotype is the expression of CD68 with a dotlike cytoplasmic pattern. This recent observation was made in 5 cases of primary cutaneous acral CD8⁺ TCL with a full set of the CD68-recognizing antibodies (PG-M1, KP1, and KiM1P).[68,69] Other forms of CD8⁺ lymphoproliferative disease with cutaneous involvement were negative. This phenomenon, however, needs to be further tested and validated in independent series with a larger numbers of cases.

## PROGNOSIS

Evidence so far supports an indolent behavior with localized disease, good response to skin-directed

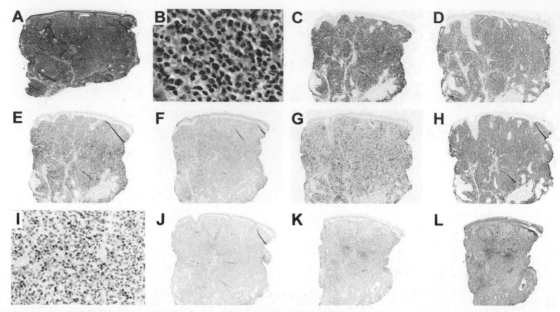

**Fig. 8.** Primary cutaneous acral CD8+ TCL. Diffuse pandermal lymphoid infiltrate. With a prominent grenz zone (*A*), the infiltrate is composed of medium-sized atypical lymphocytes with irregular nuclear margins and small nucleoli (*B*). Atypical cells are diffusely positive for CD3, CD2, and CD5 (*C–E*), with loss of expression of CD7 (*F*). CD4 is positive in histiocytes and small reactive lymphocytes (*G*). The neoplastic population is positive for CD8 and TIA-1 (*H, I*) and negative for CD30, CD56, and EBER (*J–L*) (H&E, original magnification, [*A*] ×20; [*B*] ×400; [*C*] ×20; [*D*] ×20; [*E*] ×20; [*F*] ×20; [*G*] ×20; [*H*] ×20; [*I*] ×200; [*J*] ×20; [*K*] ×20; [*L*] ×20).

treatments (topical corticosteroids, surgery, or radiotherapy), and even occasional spontaneous regression.[3,58,62,67] Approximately 20% of patients have cutaneous relapses, but systemic dissemination resulting in morbidity and mortality has not been reported.

## DIFFERENTIAL DIAGNOSIS

Distinguishing primary cutaneous acral CD8+ TCL from other cytotoxic CD8+ lymphomas with more aggressive behavior is an important and challenging task. Clinical information is crucial to reach a diagnosis. When detailed clinical data, such as location (ear, nose, and extremities), history of slow growth, and the presence of solitary/localized lesion(s) are provided and coupled with histologic and immunohistochemical features, including the presence of a monotonous, diffuse, nonepidermotropic diffuse dermal infiltrate of intermediate-to-large CD8+ nonactivated cytotoxic cells lymphoid cells with blastlike morphology, a diagnosis of primary cutaneous acral CD8+ TCL is not difficult.

The preferential dermal involvement, with absence of CD30 expression and negativity for CD56 and EBER, distinguishes these cases from SPTCL, CD30+ LPDs, and NK/T-cell LPD, respectively. Careful consideration of unusual CD8+ peripheral TCLs, not otherwise specified,

presenting in the skin is essential in the differential diagnosis.[69] Clinicopathologic correlation is, therefore, paramount.

## MYCOSIS FUNGOIDES WITH CD8 PHENOTYPE

### OVERVIEW

MF and its variants represent the most common type of cutaneous TCLs (approximately 50% of all primary cutaneous lymphomas). According to the WHO-EORTC classification of these neoplasm, the term MF should be used only for the classic Alibert-Bazin type, characterized by the evolution of patches, plaques, and tumors, or for variants showing a similar clinical course.[8] Usually, MF is derived from mature CD4+ memory T cells; however, as many as 20% of cases of early MF display a cytotoxic phenotype with CD8+ expression.[70,71] The cytotoxic phenotype is more commonly associated with unusual variants typified by pigmentary changes, namely, poikilodermatous, hyperpigmented, hypopigmented, and chronic purpuric MF, and occurs more frequently in children and young adults.[72–79] PR is a variant of MF characterized by the presence of localized lesions with an intraepidermal proliferation of neoplastic T cells, with common expression of CD8.[32,38,80] In addition, few cases of immunophenotypical shift between CD4 and CD8 have been reported and association with disease progression has been proposed.[81,82] Likewise, the expression of cytotoxic proteins by neoplastic CD4[+] T cells has been detected more often in tumors showing blastic transformation.[83]

## CLINICAL FEATURES

Clinically, MF mostly presents with slowly progressive erythematous patches and plaques, preferentially on sun-protected areas of the skin. Most of the CD8[+] MF cases in adults show a long history of poikilodermatous or hyperpigmented plaques. Hyperpigmented MF has a predilection for dark-complexioned individuals (Fitzpatrick skin type IV),[77] whereas pediatric patients present more commonly with hypopigmented lesions (73% of the pediatric cases).[75,76,78] Patients with the

hypopigmented variant of MF usually present with clinical findings in the first or second decade of life. Lesions are multiple, especially on the trunk, buttocks, and extremities (**Fig. 9**). By contrast, the typical presentation of PR (Woringer-Kolopp type) is as a solitary/localized psoriasiform or hyperkeratotic patch or plaque, which is usually localized on the extremities and is slowly progressive (see **Fig. 11**A).[32,38,80]

## HISTOLOGIC FEATURES

Morphologically, the neoplastic lymphoid infiltrate in MF is epidermotropic and composed predominantly of small to intermediate-sized atypical lymphocytes with hyperchromatic, cerebriform nuclei and clear cytoplasm (haloed cells) (**Fig. 10**A and B where A is).[70–79] These atypical lymphocytes often colonize the basal layer of epidermis singly

*Fig. 9.* Hypopigmented MF: a 9-year-old girl with history of long-standing hypopigmented scattered macules coalescing into patches over trunk and buttocks.

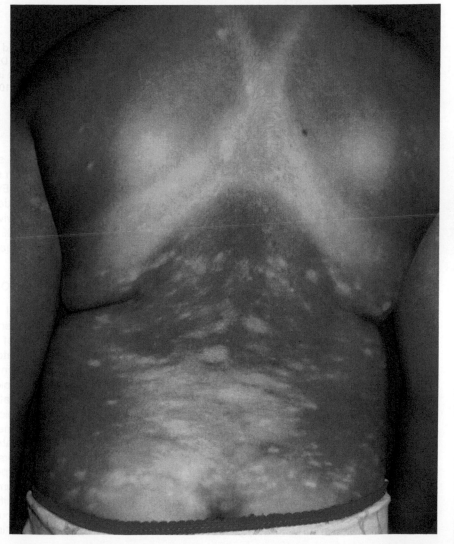

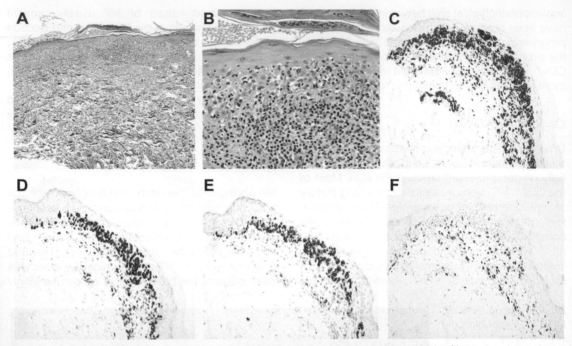

*Fig. 10.* MF with CD8 phenotype. Biopsy specimen demonstrates an atypical lymphoid infiltrate involving the superficial dermis (*A, B* where *A* is). Immunohistochemical studies highlight CD3 and CD5$^+$ T cells (*C, D*) expressing CD8, focally lining up at the basal epidermis and forming a string of pearls (*E*). There is significant loss of CD7 (*F*) (H&E, original magnification, [*A*] ×40; [*B*] ×200; [*C*] ×100; [*D*] ×100; [*E*] ×100; [*F*] ×100).

or in a linear fashion, forming a string of pearls (tagging) (see **Fig. 10**E). Pautrier microabscesses, which consist of small aggregates of atypical lymphocytes often in association with Langerhans cells, can be helpful in the diagnosis but are seen in less than 25% of cases.[71,75] In PR, epidermotropism is extensive. Neoplastic cells in cases of PR are larger than mature lymphoid cells with large nuclei with irregular borders, surrounded by a clear halo that replaces most of the cytoplasm. These cytomorphologic features prompted Braun-Falco and colleagues[38] to introduce the term, PR, to acknowledge the similarity of the epidermotropic atypical lymphoid cells to the intraepidermal adenocarcinoma cells found in Paget disease (**Fig. 11**B–I).[38]

Hyperpigmented and hypopigmented MF display changes of ordinary MF and are also characterized by interface changes along with epidermotropism of atypical melanocytes and papillary dermal melanophages.[77]

T-cell aberrancies, such as loss of CD7 in a significant percentage (eg, >50% at the least), of the epidermotropic lymphocytes and/or loss of CD5, CD2, or CD3 are an important adjunct in the diagnosis of CD8$^+$ MF as in other variants of the disease (see **Fig. 10**F). Some loss of CD7 expression, however, is often seen in inflammatory processes.[84]

## PROGNOSIS

From the prognostic standpoint, the clinical behavior of CD8$^+$ MF in early stages is similar to that of the CD4 type. Even hypopigmented MF and juvenile and poikilodermatous MF are associated with improved survival (disease-specific survival at 20 years is 98% and 73%, respectively) and reduced risk of disease progression.[70,75,84]

## DIFFERENTIAL DIAGNOSIS

The clinical differential diagnosis of hypopigmented and hyperpigmented MF is wide. The differential diagnosis of hyperpigmented MF includes postinflammatory hyperpigmentation, erythema dyschromicum perstans (ashy dermatosis), cutaneous amyloidosis, atrophoderma of Pasini-Pierini, and idiopathic eruptive macular hyperpigmentation.[77] Clinical entities that can be confused with hypopigmented MF include vitiligo, leprosy, postinflammatory hypopigmentation, pityriasis alba, tinea versicolor, sarcoidosis, and progressive macular hypomelanosis. In comparison with other hypopigmented disorders, hypopigmented MF is significantly associated with progressive disease course (increasing number of lesions); involvement of distal upper limbs and

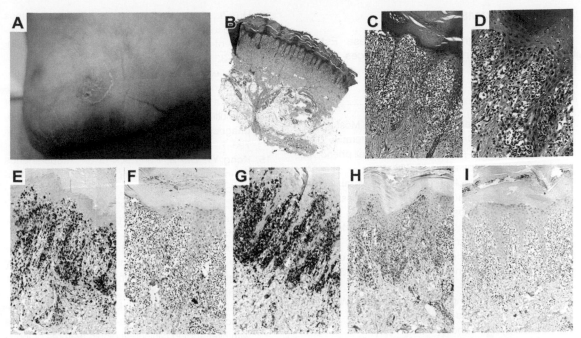

*Fig. 11.* PR: solitary hyperkeratotic plaque on the foot (*A*). There is epidermal hyperplasia with hyperkeratosis and parakeratosis (*B*). Prominent epidermotropism (*C*) of large atypical lymphoid cells with abundant clear cytoplasm (*D*). Neoplastic cells are positive for CD3 (*E*) with loss of expression of CD7 (*F*). Diffuse and intense positivity for CD8 (*G*) is observed, associated with weak staining for betaF1 (*H*) and negativity for CD45RA (*I*) (H&E, original magnification, [*B*] ×20; [*C*] ×100; [*D*] ×200; [*E*] ×200; [*F*] ×200; [*G*] ×200; [*H*] ×200; [*I*] ×200).

proximal lower limbs, including limb girdles; large-sized lesions (>5 cm); scaliness; erythema; atrophy; and mottled pigmentation.[79]

A recently described entity, initially named annular lichenoid dermatitis of youth, is an important clinical and histologic simulator of MF.[85] Because cases may occur rarely in adults, the condition is now known as annular lichenoid dermatosis. Clinically, annular lichenoid dermatosis presents with asymptomatic, solitary localized annular plaques/patches usually localized to the groin and the trunk. Histologic findings in the disease an interface reaction with hydropic degeneration of basal cells and a bandlike lymphocytic infiltrate, mainly affecting rete tips, which have a characteristic quadrangular-shaped and associated with collections of apoptotic keratinocytes. Intraepidermal lymphocytes express mainly CD8. Hypopigmented MF lesions are not usually annular and tend to be more generalized, and histologic evaluation usually displays epidermal atrophy, more prominent epidermotropism, cytologic atypia, tagging, and lack of colloid bodies. In addition, demonstration of an aberrant phenotype and evidence of clonal TCR rearrangement str often seen in MF.

As discussed previously, PR should always be considered in the differential diagnosis of strikingly epidermotropic forms of cutaneous TCL. Because PR is characterized by a T-cell infiltrate with variable + phenotype that include cases that are, βF1+, CD3+, CD8+, or rarely CD3+, CD4−, and CD8− (some of them with proved γδ expression),[86] the differential with CD8+ AECTCL or PCGDTCL is highly relevant and rigorous clinicopathologic correlation is pivotal to avoid a misdiagnosis.

## SUMMARY

In this review, the group of primary cutaneous cytotoxic TCLs is described. These lymphomas can be broadly divided into 2 groups. The first group includes CD8+ MF, primary acral CD8+ lymphoma, SPTCL, and CD30+ LPDs with cytotoxic phenotype. These are lymphoid neoplasm with indolent behavior. A second group characterized by dismal prognosis, comprises PCGDTCL, CD8+ AECTCL, and NK/T-cell LPDs. When dealing with cytotoxic lymphomas in particular and with cutaneous lymphomas in general, it is crucial to adopt a unifying approach, including thorough clinical data, laboratory findings, and histologic, and immunohistochemical, and gene analysis results. This is paramount to reaching a correct diagnosis with prognostically relevant subtype attribution.

## ACKNOWLEDGMENTS

We are very grateful to Dr Teresa Estrach Panella for providing the clinical images showed in this work.

## REFERENCES

1. Kummer J, Vermeer H, Dukers D, et al. Most primary cutaneous CD30-positive lymphoproliferative disorders have a CD4-positive cytotoxic T-cell phenotype. J Invest Dermatol 1997;109:636–40.

2. Boulland ML, Wechsler J, Bagot M, et al. Primary CD30-positive cutaneous T-cell lymphomas and lymphomatoid papulosis frequently express cytotoxic proteins. Histopathology 2000;36(2):136–44.

3. Swerdlow SH, Campo E, Pileri SA, et al. The 2016 revision of the World Health Organization classification of lymphoid neoplasms. Blood 2016;127(20): 2375–90.

4. Swerdlow SH, Campo E, Harris NL, et al. WHO classification of tumors of hematopoietic and lymphoid tissues. Lyon (France): IARC Press; 2008.

5. Taghon T, Rothenberg EV. Molecular mechanisms that control mouse and human TCR-alphabeta and TCR-gammadelta T cell development. Semin Immunopathol 2008;30:383–98.

6. Sun JC, Lanier LL. NK cell development, homeostasis and function: parallels with CD8(+) T cells. Nat Rev Immunol 2011;11(10):645–57.

7. Krzywinska E, Cornillon A, Allende-Vega N, et al. CD45 Isoform Profile Identifies Natural Killer (NK) Subsets with Differential Activity. PLoS One 2016; 11(4):e0150434.

8. Willemze R, Jaffe ES, Burg G, et al. WHO-EORTC classification for cutaneous lymphomas. Blood 2005;105:3768–85.

9. Go RS, Wester SM. Immunophenotypic and molecular features, clinical outcomes, treatments, and prognostic factors associated with subcutaneous panniculitis-like T-cell lymphoma: a systematic analysis of 156 patients reported in the literature. Cancer 2004;101:1404–13.

10. Willemze R, Jansen PM, Cerroni L, et al. Subcutaneous panniculitis-like T-cell lymphoma: definition, classification, and prognostic factors: an EORTC Cutaneous Lymphoma Group Study of 83 cases. Blood 2008;111:838–45.

11. Huppmann AR, Xi L, Raffeld M, et al. Subcutaneous panniculitis-like T-cell lymphoma in the pediatric age group: a lymphoma of low malignant potential. Pediatr Blood Cancer 2013;60(7):1165–70.

12. Johnston EE, LeBlanc RE, Kim J, et al. Subcutaneous panniculitis-like T-cell lymphoma: Pediatric case series demonstrating heterogeneous presentation and option for watchful waiting. Pediatr Blood Cancer 2015;62(11):2025–8.

13. Hu ZL, Sang H, Deng L, et al. Subcutaneous panniculitis-like T-cell lymphoma in children: a review of the literature. Pediatr Dermatol 2015;32(4): 526–32.

14. Oschlies I, Simonitsch-Klupp I, Maldyk J, et al. Subcutaneous panniculitis-like T-cell lymphoma in children: a detailed clinicopathological description of 11 multifocal cases with a high frequency of haemophagocytic syndrome. Br J Dermatol 2015;172(3): 793–7.

15. Kong YY, Dai B, Kong JC, et al. Subcutaneous panniculitis-like T-cell lymphoma: a clinicopathologic, immunophenotypic, and molecular study of 22 Asian cases according to WHO-EORTC classification. Am J Surg Pathol 2008;32(10): 1495–502.

16. Yokota K, Akiyama Y, Adachi D, et al. Subcutaneous panniculitis-like T-cell lymphoma accompanied by Sjogren's syndrome. Scand J Rheumatol 2009; 38(6):494–5.

17. Pincus LB, LeBoit PE, McCalmont TH, et al. Subcutaneous panniculitis-like T-cell lymphoma with overlapping clinicopathologic features of lupus erythematosus: coexistence of 2 entities? Am J Dermatopathol 2009;31(6):520–6.

18. Michot C, Costes V, Gerard-Dran D, et al. Subcutaneous panniculitis-like T-cell lymphoma in a patient receiving etanercept for rheumatoid arthritis. Br J Dermatol 2009;160(4):889–90.

19. Lozzi GP, Massone C, Citarella L, et al. Rimming of adipocytes by neoplastic lymphocytes: a histopathologic feature not restricted to subcutaneous T-cell lymphoma. Am J Dermatopathol 2006;28(1):9–12.

20. Massone C, Kodama K, Salmhofer W, et al. Lupus erythematosus panniculitis (lupus profundus): clinical, histopathological, and molecular analysis of nine cases. J Cutan Pathol 2005;32(6):396–404.

21. Liau JY, Chuang SS, Chu CY, et al. The presence of clusters of plasmacytoid dendritic cells is a helpful feature for differentiating lupus panniculitis from subcutaneous panniculitis-like T-cell lymphoma. Histopathology 2013;62(7):1057–66.

22. Bosisio F, Boi S, Caputo V, et al. Lobular panniculitic infiltrates with overlapping histopathologic features of lupus panniculitis (lupus profundus) and subcutaneous T-cell lymphoma: a conceptual and practical dilemma. Am J Surg Pathol 2015;39(2):206–11.

23. LeBlanc RE, Tavallaee M, Kim YH, et al. Useful parameters for distinguishing subcutaneous panniculitis-like T-cell lymphoma from lupus erythematosus panniculitis. Am J Surg Pathol 2016;40(6): 745–54.

24. Magro CM, Crowson AN, Kovatich AJ, et al. Lupus profundus, indeterminate lymphocytic lobular panniculitis and subcutaneous T-cell lymphoma: a spectrum of subcuticular T-cell lymphoid dyscrasia. J Cutan Pathol 2001;28:235–8.

25. Park HS, Choi JW, Kim BK, et al. Lupus erythematosus panniculitis: clinicopathological, immunophenotypic, and molecular studies. Am J Dermatopathol 2010;32:24–30.
26. Berti E, Tomasini D, Vermeer MH, et al. Primary cutaneous CD8-positive epidermotropic cytotoxic T cell lymphomas. A distinct clinicopathological entity with an aggressive clinical behavior. Am J Pathol 1999;155:483–92.
27. Santucci M, Pimpinelli N, Massi D, et al. Cytotoxic/natural killer cell cutaneous lymphomas: report of EORTC cutaneous lymphoma task forcé workshop. Cancer 2003;97:610–27.
28. Bekkenk MW, Vermeer MH, Jansen PM, et al. Peripheral T-cell lymphomas unspecified presenting in the skin: analysis of prognostic factors in a group of 82 patients. Blood 2003;102:2213–9.
29. Massone C, Chott A, Metze D, et al. Subcutaneous, blastic natural killer (NK), NK/T-cell, and other cytotoxic lymphomas of the skin: a morphologic, immunophenotypic, and molecular study of 50 patients. Am J Surg Pathol 2004;28:719–35.
30. Gormley RH, Hess SD, Anand D, et al. Primary cutaneous aggressive epidermotropic CD8+ T-cell lymphoma. J Am Acad Dermatol 2010;62(2):300–7.
31. Nofal A, Abdel-Mawla MY, Assaf M, et al. Primary cutaneous aggressive epidermotropic CD8(+) T-cell lymphoma: proposed diagnostic criteria and therapeutic evaluation. J Am Acad Dermatol 2012;67:748–59.
32. Robson A, Assaf C, Bagot M, et al. Aggressive epidermotropic cutaneous CD8+ lymphoma: a cutaneous lymphoma with distinct clinical and pathological features. Report of an EORTC Cutaneous Lymphoma Task Force Workshop. Histopathology 2015;67(4):425–41.
33. Saggini A, Gulia A, Argenyi Z, et al. A variant of lymphomatoid papulosis simulating primary cutaneous aggressive epidermotropic CD8+ cytotoxic T-cell lymphoma. Description of 9 cases. Am J Surg Pathol 2010;34:1168–75.
34. Cardoso J, Duhra P, Thway Y, et al. Lymphomatoid papulosis type D: a newly described variant easily confused with cutaneous aggressive CD8- positive cytotoxic T-cell lymphoma. Am J Dermatopathol 2012;34:762–5.
35. Plaza JA, Feldman AL, Magro C. Cutaneous CD30-positive lymphoproliferative disorders with CD8 expression: a clinicopathologic study of 21 cases. J Cutan Pathol 2013;40:236–47.
36. McQuitty E, Curry JL, Tetzlaff MT, et al. The differential diagnosis of CD8-positive ("type D") lymphomatoid papulosis. J Cutan Pathol 2014;41:88–100.
37. Martires KJ, Ra S, Abdulla F, et al. Characterization of primary cutaneous CD8+/CD30+ lymphoproliferative disorders. Am J Dermatopathol 2015;37(11):822–33.
38. Haghighi B, Smoller BR, LeBoit PE, et al. Pagetoid reticulosis (Woringer-Kolopp disease): an immunophenotypic, molecular, and clinicopathologic study. Mod Pathol 2000;13:502–10.
39. Kempf W, Kazakov DV, Palmedo G, et al. Pityriasis lichenoides et varioliformis acuta with numerous CD30+ cells: a variant mimicking lymphomatoid papulosis and other cutaneous lymphomas. A clinicopathologic, immunohistochemical, and molecular biological study of 13 cases. Am J Surg Pathol 2012;36:1021–9.
40. Fierro MT, Novelli M, Savoia P, et al. CD45RA+ immunophenotype in mycosis fungoides: clinical, histological and immunophenotypical features in 22 patients. J Cutan Pathol 2001;28:356–62.
41. Roullet M, Gheith SM, Mauger J, et al. Percentage of gamma-delta T cells in panniculitis by paraffin immunohistochemical analysis. Am J Clin Pathol 2009;131:820–6.
42. Garcia-Herrera A, Song JY, Chuang SS, et al. Nonhepatosplenic gammadelta T-cell ymphomas represent a spectrum of aggressive cytotoxic T-cell lymphomas with a mainly extranodal presentation. Am J Surg Pathol 2011;35:1214–25.
43. Guitart J, Weisenburger DD, Subtil A, et al. Cutaneous gammadelta T-cell lymphomas: a spectrum of presentations with overlap with other cytotoxic lymphomas. Am J Surg Pathol 2012;36(11):1656–65.
44. Magro CM, Wang X. Indolent primary cutaneous gamma/delta T-cell lymphoma localized to the subcutaneous panniculus and its association with atypical lymphocytic lobular panniculitis. Am J Clin Pathol 2012;138:50.
45. Endly DC, Weenig RH, Peters MS, et al. Indolent course of cutaneous gamma-delta T-cell lymphoma. J Cutan Pathol 2013;40(10):896–902.
46. Kempf W, Kazakov DV, Scheidegger PE, et al. Two cases of primary cutaneous lymphoma with a γ/δ+ phenotype and an indolent course: further evidence of heterogeneity of cutaneous γ/δ+ T-cell lymphomas. Am J Dermatopathol 2014;36(7):570–7.
47. Toro JR, Beaty M, Sorbara L, et al. Gamma delta T-cell lymphoma of the skin: a clinical, microscopic, and molecular study. Arch Dermatol 2000;136:1024–32.
48. Toro JR, Liewehr DJ, Pabby N, et al. Gamma-delta T-cell phenotype is associated with significantly decreased survival in cutaneous T-cell lymphoma. Blood 2003;101:3407–12.
49. Alexander RE, Webb AR, Abuel-Haija M, et al. Rapid progression of primary cutaneous gamma-delta T-cell lymphoma with an initial indolent clinical presentation. Am J Dermatopathol 2014;36(10):839–42.
50. Rodríguez-Pinilla SM, Ortiz-Romero PL, Monsalvez V, et al. TCR-γ expression in primary cutaneous T-cell lymphomas. Am J Surg Pathol 2013;37(3):375–84.

51. Kash N, Massone C, Fink-Puches R, et al. Phenotypic variation in different lesions of mycosis fungoides biopsied within a short period of time from the same patient. Am J Dermatopathol 2016;38(7):541–5.

52. Martinez-Escala ME, Sidiropoulos M, Deonizio J, et al. γδ T-cell-rich variants of pityriasis lichenoides and lymphomatoid papulosis: benign cutaneous disorders to be distinguished from aggressive cutaneous γδT-cell lymphomas. Br J Dermatol 2015;172(2):372–9.

53. Quintanilla-Martinez L, Ridaura C, Nagl F, et al. Hydroa vacciniforme-like lymphoma: a chronic EBV+ lymphoproliferative disorder with risk to develop a systemic lymphoma. Blood 2013;122(18):3101–10.

54. Pongpruttipan T, Sukpanichnant S, Assanasen T, et al. Extranodal NK/T-cell lymphoma, nasal type, includes cases of natural killer cell and alphabeta,-gammadelta, and alphabeta/gammadelta T-cell origin: a comprehensive clinicopathologic and phenotypic study. Am J Surg Pathol 2012;36:481–99.

55. Lee WJ, Jung JM, Won CH, et al. Cutaneous extranodal natural killer/T-cell lymphoma: a comparative clinicohistopathologic and survival outcome analysis of 45 cases according to the primary tumor site. J Am Acad Dermatol 2014;70(6):1002–9.

56. Takata K, Hong ME, Sitthinamsuwan P, et al. Primary cutaneous NK/T-cell lymphoma, nasal type and CD56-positive peripheral T-cell lymphoma: a cellular lineage and clinicopathologic study of 60 patients from Asia. Am J Surg Pathol 2015;39(1):1–12.

57. Iqbal J, Wright G, Wang C, et al. Gene expression signatures delineate biological and prognostic subgroups in peripheral T-cell lymphoma. Blood 2014;123(19):2915–23.

58. Petrella T, Maubec E, Cornillet-Lefebvre P, et al. Indolent CD8-positive lymphoid proliferation of the ear. A distinct primary cutaneous T-cell lymphoma? Am J Surg Pathol 2007;31:1887–92.

59. Li XQ, Zhou XY, Sheng WQ, et al. Indolent CD8+ lymphoid proliferation of the ear: a new entity and possible occurrence of signet ring cells. Histopathology 2009;55:468–70.

60. Suchak R, O'Connor S, McNamara C, et al. Indolent CD8-positive lymphoid proliferation on the face: part of the spectrum of primary cutaneous small-/medium-sized pleomorphic T-cell lymphoma or a distinct entity? J Cutan Pathol 2010;37:977–81.

61. Beltraminelli H, Mullegger R, Cerroni L. Indolent CD8+ lymphoid proliferation of the ear: a phenotypic variant of the small–medium pleomorphic cutaneous T-cell lymphoma? J Cutan Pathol 2010;37:81–4.

62. Swick BL, Baum CL, Venkat AP, et al. Indolent CD8+ lymphoid proliferation of the ear: report of two cases and review of the literature. J Cutan Pathol 2011;38:209–15.

63. Zeng W, Nava VE, Cohen P, et al. Indolent CD8-positive T-cell lymphoid proliferation of the ear: a report of two cases. J Cutan Pathol 2012;39:696–700.

64. Li JY, Guitart J, Pulitzer MP, et al. Multicenter case series of indolent small/medium-sized CD8+ lymphoid proliferations with predilection for the ear and face. Am J Dermatopathol 2014;36:402–8.

65. Greenblatt D, Ally M, Child F, et al. Indolent CD8(+) lymphoid proliferation of acral sites: a clinicopathologic study of six patients with some atypical features. J Cutan Pathol 2013;40:248–58.

66. Wobser M, Petrella T, Kneitz H, et al. Extrafacial indolent CD8-positive cutaneous lymphoid proliferation with unusual symmetrical presentation involving both feet. J Cutan Pathol 2013;40:955.

67. Kluk J, Kai A, Koch D, et al. Indolent CD8-positive lymphoid proliferation of acral sites: three further cases of a rare entity and an update on a unique patient. J Cutan Pathol 2016;43(2):125–36.

68. Wobser M, Roth S, Reinartz T, et al. CD68 expression is a discriminative feature of indolent cutaneous CD8-positive lymphoid proliferation and distinguishes this lymphoma subtype from other CD8-positive cutaneous lymphomas. Br J Dermatol 2014;172:1573.

69. Wobser M, Reinartz T, Roth S, et al. Cutaneous CD8+ Cytotoxic T-Cell Lymphoma infiltrates: clinicopathological correlation and outcome of 35 cases. Oncol Ther 2016;4:199–210.

70. Massone C, Crisman G, Kerl H, et al. The prognosis of early mycosis fungoides is not influenced by phenotype and T-cell clonality. Br J Dermatol 2008;159:881–6.

71. Massone C, Kodama K, Kerl H, et al. Histopathologic features of early (patch) lesions of mycosis fungoides: a morphologic study on 745 biopsy specimens from 427 patients. Am J Surg Pathol 2005;29:550.

72. Whittam LR, Calonje E, Orchard G, et al. CD8-positive juvenile onset mycosis fungoides: an immunohistochemical and genotypic analysis of six cases. Br J Dermatol 2000;143:1199–204.

73. El Shabrawi-Caelen L, Cerroni L, Medeiros LJ, et al. Hypopigmented mycosis fungoides. Frequent expression of a CD8+ T-cell phenotype. Am J Surg Pathol 2002;26:450.

74. Nikolaou VA, Papadavid E, Katsambas A, et al. Clinical characteristics and course of CD8+ cytotoxic variant of mycosis fungoides: a case series of seven patients. Br J Dermatol 2009;161:826–30.

75. Pope E, Weitzman S, Ngan B, et al. Mycosis fungoides in the pediatric population: report from an international Childhood Registry of Cutaneous Lymphoma. J Cutan Med Surg 2010;14:1.

76. Nanda A, AlSaleh QA, Al-Ajmi A, et al. Myoocis fungoides in Arab children and adolescents: a report

of 36 patients from Kuwait. Pediatr Dermatol 2010; 27:607.

77. Pavlovsky L, Mimouni D, Amitay-Laish I, et al. Hyper-pigmented mycosis fungoides: an unusual variant of cutaneous T-cell lymphoma with a frequent CD8+ phenotype. J Am Acad Dermatol 2012;67:69–75.

78. Castano E, Glick S, Wolgast L, et al. Hypopigmented mycosis fungoides in childhood and adolescence: a long-term retrospective study. J Cutan Pathol 2013; 40:924–34.

79. Abdel-Halim M, El-Nabarawy E, El Nemr R, et al. Frequency of Hypopigmented Mycosis Fungoides in Egyptian Patients Presenting With Hypopig-mented Lesions of the Trunk. Am J Dermatopathol 2015;37:834–40.

80. Burns MK, Chan LS, Cooper KD. Woringer-Kolopp disease (localized pagetoid reticulosis) or unile-sional mycosis fungoides? An analysis of eight cases with benign disease. Arch Dermatol 1995; 131(3):325–9.

81. Aung PP, Climent F, Muzzafar T, et al. Immunophe-notypic shift of CD4 and CD8 antigen expression in primary cutaneous T-cell lymphomas: a clinicopathologic study of three cases. J Cutan Pathol 2014;41(1):51–7.

82. Endo C, Naka Y, Miyagaki T, et al. Immunopheno-typic shift from CD4(+) to CD8(+) in mycosis fun-goides. Br J Dermatol 2016;175(4):830–3.

83. Vermeer MH, Geelen FA, Kummer JA, et al. Expres-sion of cytotoxic proteins by neoplastic T cells in mycosis fungoides increases with progression from plaque stage to tumor stage disease. Am J Pathol 1999;154(4):1203–10.

84. Song SX, Willemze R, Swerdlow SH, et al. Mycosis fungoides: report of the 2011 Society for Hematopa-thology/European Association for Haematopathology workshop. Am J Clin Pathol 2013;139(4):466–90.

85. Kazlouskaya V, Trager JD, Junkins-Hopkins JM. Annular lichenoid dermatitis of youth: a separate en-tity or on the spectrum of mycosis fungoides? Case report and review of the literature. J Cutan Pathol 2015;42(6):420–6.

86. Tomasini D, Niccoli A, Crivelli F. Pagetoid reticulosis tumor cells with double expression of TCRγδ and TCRαβ: an off-target phenomenon or genuine expression? J Cutan Pathol 2015;42(6):427–34.

# Epstein-Barr Virus–associated Lymphoproliferative Disorders in the Skin

John R. Goodlad, MBChB, MD

## KEYWORDS

- Skin • EBV • Mucocutaneous ulcer • Lymphomatoid granulomatosis
- Diffuse large B-cell lymphoma • Hydroa vacciniforme • Extranodal NK/T-cell lymphoma
- Immunosuppression

## Key points

- Epstein-Barr virus (EBV)–associated lymphoproliferations involving the skin are rare, may be of B, T, or natural killer (NK) cell lineage, and encompass a spectrum of clinical behavior requiring different approaches to treatment.
- EBV-positive B-cell lymphoproliferations that frequently involve the skin include EBV-positive mucocutaneous ulcer, lymphomatoid granulomatosis, and EBV-positive diffuse large B-cell lymphoma.
- These show overlapping pathologic features but can be separated with close attention to pathologic detail and clinical features.
- The most frequently encountered cutaneous EBV-positive lymphoproliferations of T or NK cell type are hydroa vacciniforme–like lymphoproliferative disorder and extranodal NK/T-cell lymphoma, nasal type.
- These disorders also share many pathologic features and clinical correlation is essential in differentiating the more indolent from the more aggressive forms of disease.

## ABSTRACT

Epstein-Barr virus (EBV)–associated lymphoproliferations involving the skin are a rare but important group of diseases with a broad spectrum of behavior, ranging from self-limiting spontaneously resolving disorders to highly aggressive malignancies. They may be of B, T, or natural killer (NK) cell type and include EBV-positive mucocutaneous ulcer, lymphomatoid granulomatosis, EBV-positive diffuse large B-cell lymphoma, hydroa vacciniforme–like lymphoproliferative disorder, and extranodal NK/T-cell lymphoma of nasal type. Recognition and distinction of these entities is important in view of their differing prognoses and treatments. An
association with EBV may be the first indication that a patient is immunosuppressed.

## OVERVIEW

Epstein-Barr virus (EBV), formally designated human herpesvirus 4, is a ubiquitous gamma herpes virus that infects approximately 90% of the population worldwide.[1] In most cases, infection occurs in childhood and is asymptomatic, although a minority who are infected in adolescence or adulthood present with infectious mononucleoisis.[2,3] Following acute infection the virus assumes a latent state in which it persists in circulating B lymphocytes without active viral production. In the

Disclosure: The author has nothing to disclose.
Haematological Malignancy Diagnostic Services (HMDS), Level 3, Bexley Wing, St James's University Hospital, Leeds LS9 7TF, UK
*E-mail address:* john.goodlad@nhs.net

Surgical Pathology 10 (2017) 429–453
http://dx.doi.org/10.1016/j.path.2017.01.001

latent state EBV is maintained through expression of a limited number of viral transcripts and proteins that affect the host cell cycle, promoting cellular proliferation and inhibiting apoptosis. In healthy individuals this proliferation is limited by the host immune system. However, when host immunity is compromised, EBV-driven cell division can go unchecked, producing a variety of lymphoproliferative disorders (LPDs).[2–4]

Immune dysregulation leading to EBV-associated LPDs is well documented in association with organ transplant, iatrogenic immunosuppression for a variety of autoimmune diseases, congenital immune deficiency, and human immunodeficiency virus (HIV) infection,[4] and age-related immune senescence has more recently been recognized as a predisposing factor.[5–7] In addition, EBV is implicated in a variety of other LPDs in apparently immune-competent patients, including classic Hodgkin lymphoma, Burkitt lymphoma, some cases of diffuse large B-cell lymphoma (DLBCL) in young patients, and extranodal natural killer (NK)/T-cell lymphoma of nasal type.[2–4,8–10]

EBV-associated LPDs encompass a broad spectrum of disease and include disorders of B, T, and NK cells. These disorders range in severity from benign self-limiting conditions to aggressive, rapidly fatal malignancies. Although most commonly encountered and recognized in lymph nodes and noncutaneous extranodal sites, the skin too may be the site of presentation, although this fact is often under-recognized. Although virtually any lymphoma can involve the skin, often as a consequence of disseminated disease, this article focuses on EBV-associated lymphoproliferations that preferentially or frequently present at cutaneous sites and that illustrate the range of behavior within this enigmatic group of diseases, highlighting the importance of accurate diagnosis to facilitate appropriate management.

## EPSTEIN-BARR VIRUS–ASSOCIATED B-CELL LYMPHOPROLIFERATIVE DISORDERS IN THE SKIN

Well-defined EBV-associated lymphomas of B-cell origin, such as Burkitt lymphoma and classic Hodgkin lymphoma, only rarely involve the skin and, when present, this is usually the result of direct extension from underlying nodal disease or a late manifestation of extensive dissemination.[11–13] This article focuses on 0 entities that are either localized to the skin at presentation or represent conditions that frequently present in

the skin, or involve cutaneous sites during the course of the disease.

## EPSTEIN-BARR VIRUS–POSITIVE MUCOCUTANEOUS ULCER

EBV-positive (EBV+) mucocutaneous ulcer (MCU) is a recently described disorder that arises on a background of immune senescence in apparently healthy elderly individuals, in patients receiving immunosuppressive therapy after organ transplant, or following treatment of autoimmune disease.[14–18] In the context of autoimmune disease, methotrexate is the most commonly implicated drug.[14,16,17,19] The pathogenesis of EBV+ MCU is not fully established but it is hypothesized that immune surveillance is reduced to a level that is only just sufficient to maintain EBV in a dormant state systemically. Additional localized factors are then thought to tip the balance toward an EBV-driven lymphoproliferation at the affected site, often corresponding with locations where EBV-infected cells are prevalent, such as Waldeyer's ring.[14]

The disease is characterized by the development of a solitary, well-circumscribed, often painful ulcerating lesion at a mucosal or cutaneous site. Oropharyngeal mucosa is the most frequent site of presentation. Cutaneous involvement is often perioral but other acral sites or the trunk may be affected.[14,16,19,20] Any part of the gastrointestinal tract may be involved and patients occasionally present with a variety of abdominal symptoms, including as abdominal emergencies.[18] There is no detectable underlying mass lesion, either on clinical examination or imaging, and no associated lymphadenopathy or splenomegaly.[18] EBV DNA is typically undetectable in peripheral blood, in contrast with many other types of EBV-associated LPDs.[18]

Biopsy reveals a circumscribed shallow ulcer, the base of which contains a polymorphous infiltrate comprising variable numbers of immunoblasts and large atypical Reed-Sternberg–like cells. An admixture of small lymphocytes, plasma cells, histiocytes, and eosinophils is present and plasmacytoid apoptotic cells are usually prominent. Vascular invasion with thrombosis and sometimes necrosis is present in a significant proportion. The base of the lesion is sharply defined by a rim of small lymphocytes (Figs. 1 and 2). In squamous mucosa and skin there may be reactive epithelial atypia, and pseudoepitheliomatous hyperplasia is often present.[14,18] The immunoblasts and Reed-Sternberg–like cells are EBV-positive B cells that are uniformly CD30 and, in some, CD15 positive. Although CD20 is downregulated in a proportion of cases, these blast cells typically

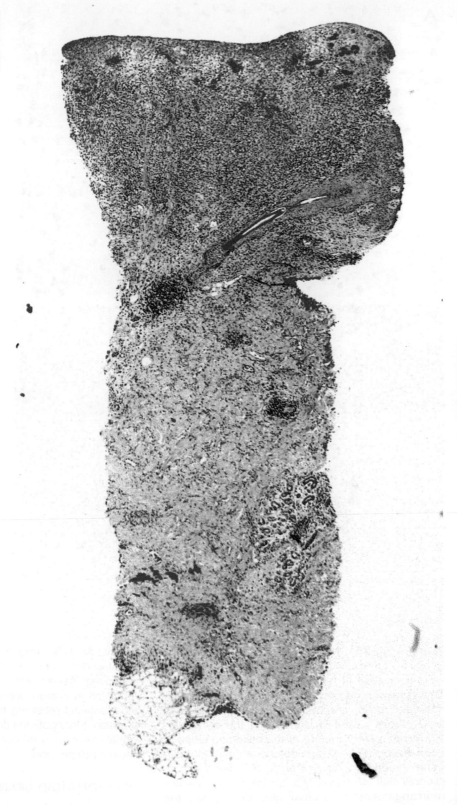

*Fig. 1.* Punch biopsy from a cutaneous EBV+ MCU showing relative circumscription in the deep aspect (H&E, original magnification ×1.25).

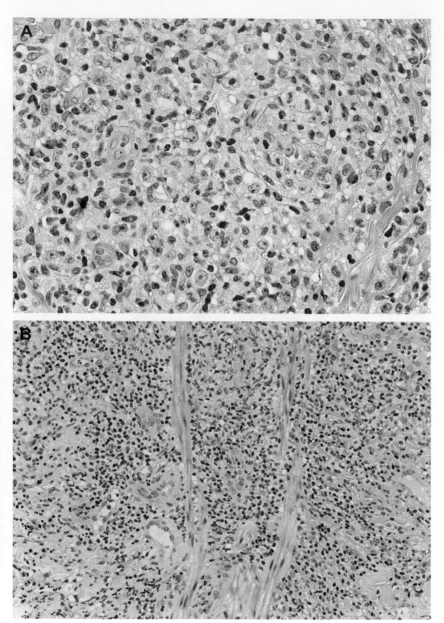

*Fig. 2.* High-power view of EBV+ MCU. (*A*) Aggregates of large immunoblastlike cells are seen superficially (H&E, original magnification ×20). (*B*) Small lymphocytes predominate at the base of the lesion (H&E, original magnification ×20).

express PAX5, MUM1, OCT2, and, usually, BOB1[14,18] (Fig. 3). Staining for EBV reveals a type II or type III latency pattern in most.[14,18,19] The background small lymphocytes, and some activated cells, are of T lineage and antibodies to CD3 are useful in highlighting the constraining rim of T lymphocytes at the base and sides of each lesion (Fig. 4). Monoclonal immunoglobulin gene rearrangement can be identified in around half of cases and clonal T-cell receptor rearrangements are often also detectable, the latter reflecting a restricted but reactive T-cell repertoire.[14,16,18]

EBV+ MCU is an indolent disease. In apparently immunocompetent elderly individuals, spontaneous regression seems to be the norm, although reduction in immunosuppression is sufficient for most patients receiving therapeutic immunosuppression. Most patients do not relapse, but occasional cases run a relapsing and remitting course without progression.[14–17,21,22]

## LYMPHOMATOID GRANULOMATOSIS

Lymphomatoid granulomatosis (LyG) is a rare angiocentric and angiodestructive EBV-driven

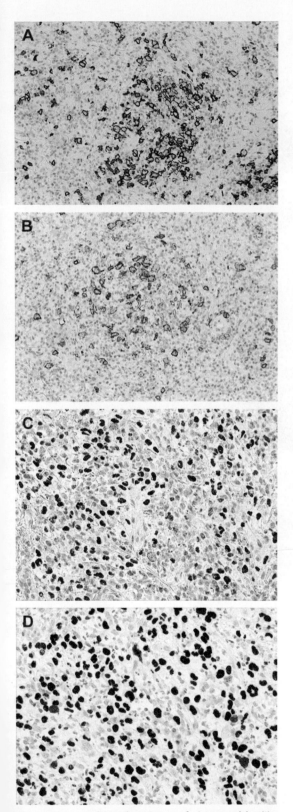

*Fig. 3.* Immunohistochemistry of immunoblastlike cells in EBV+ MCU. These cells are positive for CD20 (*A*), CD30 (*B*), OCT2 (*C*), and EBV (EBER) (*D*) (H&E, original magnification [*A*] ×20, [*B*] ×20, [*C*] ×20, [*D*] ×20).

B-cell LPD with a prominent reactive T-cell component. It most frequently affects men (male/female ratio, 2:1; mean age, 46–48 years), although it may be encountered in the pediatric age group.[23–26] Some cases are associated with overt immunosuppression that may be hereditary; for example, Wiskott-Aldrich syndrome, X-linked lymphoproliferative syndrome, and common variable immune deficiency. Other cases are associated with HIV infection or iatrogenic immunosuppression following allogeneic organ transplant or as treatment of autoimmune disease.[27–29] Some patients have a history of concurrent or treated malignancy.[30] In patients with no obvious immune dysregulation it may still be possible to identify evidence of impaired immunity on specific testing in the form of abnormal T-cell subsets in the peripheral blood or impaired responses to skin tests for antigens.[31,32]

LyG presents at extranodal sites and it is very unusual for there to be lymph node or splenic involvement. Most, if not all, cases involve the lung, and some investigators argue against a diagnosis of LyG in the absence of pulmonary disease. Other sites typically affected include skin (20%–50% of cases), central nervous system (CNS) (approximately 30%), kidney (30%), and liver (30%).[23,25,26] Signs and symptoms are related to the site of involvement but most patients have respiratory symptoms in the form of cough, dyspnea, and/or chest pain.[26,33,34] Chest radiograph typically shows multiple nodules bilaterally, principally in the lower lobes.[26] Cutaneous manifestations are variable and lesions may manifest as erythematous papules and nodules, indurated plaques, folliculitis-like eruptions, or superficial ulcerations.[30,34–38]

In the skin, biopsies of nodular lesions are most informative. There is a perivascular infiltrate that may be present throughout the dermis and involve the subcutaneous fat (**Fig. 5**). Small lymphocytes typically predominate with variable numbers of large atypical immunoblast-like cells also being present (**Fig. 6**). The latter occasionally resemble Reed-Sternberg cells. There is infiltration and destruction of blood vessel walls with necrosis of surrounding parenchyma. Histiocytes and plasma cells may also be present within the infiltrate, but neutrophils and eosinophils are typically inconspicuous. Granulomas are not a feature of LyG, although they may be seen in lesional skin as part of a reaction to fat necrosis.[23,24,36] The large atypical blast cells are EBV-positive B cells that often express CD30 but not usually CD15. The background small lymphocytes are of T lineage and include CD4-positive and CD8-positive subsets [23,24] (**Figs. 7** and **8**).

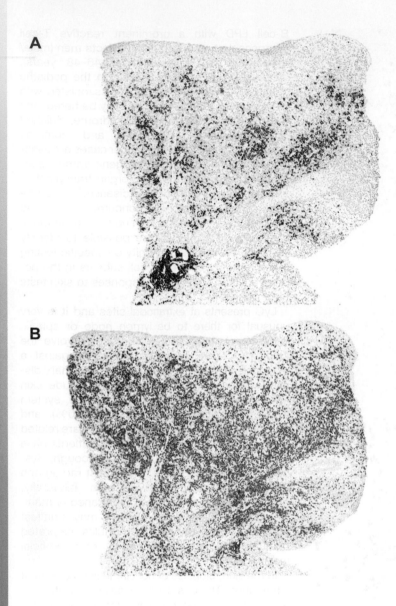

**Fig. 4.** (A) Antibodies to CD20 highlight aggregates of immunoblastlike cells in an EBV+ MCU. (B) The small lymphocytes at the base of the lesion are CD3+ T cells (H&E, original magnification [A] ×1.25, [B] ×1.25)].

Lesions can and should be graded by the number of large EBV-positive B cells. In grade I lesions there are fewer than 5 per high-power field (hpf) identifiable by in situ hybridization for EBER, with little or no necrosis. Blasts are more conspicuous in grade II LyG, numbering up to 50/hpf and may be seen in small clusters. Necrosis is more common. A polymorphic background is still discernible in grade III lesions but there are more than 50 EBV+ blast cells/hpf with formation of small confluent sheets. Extensive necrosis is usually also present.[23,26]

Most cases of LyG pursue an aggressive clinical course with a median survival of less than 2 years quoted in some historical series. Treatment is currently dictated by grade. Interferon alfa is recommended for grades I and II LyG, with more aggressive multiagent chemotherapy (eg, DA-EPOCH-R) reserved for grade III disease.[23,26]

## EPSTEIN-BARR VIRUS–POSITIVE DIFFUSE LARGE B-CELL LYMPHOMA, NOT OTHERWISE SPECIFIED

In the updated World Health Organization (WHO) classification, EBV-positive DLBCL, not otherwise specified is used to distinguish EBV+ large B-cell

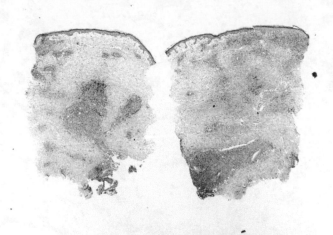

*Fig. 5.* A case of LyG showing a perivascular lymphoid infiltrate that is present throughout the dermis (H&E, original magnification ×1.25).

proliferations from other more specific entities with neoplastic large EBV+ cells, including EBV+ MCU, LyG, and posttransplant LPDs.[39] These tumors occur in apparently immunocompetent individuals, usually more than 50 years of age, and have a poorer prognosis than EBV-negative DLBCL in the same age group. They were originally designated EBV+ DLBCL of the elderly and are thought to arise as a consequence of immune senescence.[7,40] However, more recent studies have reported pathologically similar lymphomas in younger patients with a better survival than previously documented in older adults.[8] In the elderly

age group there is a slight male predominance (male/female ratio, 1.4:1) and a higher incidence has been reported among east Asian than Western populations (8.7%–11.4% vs <5%) in some studies.[6,7,40] EBV+ DLBCL presents at extranodal sites in 70% of patients, although there is often concurrent lymph node involvement. Virtually any extranodal site, including the skin, can be involved.[5,7,40–45]

Morphologically there are 2 main patterns recognized. In the polymorphic subtype there are centroblast, immunoblast, and plasmablastlike cells together with a variable component of

*Fig. 6.* The perivascular lymphoid infiltrate in a case of LyG showing scattered large blastlike cells (*arrows*) against a background of small lymphocytes (H&E, original magnification ×20).

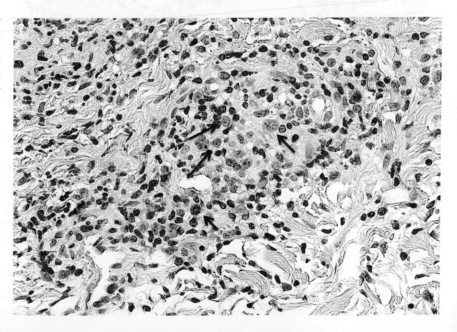

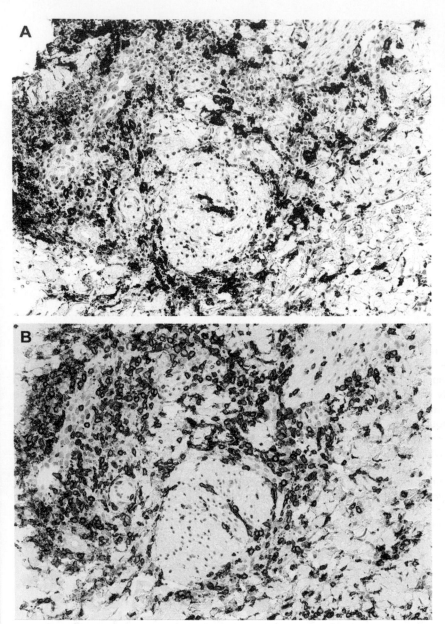

A

B

*Fig. 7.* Antibodies to CD20 (*A*) highlight the scattered blasts in a case of LyG (H&E, original magnification ×20). The background small lymphocytes are CD3+ small T cells (*B*) (H&E, original magnification ×20).

reactive cells, including lymphocytes, plasma cells, and histiocytes. Other cases have a more monomorphic appearance, comprising monotonous sheets of large transformed B cells.[5,7,40,45] Both subtypes may contain large atypical Reed-Sternberg–like cells and both patterns may be seen within the same lesion[46] (**Figs. 9** and **10**). Foci of geographic necrosis are common (**Fig. 11**). The neoplastic cells express B-cell antigens and usually have a post–germinal center phenotype, lacking CD10 and expressing IRF4. There is also frequent expression of CD30 and BCL2 and a type III latency pattern (EBER/LMP1/ EBNA2+) is present in greater than 90% of cases[46] (**Fig. 12**).

EBV+ DLBCL is an aggressive disease when presenting in patients more than 50 years of age, responding less well to conventional therapies than EBV-negative DLBCL in cohorts of equivalent age. Novel therapies for treating this type of lymphoma are therefore currently under investigation.[5]

## DIFFERENTIAL DIAGNOSIS

Distinction of the 3 entities discussed earlier from one another is paramount in view of their

*Fig. 8.* Staining for LMP1 in a case of LyG showing a positive reaction in large blastlike cells infiltrating a vessel wall (H&E, original magnification ×20).

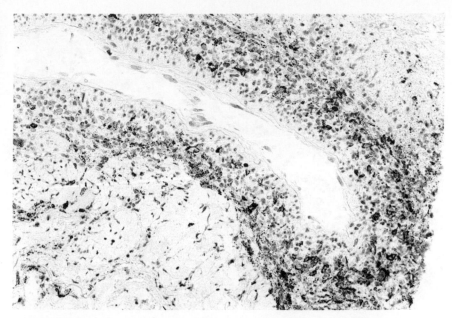

contrasting clinical courses and requirement for different treatment approaches. This distinction can be extremely difficult on purely pathologic grounds in view of the considerable overlap in morphology and immunophenotype. This difficulty is frequently further compounded when only small and fragmented biopsies, often containing only part of the lesion, are available and when clinical information is limited.

The differential diagnosis of EBV+ MCU includes LyG, EBV+ DLBCL, and EBV+ classic Hodgkin lymphoma. The cytologic composition and phenotype of MCU, EBV+ can be indistinguishable from LyG, and in some cases is identical to EBV+ DLBCL. Clinical features are paramount in making the distinction. Most important is the localized nature of EBV+ MCU and absence of a mass lesion.[14,16–18,47] Peripheral blood EBV DNA load may also be useful and a putative diagnosis of EBV+ MCU should be questioned if it is increased.[18] Pathologic features can also be helpful in adequate biopsies. EBV+ MCU is always sharply circumscribed with a band of small T cells at the base of the lesion, and this should help differentiate from the more infiltrative patterns seen with LyG and EBV+ DLBCL.

*Fig. 9.* Low-power view of a case of EBV+ DLBCL showing a perivascular and diffuse lymphoid infiltrate (H&E, original magnification ×4).

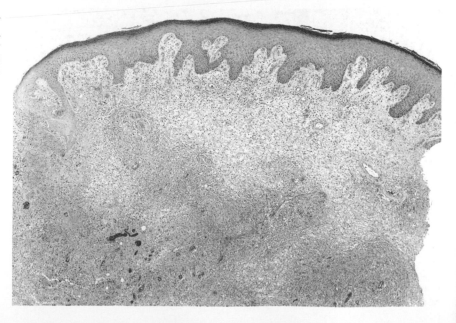

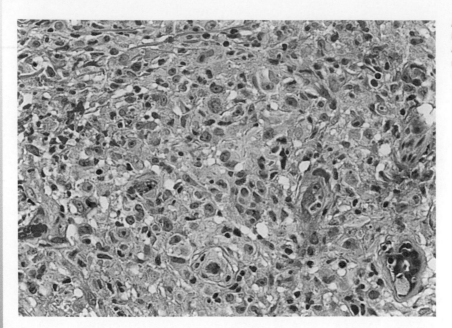

*Fig. 10.* Blasts in EBV+ DLBCL with a polymorphic appearance (H&E, original magnification ×40).

EBV+ MCU may also resemble classic Hodgkin lymphoma morphologically and phenotypically, with the Reed-Sternberg–like cells expressing CD30 and CD15. However, the clinical criteria described earlier, the extreme rarity of classic Hodgkin lymphoma presenting as extranodal disease in the absence of nodal involvement, and the presence of an intact B-cell program with CD45 expression in EBV+ MCU should allow distinction.

Distinguishing LyG from EBV+ DLBCL can be problematic, particularly in higher grade lesions,

although in practice the approach to managing grade III LyG is similar, if not identical, to that for EBV+ DLBCL. Clinical features are again important, in particular the presence of characteristic lung lesions in LyG and absence of lymph node involvement.[23] Pathologically, LyG always has a rich background of reactive T cells, which are not always prominent in EBV+ DLBCL.

Other diagnostic considerations include Wegener granulomatosis, extranodal nasal-type NK/T-cell lymphoma, and subcutaneous panniculitislike

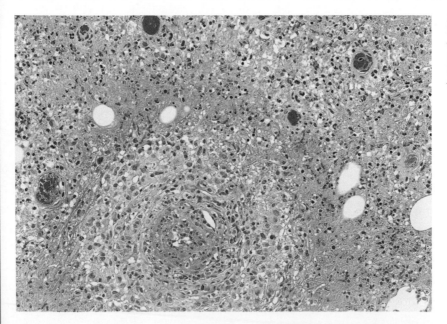

*Fig. 11.* Angioinvasion and angiodestruction with secondary necrosis in a case of EBV+ DLBCL (H&E, original magnification ×20).

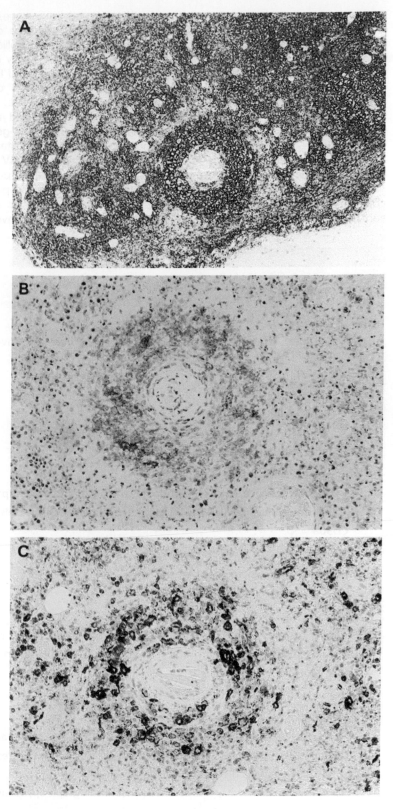

**Fig. 12.** Staining with antibodies to CD20 (H&E, original magnification ×10) (*A*), CD30 (H&E, original magnification ×10) (*B*), and LMP1 (H&E, original magnification ×10) (*C*) in a case of EBV+ DLBCL.

T-cell lymphoma. Wegener granulomatosis differs clinically by its involvement of the upper rather than lower respiratory tract and the presence of necrotizing vasculitis accompanied by granulomatous inflammation. Pulmonary involvement is uncommon in NK/T-cell lymphoma, and, although also associated with EBV infection, this neoplasm is characterized by a CD3–, CD20–, CD3ε+, CD56+ phenotype. The infiltrate in subcutaneous panniculitislike T-cell lymphoma is more monotonous than that seen in LyG, it is EBV negative, and consists predominantly of CD8+ T cells.

Primary cutaneous B-cell lymphomas with large cell morphology are by definition stage 1E at presentation, unlike EBV+ DLBCL, which is often of advance stage, cutaneous involvement reflecting the presence of disseminated disease. Primary cutaneous follicle center lymphoma, even when predominantly of large cell type, contains a predominance of large cleaved cells rather than the immunoblast or centroblastlike cells seen in EBV+ DLBCL. The neoplastic cells are also EBV negative and display a germinal center rather than a post–germinal center phenotype. In the absence of staging information, staining for EBV separates EBV+ DLBCL from primary cutaneous DLBCL-leg type, which may otherwise be morphologically and phenotypically identical; this is also the case for DLBCL of activated B-cell type secondarily involving the skin.

## Key Points

*Cutaneous B-cell LPDs*

EBV+ B-cell LPDs that present primarily in the skin, or frequently involve the skin during the course of the disease, include:

- EBV-positive MCU

- LyG

- EBV-positive DLBCL

These disorders display a spectrum of behavior:

- Benign, self-limiting (eg, EBV+ MCU)

- Aggressive malignancy (eg, EBV+ DLBCL)

The pathologic features of these entities show considerable overlap:

- EBV+ immunoblastlike B cells, including Reed-Sternberg–like cells
  - CD30+
  - OCT2+
  - Post–germinal center phenotype
  - Type II or type III latency pattern (LMP1+)
- Background of small T cells and histiocytes

- Angiocentric and angiodestructive growth pattern with necrosis frequently encountered

EBV+ mucocutaneous differentiated from LyG and EBV+ DLBCL on the basis of:

- Solitary nature

- Absence of mass lesion

- Absence of EBV DNA in peripheral blood

- Circumscribed lesion with confining rim of small T cells at edges and base

LyG differs from EBV+ DLBCL largely on the basis of clinical features:

- LyG has more limited distribution:
  - Lung involvement with characteristic chest radiograph appearances should always be present
  - CNS, kidney, and liver also frequently involved
  - Absence of lymphadenopathy and splenomegaly

- LyG always has background of small T cells

Important to recognize and separate these entities because:

- Identification of EBV+ B-cell LPDs may be the first indication that the patient is immunosuppressed

- Prognosis and treatment differ:
  - EBV+ MCU; reduction in immunosuppression (if applicable), excision and/or single-agent rituximab
  - LyG grades I and II; interferon alfa
  - LyG grade III; R-CHOP/DA-EPOCH-R plus or minus a reduction in immunosuppression (if applicable)
  - EBV+ DLBCL; R-CHOP plus or minus a reduction in immunosuppression (if applicable)

## EPSTEIN-BARR VIRUS–ASSOCIATED T-CELL/NATURAL KILLER–CELL PROLIFERATIONS ENCOUNTERED IN THE SKIN

B cells are the natural hosts for EBV, and most EBV-associated LPDs are of B lineage. However, EBV can also infect T and NK cells in some patients during acute infection and EBV-associated T-cell and NK-cell LPDs are well documented.[2,4,48–50] Most of these occur in patients from east Asia and Latin America and include chronic active EBV (CAEBV) infection and the T-cell lymphomas that may follow, extranodal NK-cell/T-cell lymphoma of nasal type,[2,49] aggressive NK-cell leukemia, and a subset of peripheral T-cell lymphomas,[39,50–55] the lymphomas often in the context of impaired immunity.

CAEBV infection of T/NK cell type shows a broad spectrum of clinical manifestations, ranging from indolent, localized, self-limiting proliferations to aggressive and often fatal systemic disease characterized by fever, hepatosplenomegaly, and lymphadenopathy.[56,57] A proportion of cases within this group, at both ends of the clinical spectrum, show a predilection for the skin and have been reported previously under a variety of different names, including hydroa vacciniforme (HV), HV-like lymphoma, and edematous scarring vasculitic panniculitis.[58–67] The current preferred terminology for this group of disorders with cutaneous manifestations is HV-like LPDs.[39,58] These will be discussed, together with extranodal NK-cell/T-cell lymphoma, which is the other EBV-positive T-cell/NK-cell proliferation that also frequently involves the skin.

## HYDROA VACCINIFORME–LIKE LYMPHOPROLIFERATIVE DISORDER

HV was historically defined in Western countries as a rare photosensitivity disorder of childhood characterized by development of papules and vesicles on sun-exposed skin of the face and dorsum of hands. Lesions evolve to crusts that heal leaving varicelliform scars.[59] In most cases the symptoms develop in childhood and resolve during early adult life. There are no associated systemic symptoms. A clinical syndrome very similar to HV but with a more aggressive clinical course was subsequently described in children from east Asia, Latin America, and Mexico under the rubric of HV-like lymphoma. These patients presented with marked facial edema together with recurring vesiculopapular rashes and development of large ulcers and crusts. Healing of these lesions is associated with severe scarring and disfigurement. Unlike classic HV, the skin lesions develop on sun-exposed and non–sun-exposed skin. Moreover, systemic symptoms are usually present in the form of fever, weight loss, hepatosplenomegaly, and lymphadenopathy. There is frequent association with severe mosquito bite hypersensitivity and the prognosis is often poor, possibly with a fatal outcome.[60–66,68] This entity was incorporated into the 2008 WHO classification and considered separate from classic HV.[69]

More recent analysis has shown considerable clinical and pathologic overlap between cases originally designated as classic HV and HV-like lymphoma.[58,68,70] Together with a lack of reproducible morphologic, immunophenotypic, and molecular findings to allow the distinction of these two putative entities, this has led to the proposal that there is a spectrum of EBV-associated T-cell/NK-cell lymphoproliferations with HV-like cutaneous manifestations; classic, self-resolving HV at one end and HV-like lymphoma with an aggressive clinical course at the other.[56–58,68] Consequently, the preferred approach is to include all such lesions under the heading of HV-like LPD, and this is the recommended nomenclature used in the 2016 update of the WHO classification.[39]

The clinical features of HV-like LPD are as described earlier and all cases run a waxing and waning course. The more severe form of the illness is characterized by extensive and disfiguring skin lesions, involvement of non–sun-exposed sites, and a potentially fatal clinical course. On histology, HV-like LPD is characterized by a perivascular and periadnexal lymphoid infiltrate (**Fig. 13**). In some cases, this is sparse, with only few reactive-appearing lymphocytes, but in others the infiltrate is dense with obvious cytologic atypia manifesting as large cells with irregular nuclei, prominent nucleoli, and abundant clear cytoplasm (**Figs. 14** and **15**). There may be associated angiodestruction with extension into the subcutaneous fat. Spongiotic vesicles are often present, and lesions are often ulcerated, but there is no epidermotropism.[58]

The infiltrating cells are by definition positive for EBV by in situ hybridization, but only rarely express LMP1 and are negative for EBNA2.[58] Typically, they only account for a proportion of the infiltrate (10%–40%), the remaining cells being reactive.[58,68] The phenotype of the EBV-positive cells varies from case to case. Some display a T-cell phenotype (60%–70% cases), which may be of $\alpha\beta$ or $\gamma\delta$ type, whereas others are proliferations of NK cells (30%–40% cases).[58,68,70,71] Most cases of T lineage show clonal rearrangement of the T-cell receptor gene.[58] Patients with severe symptoms tend to have larger and deeper infiltrates, often with involvement of the subcutis. Cases with an NK phenotype seem to more often involve severe hypersensitivity to mosquito bite, more often have a prominent eosinophil component to the infiltrate, and show a tendency toward

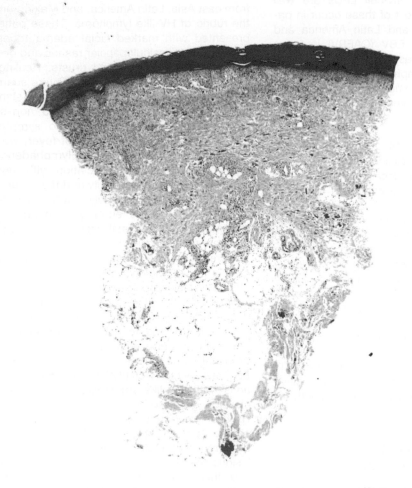

**Fig. 13.** Low-power view of a case of HV-like LPD showing a perivascular infiltrate throughout the dermis with involvement of subcutaneous fat (H&E, original magnification ×1.25).

*Fig. 14.* In this case of HV-like LPD there is incipient epidermal necrosis (*A*). A mild perivascular lymphocytic infiltrate is present in the underlying dermis (*B*) (H&E, original magnification [*A*] ×10, [*B*] ×10).

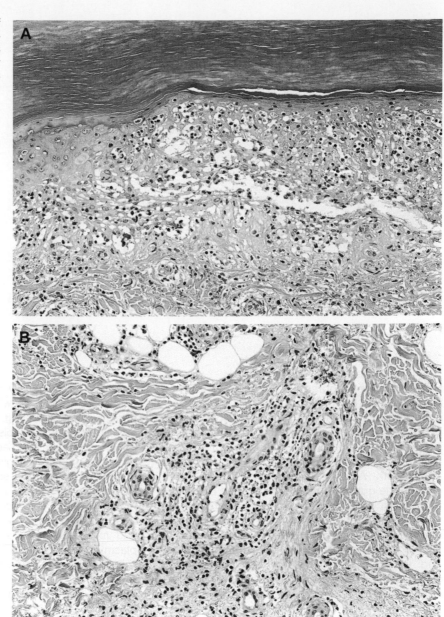

panniculitic lesions,[58,72,73] but there are no pathologic features that reliably predict clinical course.

Aggressive cases typically have severe symptoms at presentation. Fatalities result from progression to T-cell or NK-cell lymphomas or leukemias, hepatic failure, or the consequences of treatment.[58] There is no standard treatment but multiagent chemotherapy and radiotherapy seem to offer little benefit, with only transient effect without sustained remission, and these modalities may also increase the chances of dying of sepsis or liver failure.[58,62,70,71,74] Immunomodulatory

therapies may offer a better alternative as front-line treatment, and have been shown to provide temporary remission or improvement of symptoms. Agents that have been used include prednisolone, interferon alfa, chloroquine, and thalidomide.[58,60,70,74]

## EXTRANODAL NATURAL KILLER/T-CELL LYMPHOMA, NASAL TYPE

Extranodal NK-cell/T-cell lymphoma of nasal type (ENKTCL) is a predominantly extranodal

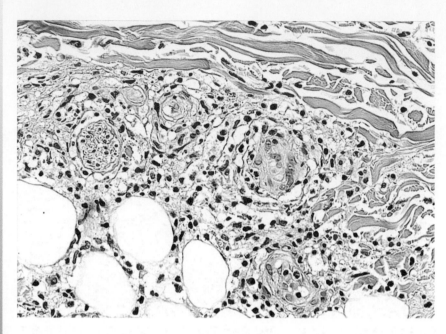

*Fig. 15.* High-power view of a case of HV-like LPD. The lymphocytes show only mild nuclear irregularities and hyperchromasia. Occasional eosinophils are also seen (H&E, original magnification ×40).

EBV-associated aggressive lymphoma that may be of NK-cell or T-cell phenotype.[39] It is rarely encountered in Western Europe and North America but accounts for more than 20% of T-cell or NK-cell lymphomas in Asian countries, as well as being frequent in Mexico and parts of Central and South America.[75–77] Most (>80%) cases involve the upper aerodigestive tract at presentation, particularly the nasal cavity, nasopharynx, paranasal sinuses, and palate.[78] However, other extranodal sites are also often involved, including skin, soft tissue, gastrointestinal tract, and testes, and in some cases disease is present in the absence of nasal involvement (so-called extranasal type).[78–82] More than half of ENKTCL present with stage I or stage II disease and in rare cases (10% of all ENKTCL) the disease is primarily cutaneous in origin.[79,83–85]

Presenting symptoms are related to sites of involvement. In most patients in whom there is nasal involvement, patients have facial edema and may complain of nasal obstruction, sinusitis, ulcers, and epistaxis. On examination, a destructive mass is often found.[78] Cutaneous involvement most commonly manifests as solitary or multiple subcutaneous masses or nodules, typically involving the upper or lower extremities, with or without ulceration. Plaques, as well as lesions resembling vasculitis, panniculitis, or cellulitis, may also occur.[83–89] Systemic symptoms such as fever, malaise, and weight loss may also be present and, in a minority of cases, there is a hemophagocytic syndrome.[79,88]

Skin biopsies typically show a dense nodular or diffuse dermal infiltrate with frequent involvement of subcutaneous fat (Fig. 16). Ulceration is common but epidermotropism is not normally a feature, although it is seen in rare cases.[82] The infiltrate is typically angiocentric with angiodestruction and extensive secondary necrosis. The constituent cells show variable morphology and may be of small, intermediate, or large size. They often have irregular nuclei, inconspicuous nucleoli, and moderate amounts of pale or clear cytoplasm[83,90–92] (see Fig. 16; Fig. 17).

By definition, the neoplastic cells are positive for EBV but may display an NK-cell or T-cell phenotype.[78,79] An NK-cell phenotype is shown by expression of CD2 and CD56 together with cytoplasmic but not surface CD3 (Fig. 18). Cytotoxic molecules are usually present but other T cell (eg, CD4, CD5, CD7, CD8) and NK cell (CD16, CD57)–associated antigens are usually absent[78] (Figs. 19 and 20). NK cells by definition show a germline pattern of T-cell receptor. A T lineage with expression of T cell–associated cell surface markers (eg, CD2, CD3, CD4, CD5, CD7, and/or CD8) and/or monoclonal T-cell receptor gene rearrangement is documented in 10% to 40% in various series.[79,83,93] These cases often also express CD56 and there is uniform expression of cytotoxic molecules.[78] They may be of αβ or γδ subtype.[93] Staining for CD30 is positive in a significant minority of biopsies.[78] Irrespective of lineage, all cases are positive for EBV by in situ

**Fig. 16.** A case of ENKTCL showing preferential involvement of the subcutaneous fat (*A*). The lymphoma is composed of fairly uniform blast cells of intermediate size (*B*) (H&E, original magnification [*A*] ×1.25, [*B*] ×40).

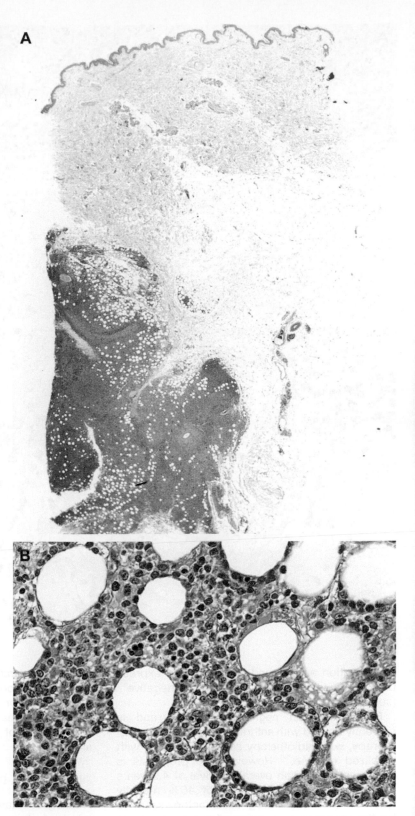

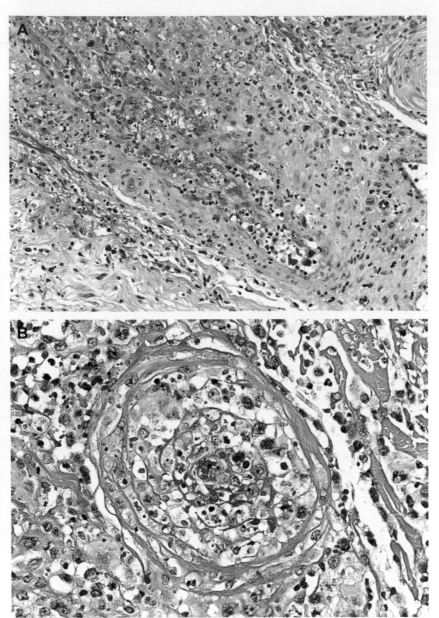

Fig. 17. Compared with Fig. 16, this case of ENKTCL shows a much more angiocentric and angiodestructive growth pattern (A, B). The constituent blast cells are large, with pleomorphic nuclei in this example (B) (H&E, original magnification [A] ×40, [B] ×40).

hybridization and around one-third also express LMP1, but staining for EBNA2 is always negative[83] (see Fig. 18).

ENKTCL is an aggressive disease and is currently treated with anthracycline-based chemotherapy, with radiotherapy added in patients with localized disease.[76] However, the prognosis is poor, with a median overall survival of 4.2 years and a 5-year overall survival of 46% recently quoted.[78] The main prognostic factors seem to be the presence or absence of nasal disease. In one Western series the 5-year overall survival for patients with nasal involvement was 5.01 years,

whereas for extranasal ENKTCL it was 0.55 years.[78] A particularly poor prognosis has also consistently been shown for ENKTCL presenting as primary cutaneous disease compared with cases with involvement of nasal or other extranasal sites.[79,83–87]

## DIFFERENTIAL DIAGNOSIS

A variety of cutaneous lymphomas may have histologic features similar to HV-like LPD and ENKTCL. An angiocentric and angiodestructive pattern of growth is often encountered in primary

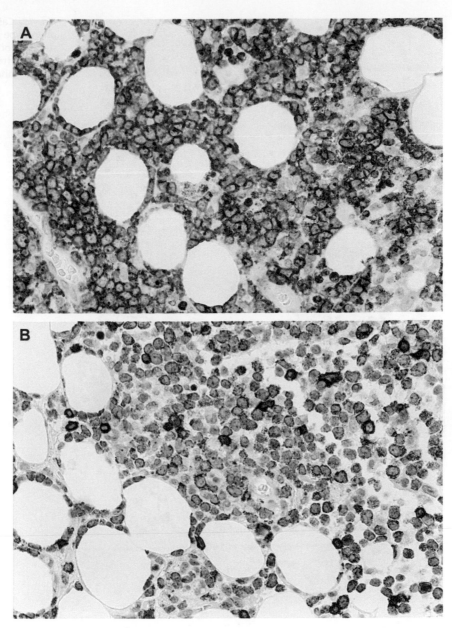

*Fig. 18.* In cases of ENKTCL with a classic NK phenotype there is strong membrane staining for CD2 (*A*), but only cytoplasmic positivity with antibodies to CD3ε (*B*) (H&E, original magnification [*A*] ×40, [*B*] ×40).

cutaneous aggressive epidermotropic CD8-positive T-cell lymphoma and primary cutaneous γδ T-cell lymphoma, whilst infiltration of subcutaneous fat is often seen in primary cutaneous γδ T-cell lymphoma as well as in subcutaneous panniculitislike T-cell lymphoma. There may also be phenotypic overlap between these entities given that HV-like LPD and ENKTCL can both show a T-cell phenotype of αβ or γδ type. Thus, demonstration of EBV in the neoplastic cells is essential in making a robust diagnosis when encountering such disorders. In these situations, the presence or absence of EBV should always be confirmed by in situ hybridization for EBER because LMP1 is only positive in a proportion of HV-like LPD and ENKTCL.

In cases in which EBV is identified, it often remains difficult to distinguish between HV-like LPD and ENKTCL. There is considerable pathologic overlap between these two entities, and separation may depend largely on clinical features. HV-like LPD tends to present in a younger age group and has a more protracted course dominated by recurring papules and vesicles, with or without systemic symptoms and organomegaly, rather than progressively destructive masses.[57,58,70,78,83]

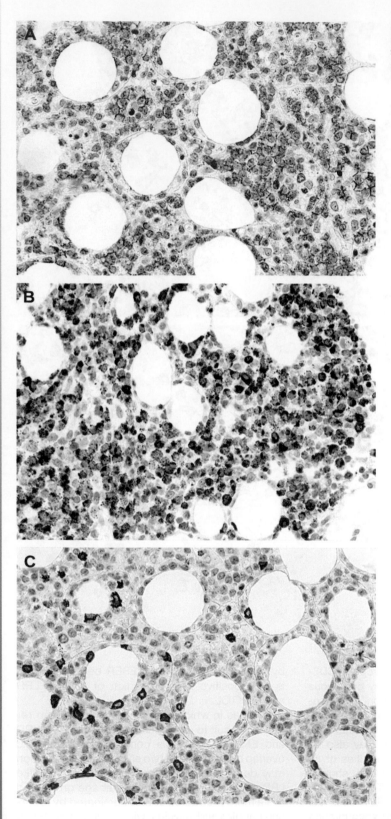

*Fig. 19.* Cases of ENKTCL with an NK phenotype typically show positive staining for CD56 (*A*) and granzyme B (*B*), but often lack CD8 (*C*) (H&E, original magnification [*A*] ×40, [*B*] ×40).

*Fig. 20.* Staining for LMP1 in a case of ENKTCL. Around one-third of cases are positive, as in this biopsy, but in situ hybridization for EBER is a much more sensitive technique for showing EBV (H&E, original magnification ×40).

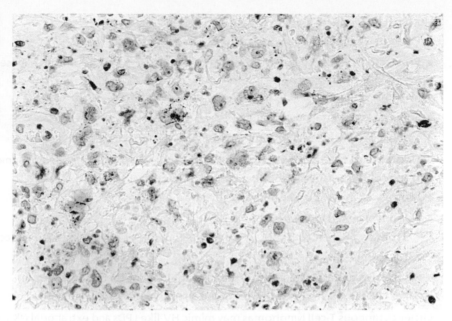

## Key points

*EBV-associated T-cell/NK-cell proliferations encountered in the skin*
EBV+ T-cell/NK-cell proliferations that present in, or frequently involve, the skin are:

- HV-like LPDs

- Extranodal NK-cell/T-cell lymphoma, nasal type

Both entities most commonly encountered in:

- East Asia

- Mexico

- Parts of Central and South America

Show overlapping pathologic features characterized by:

- Angiocentric and angiodestructive infiltrates of NK or T cells, often with involvement of subcutis

- EBV positive
    - Type I latency (EBER only) in most
    - Some cases type II (EBER and LMP1+)

- Cases with NK phenotype characterized by:
    - Positive for CD2, CD56, cytoplasmic CD3, cytotoxic molecules
    - Frequent lack of other T cell–associated surface antigens
    - Germline T-cell receptor gene

- Cases with T-cell phenotype:
    - αβ or γδ T-cell receptor expression
    - Clonal T-cell receptor gene rearrangement

HV-like LPDs, clinical features:

- Presents in children and young adults
- Protracted clinical course with recurring papules and vesicles on sun-exposed and, in more severe cases, non–sun-exposed regions
- Systemic symptoms and hepatomegaly present in some
- Some cases spontaneously remit
- Some cases progress to systemic NK-cell or T-cell lymphoma or leukemia
- No standard treatment; immunomodulatory therapies recommended by some clinicians

Extranodal NK-cell/T-cell lymphoma, nasal type, clinical features:

- Most cases involve upper aerodigestive tract
- Skin involvement frequent
  - Typically present with solitary or multiple masses or nodules on extremities
  - Ulceration common
- Aggressive disease with poor response to multiagent chemotherapy

HV-like LPDs and extranodal NK-cell/T-cell lymphoma largely distinguished on clinical grounds

Other cutaneous T-cell lymphomas may mimic HV-like LPDs and extranodal NK-cell/T-cell lymphoma but distinguished by presence or absence of EBV; for example:

- Primary cutaneous CD8-positive aggressive epidermotropic T-cell lymphoma
- Subcutaneous panniculitislike T-cell lymphoma
- Primary cutaneous γδ T-cell lymphoma

## SUMMARY

EBV-positive cutaneous LPDs may be of B, T, or NK cell type and encompass a broad spectrum of disease. They are rare, and there may be considerable pathologic overlap between cases with shared cells of origin; that is, those of B-cell lineage often resemble one another, as do those of T/NK type. Nonetheless, separation of these entities is important, in view of their different clinical courses and treatments. As is often the case with cutaneous lymphomas, clinicopathologic correlation is key because reliable distinction depends heavily on clinical features in the context of appropriate pathology.

## REFERENCES

1. Rickinson A. Epstein-Barr virus. Virus Res 2002;82: 109–13.
2. Rezk SA, Weiss LM. Epstein-Barr virus-associated lymphoproliferative disorders. Hum Pathol 2007;38: 1293–304.
3. Williams H, Crawford DH. Epstein-Barr virus: the impact of scientific advances on clinical practice. Blood 2006;107:802–9.
4. Tran H, Nourse J, Hall S, et al. Immunodeficiency-associated lymphomas. Blood Rev 2008;22:261–81.
5. Castillo JJ, Beltran BE, Miranda RN, et al. EBV-positive diffuse large B-cell lymphoma of the elderly: 2016 update on diagnosis, risk stratification and management. Am J Hematol 2016;91:530–7.
6. Ok CY, Paapathomas TG, Medeiros LJ, et al. EBV-positive diffuse large B-cell lymphoma of the elderly. Blood 2013;122:328–40.
7. Oyama T, Yamamoto K, Asano N, et al. Age-related EBV-associated B-cell lymphoproliferative disorders constitute a distinct clinicopathological group: a study of 96 patients. Cancer Res 2007; 13:5124–32.
8. Nicolae A, Pittaluga S, Abdullah S, et al. EBV-positive large B-cell lymphomas in young patients: a nodal lymphoma with evidence for a tolerogenic immune environment. Blood 2015;126:863–72.
9. Gromminger S, Mauter J, Bornkamm GW. Burkitt lymphoma: the role of Epstein-Barr virus revisited. Br J Haematol 2012;156:719–29.
10. Huang Y, de Leval L, Gaulard P. Molecular underpinning of extranodal NK/T-cell lymphoma. Best Pract Res Clin Haematol 2013;26:57–74.
11. Tassies D, Sierra J, Montserrat E, et al. Specific cutaneous involvement in Hodgkin's disease. Hematol Oncol 1992;10:75–9.
12. Baohmoyor C, Bazarbachi A, Rio B, et al. Specific cutaneous involvement indicating relapse of Burkitt's lymphoma. Am J Hematol 1997;54:176.

13. Banks PM, Arseneau JC, Gralink HR, et al. American Burkitt's lymphoma: a clinicopathologic study of 30 cases. II. Pathologic considerations. Am J Med 1975;58:322–9.

14. Dojcinov SD, Venkataraman G, Raffeld M, et al. EBV positive mucocutaneous ulcer—a study of 26 cases associated with various sources of immunosuppression. Am J Surg Pathol 2010;34:405–17.

15. Curry JL, Prieto VG, Jones DM, et al. Transient iatrogenic immunodeficiency-related B-cell lymphoproliferative disorder of the skin in a patient with mycosis fungoides/Sezary syndrome. J Cutan Pathol 2011;38:295–7.

16. Au W-Y, Ma ESK, Choy C, et al. Therapy-related lymphomas in patients with autoimmune diseases after treatment with disease-modifying anti-rheumatic drugs. Am J Hematol 2006;81:5–11.

17. Kalantzis A, Marshman Z, Falconer DT, et al. Oral effects of low-dose methotrexate treatment. Oral Surg Oral Med Oral Pathol Oral Radiol Endod 2005;100: 52–62.

18. Hart M, Thakral B, Yohe S, et al. EBV-positive mucocutaneous ulcer in organ transplant recipients. A localized indolent posttransplant lymphoproliferative disorder. Am J Surg Pathol 2014;38:1522–9.

19. Yamakawa N, Fujimoto M, Kawabata D, et al. A clinical, pathological and genetic characterization of methotrexate-associated lymphoproliferative disorders. J Rheumatol 2014;41:293–9.

20. McGinness JL, Spicknall KE, Mustasim DF. Azathioprine-induced EBV-positive mucocutaneous ulcer. J Cutan Pathol 2012;39:377–81.

21. Sadasivam N, Johnson RJ, Owen RG. Resolution of methotrexate-induced EBV-positive mucocutaneous ulcer. Br J Haematol 2014;165:584.

22. Tanaka A, Shigematsu H, Kojima M, et al. Methotrexate-associated lymphoproliferative disorder arising in a patient with adult Still's disease. J Oral Maxillofac Surg 2008;66:1492–5.

23. Song JY, Pittaluga S, Dunleavy K, et al. Lymphomatoid granulomatosis –a single institution experience. Am J Surg Pathol 2015;39:141–56.

24. Pittaluga S, Wilson WH, Jaffe ES. Lymphomatoid granulomatosis. In: Swerdlow SH, Campo E, Harris N, et al, editors. WHO classification of tumors of hematopoietic and lymphoid tissues. Lyons (France): IARC Press; 2008. p. 247–9.

25. Dunleavy K, Roschewski M, Wilson WW. Lymphomatoid granulomatosis and other Epstein-Barr virus associated lymphoproliferative processes. Curr Hematol Malig Rep 2012;7:208–15.

26. Katzenstein A-L, Doxtader E, Narenda S. Lymphomatoid granulomatosis. Insights gained over 4 decades. Am J Surg Pathol 2010;34:e35–48.

27. Lehman TJA, Church JA, Isaacs H. Lymphomatoid granulomatosis in a 13-month-old infant. J Rheumatol 1989;16:235–8.

28. Fassas A, Jagannath S, Desikan KR, et al. Lymphomatoid granulomatosis following autologous stem cell transplantation. Bone Marrow Transplant 1999; 23:79–81.

29. Sebire NJ, Haselden S, Malone M, et al. Isolated EBV lymphoproliferative disease in a child with Wiskott-Aldrich syndrome manifesting as cutaneous lymphomatoid granulomatosis and responsive to anti-CD20 immunotherapy. J Clin Pathol 2003;56: 555–7.

30. Muller FM, Lewis-Jones S, Morley S, et al. Lymphomatoid granulomatosis complicating other haematological malignancies. Br J Dermatol 2007;157: 426–9.

31. Wilson WH, Kingma DW, Raffeld M, et al. Association of lymphomatoid granulomatosis with Epstein-Barr virus infection of B-lymphocytes and response to interferon-alpha 2b. Blood 1996;87:4531–7.

32. Sordillo PP, Epremian B, Koziner B, et al. Lymphomatoid granulomatosis: an analysis of clinical and immunologic characteristics. Cancer 1982;49: 2070–6.

33. Liebow AA, Carrington CRB, Friedman PJ. Lymphomatoid granulomatosis. Hum Pathol 1972;3: 457–558.

34. Katzenstein AA, Carrington CRB, Liebow AA. Lymphomatoid granulomatosis. A clinicopathologic study of 152 cases. Cancer 1979;43:360–73.

35. Carlson KC, Gibson LE. Cutaneous signs of lymphomatoid granulomatosis. Arch Dermatol 1991;127: 1693–8.

36. Beaty MW, Toro J, Sorbara L, et al. Cutaneous lymphomatoid granulomatosis: correlation of clinical and biologic features. Am J Surg Pathol 2001;25: 1111–20.

37. Tong MM, Cooke B, Barnetson RS. Lymphomatoid granulomatosis. J Am Acad Dermatol 1992;27: 872–6.

38. Camisa C. Lymphomatoid granulomatosis: two cases with skin involvement. J Am Acad Dermatol 1989;20(4):571–8.

39. Swerdlow SH, Campo E, Pileri SA, et al. The 2016 revision of the World Health Organization classification of lymphoid neoplasms. Blood 2016;127: 2375–90.

40. Oyama T, Ichimura K, Suzuki R, et al. Senile EBV+ B-cell lymphoproliferative disorders. Am J Surg Pathol 2003;27:16–26.

41. Beltran BE, Castillo JJ, Morales D, et al. EBV-positive diffuse large B-cell lymphoma of the elderly: a case series from Peru. Am J Hematol 2011;86:663–7.

42. Hoeller S, Tzankov A, Pileri SA, et al. Epstein-Barr virus-positive diffuse large B-cell lymphoma in elderly patients is rare in Western populations. Hum Pathol 2010;41:352–7.

43. Hofscheier A, Ponciano A, Bonzheim I, et al. Geographic variation in the prevalence of

Epstein-Barr virus-positive diffuse large B-cell lymphoma of the elderly: a comparative analysis of a Mexican and a German population. Mod Pathol 2011;24:1046–54.

44. Park S, Lee J, Ko YH, et al. The impact of Epstein-Barr virus status on clinical outcome in diffuse large B-cell lymphoma. Blood 2007;110:972–8.

45. Nakamura S, Jaffe ES, Swerdlow SH. EBV positive diffuse large B-cell lymphoma of the elderly. In: Swerdlow SH, Campo E, Harris NL, et al, editors. WHO classification of tumours of haematopoietic and lymphoid tissues. Lyon (France): International Agency for Research on Cancer; 2008. p. 243–4.

46. Montes-Moreno S, Odqvist L, Diaz-Perez JA, et al. EBV-positive diffuse large B-cell lymphoma of the elderly is an aggressive post germinal center B-cell neoplasm characterized by prominent nuclear factor-kB activation. Mod Pathol 2012;25:968–82.

47. Attard AA, Praveen P, Dunn PJS, et al. EBV-positive mucocutaneous ulcer of the oral cavity: the importance of having a detailed clinical history to reach a diagnosis. Oral Surg Oral Med Oral Pathol Oral Radiol 2012;114:e37–9.

48. Mitarnun W, Suwiwat S, Pradutkanchana J, et al. Epstein-Barr virus-associated peripheral T-cell and NK-cell proliferative disease/lymphoma: clinicopathologic, serologic, and molecular analysis. Am J Hematol 2002;70:31–8.

49. Chan AC, Ho JW, Chiang AK, et al. Phenotypic and cytotoxic characteristics of peripheral T-cell and NK-cell lymphomas in relation to Epstein-Barr virus association. Histopathology 1999;34:16–24.

50. Swerdlow SH. T-cell and NK-cell post transplant lymphoproliferative disorders. Am J Clin Pathol 2007; 127:887–95.

51. Tan BT, Warnke RA, Arber DA. The frequency of B- and T-cell gene rearrangements and Epstein Barr virus in T-cell lymphomas: a comparison between angioimmunoblastic T-cell lymphoma and peripheral T-cell lymphoma, unspecified with and without associated B-cell proliferations. J Mol Diagn 2006;8: 466–75.

52. Dupuis J, Emile JF, Mounier N, et al. Prognostic significance of Epstein-Barr virus in nodal peripheral T-cell lymphoma, unspecified: a Groupe d'Etude des Lymphomes de l'Adulte (GELA) study. Blood 2006; 108:4163–9.

53. Chan J, Wong KF, Jaffe ES, et al. Aggressive NK-cell leukemia. In: Jaffe ES, Harris NL, Stein H, et al, editors. World Health Organization classification of tumors. Pathology and genetics of tumors of hematopoietic and lymphoid tissues. Lyon (France): IARC Press; 2001. p. 198–200.

54. Attygalle AD, Cabeçadas J, Gaulard P, et al. Peripheral T-cell and NK-cell lymphomas and their mimics; taking a step forward - report on the Lymphoma Workshop of the XVIth meeting of the European Association for Haematopathology and the Society for Hematopathology. Histopathology 2014;64: 171–99.

55. Kato S, Asano N, Miyata-Takata T, et al. T-cell receptor (TCR) phenotype of nodal Epstein-Barr virus (EBV)-positive cytotoxic T-cell lymphoma (CTL): a clinicopathologic study of 39 cases. Am J Surg Pathol 2015;39(4):462–71.

56. Oshima K, Kimura H, Yoshino T, et al. Proposed categorization of pathological states of EBV-associated T/natural killer-cell lymphoproliferative disorder in children and young adults: overlap with chronic active EBV infection and infantile fulminant EBV T-LPD. Pathol Int 2008;58(4):209–17.

57. Cohen JI, Kimura H, Nakamura S, et al. Epstein-Barr virus-associated lymphoproliferative disease in non-immunocompromised hosts: a status report and summary of an international meeting, 8-9 September 2008. Ann Oncol 2009;20:1472–82.

58. Quintanilla-Martinez L, Ridaura C, Nagl F, et al. Hydroa vacciniforme-like lymphoma: a chronic EBV+ lymphoproliferative disorder with risk to develop a systemic lymphoma. Blood 2013;122:3101–10.

59. Gupta G, Man I, Kemmett D. Hydroa vacciniforme: a clinical and follow-up study of 17 cases. J Am Acad Dermatol 2000;42:208–13.

60. Ruiz-Maldonado R, Parrilla FM, Orozco-Covarrubias ML, et al. Edematous, scarring vasculitic panniculitis: a new multisystemic disease with malignant potential. J Am Acad Dermatol 1995;32:37–44.

61. Magana M, Sangueza P, Gil-Beristain J, et al. Angiocentric cutaneous T-cell lymphoma of childhood (hydroa-like lymphoma): a distinctive type of cutaneous T-cell lymphoma. J Am Acad Dermatol 1998;38:574–9.

62. Barrionuevo C, Anderson VM, Zevallos-Giampietri E, et al. Hydroa-like cutaneous T-cell lymphoma: a clinicopathologic and molecular genetic study of 16 pediatric cases from Peru. Appl Immunohistochem Mol Morphol 2002;10:7–14.

63. Tabata N, Aiba S, Ichinohazama R, et al. Hydroa vacciniforme-like lymphomatoid papulosis in a Japanese child: a new subset. J Am Acad Dermatol 1995;32:378–81.

64. Gu H, Chang B, Qian H, et al. A clinical study on severe hydroa vacciniforme. Chin Med J (Engl) 1996; 109:645–7.

65. Iwatsuki K, Ohtsuka M, Akiba H, et al. Atypical hydroa vacciniforme in childhood: from a smoldering stage to Epstein-Barr virus-associated lymphoid malignancy. J Am Acad Dermatol 1999;40:283–4.

66. Cho KH, Kim CW, Lee DY, et al. An Epstein-Barr virus-associated lymphoproliferative lesion of the skin presenting as recurrent necrotic papulovesicles of the face. Br J Dermatol 1996;134:791–6.

67. Goldgeier MH, Nordlund JJ, Lucky AW, et al. Hydroa vacciniforme: diagnosis and therapy. Arch Dermatol 1982;118:588–91.

68. Iwatsuki K, Satoh M, Yamamoto T, et al. Pathogenic link between hydroa vacciniforme and Epstein-Barr virus-associated hematologic disorders. Arch Dermatol 2006;142(5):587–95.

69. Quintanilla-Martinez L, Kimura H, Jaffe ES. EBV positive T-cell lymphoproliferative disorders of childhood. In: Swerdlow SH, Campo E, Harris NL, et al, editors. WHO classification of tumours of haematopoietic and lymphoid tissues. 4th edition. Lyon (France): International Agency for Research on Cancer (IARC); 2008. p. 278–80.

70. Kimura H, Ito Y, Kawabe S, et al. EBV-associated T/NK-cell lymphoproliferative diseases in non-immunocompromised hosts: prospective analysis of 108 cases. Blood 2012;119:673–86.

71. Rodrıguez-Pinilla SM, Barrionuevo C, Garcia J, et al. EBV-associated cutaneous NK/T-cell lymphoma: review of a series of 14 cases from Peru in children and young adults. Am J Surg Pathol 2010;34(12):1773–82.

72. Kawa K, Okamura T, Yagi K, et al. Mosquito allergy and Epstein-Barr virus associated T/natural killer-cell lymphoproliferative disease. Blood 2001;98:3173–4.

73. Kimura H, Hoshino Y, Kanegane H, et al. Clinical and virologic characteristics of chronic active Epstein-Barr virus infection. Blood 2001;98:280–6.

74. Xu Z, Lian S. Epstein-Barr virus-associated hydroa vacciniforme-like cutaneous lymphoma in seven Chinese children. Pediatr Dermatol 2010;27:463–9.

75. Vose J, Armitage J, Weisenburger D, International T-cell Lymphoma Project. International T-cell and natural killer/T-cell lymphoma study: pathology findings and clinical outcomes. J Clin Oncol 2008;26:4124–30.

76. Tse E, Kwong Y-K. How I treat NK/T-cell lymphoma. Blood 2013;121:4997–5005.

77. Laurini JA, Perry AM, Boilesen E, et al. Classification of non-Hodgkin lymphoma in Central and South America: a review of 1028 cases. Blood 2012;120:4795–801.

78. Li S, Feng X, Li T, et al. Extranodal NK/T-cell lymphoma, nasal type. A report of 73 cases at MD Anderson Cancer Center. Am J Surg Pathol 2013;37:14–23.

79. Au WY, Weisenburger DD, Intragumtornchai T, et al. Clinical differences between nasal and extranasal natural killer/T-cell lymphoma: a study of 136 cases from the International Peripheral T-Cell Lymphoma Project. Blood 2009;113:3931–7.

80. Lee J, Suh C, Park YH, et al. Extranodal natural killer T-cell lymphoma, nasal-type: a prognostic model from a retrospective multicenter study. J Clin Oncol 2006;24:612–8.

81. Panano L, Gallamini A, Trape G, et al. NK/T-cell lymphomas 'nasal type': an Italian multicentric retrospective survey. Ann Oncol 2006;17:794–800.

82. Oshimi K, Kawa K, Nakamura S, et al. NK-cell neoplasms in Japan. Hematology 2005;10:237–45.

83. Takata K, Hong ME, Sitthinamsuwan P, et al. Primary cutaneous NK/T-cell lymphoma, nasal type and CD56-positive peripheral T-cell lymphoma. A cellular lineage and clinicopathologic study of 60 patients from Asia. Am J Surg Pathol 2015;39:1–12.

84. Kim TM, Lee SY, Jeon YK, et al. Clinical heterogeneity of extranodal NK/T-cell lymphoma, nasal type: a national survey of the Korean Cancer Study Group. Ann Oncol 2008;19:1477–84.

85. Suzuki R, Suzumiya J, Yamaguchi M, et al. Prognostic factors for mature natural killer (NK) cell neoplasms: aggressive NK cell leukemia and extranodal NK cell lymphoma, nasal type. Ann Oncol 2010;21:1032–40.

86. Choi Y-L, Park J-H, Namkung J-H, et al. Extranodal NK/T-cell lymphoma with cutaneous involvement: 'nasal' vs. 'nasal-type' subgroups – a retrospective study of 18 patients. Br J Dermatol 2009;160:333–7.

87. Massone C, Chott A, Metze D, et al. Subcutaneous blastic natural killer (NK), NK/T-cell, and other cytotoxic lymphomas of the skin. Am J Surg Pathol 2004;28:719–35.

88. Jang K-A, Choi J-H, Sung K-J, et al. Primary CD56+ nasal-type T/natural killer-cell subcutaneous panniculitic lymphoma: presentation as haemophagocytic syndrome. Br J Dermatol 1999;141:706–9.

89. Jia H, Sun T. Extranodal NK/T-cell lymphoma mimicking cellulitis. Leuk Lymphoma 2007;45:1467–70.

90. Chang S-E, Huh J, Choi J-H, et al. Clinicopathological features of CD56+ nasal-type T/natural killer cell lymphomas with lobular panniculitis. Br J Dermatol 2000;142:924–30.

91. Santucci M, Pimpinelli N, Massi D, et al. Cytotoxic/natural killer cell cutaneous lymphomas. Report of the EORTC Cutaneous Lymphoma Task Force Workshop. Cancer 2003;97:610–27.

92. Chan JKC, Quintanilla-Martinez L, Ferry JA, et al. Extranodal NK/T-cell lymphoma, nasal type. In: Swerdlow SH, Campo E, Harris N, et al, editors. WHO classification of tumors: pathology and genetics of tumors of hematopoietic and lymphoid tissues. Lyons (France): IARC Press; 2008. p. 285–8.

93. Pongruttipan T, Sukpanichnant S, Assanasen T, et al. Extranodal NK/T-cell lymphoma, nasal type, includes cases of natural killer cell and αβ, γδ, and αβ/γδ T-cell origin: a comprehensive clinicopathologic and phenotypic study. Am J Surg Pathol 2012;36:481–99.

# Cutaneous Pseudolymphoma

Christina Mitteldorf, MD[a],*, Werner Kempf, MD[b,c]

## KEYWORDS

- Cutaneous pseudolymphoma • T-cell • B-cell • Borreliosis • Tattoo • Histology

## Key Points

- Cutaneous pseudolymphoma (PSLs) are a heterogeneous group of lymphocyte-rich infiltrates, simulating clinically and/or histologically cutaneous lymphoma.
- Numerous causative agents can induce PSLs.
- Clinicopathologic correlation is essential to achieve the correct diagnosis.
- PSLs can be split based on clinical and/or histologic presentation into 4 groups.

## ABSTRACT

The term, *cutaneous pseudolymphoma (PSL)*, refers to a group of lymphocyte-rich infiltrates, which either clinically and/or histologically simulate cutaneous lymphomas. Clinicopathologic correlation is essential to achieve the final diagnosis in cutaneous PSL and to differentiate it from cutaneous lymphomas. A wide range of causative agents (eg, *Borrelia*, injections, tattoo, and arthropod bite) has been described. Based on clinical and/or histologic presentation, 4 main groups of cutaneous PSL can be distinguished: (1) nodular PSL, (2) pseudo–mycosis fungoides, (3) other PSLs (representing distinct clinical entities), and (4) intravascular PSL. The article gives an overview of the clinical and histologic characteristics of cutaneous PSLs.

## OVERVIEW

### DEFINITION

Cutaneous PSL refers to a group of skin diseases, which are defined as benign lymphoproliferative processes that clinically and/or histologically simulate cutaneous lymphomas. A wide range of causative agents (**Box 1**) has been described. Nevertheless a causative factor for PSL can often not be found. Those cases are referred to as idiopathic PSL.

## CLASSIFICATION

Various approaches have been proposed to categorize cutaneous PSL, for example, according to the cause, the predominating component in the lymphocytic infiltrate (T-cell, B-cell, or mixed), or distinct clinical features (reviewed by Rijlaarsdam and Willemze,[1] Ploysangam and colleagues,[2] and Gilliam and Wood[3]). In daily work, clinicians or pathologists encountering infiltrates suspicious as a PSL cannot recognize the cause and the phenotype at first glance without further diagnostic work-up. Moreover, the composition of the infiltrate is determined mostly by genetic and immunologic factors of the host rather than the causative agent per se, because the same agents can in many instances induce B-cell PSL (B-PSL) and T-cell PSL (T-PSL) as well.

From a practical point of view, cutaneous PSL can be split into 4 main groups based on clinical and/or histologic presentation:

1. Nodular PSL: solitary or multiple nodule(s), which resemble clinically and histologically lymphoma

Disclosure Statement: The authors have nothing to disclose.
[a] Department of Dermatology, HELIOS Klinikum Hildesheim, Senator-Braun-Allee 33, Hildesheim 31134, Germany; [b] Kempf & Pfaltz, Histologische Diagnostik, Seminarstrasse 1, 8057 Zürich, Zurich, Switzerland; [c] Department of Dermatology, University Hospital Zurich, Gloriastrassse 31, 8091 Zürich, Switzerland
* Corresponding author.
*E-mail address:* Christina.mitteldorf@helios-kliniken.de

Surgical Pathology 10 (2017) 455–476
http://dx.doi.org/10.1016/j.path.2017.01.002
1875-9181/17/

---

**Box 1**
**Causes of pseudolymphoma**

Infectious agents

Spirochetal bacteria (*Borrelia* species and *Treponema pallidum*), viruses (eg, herpesvirus species, *Molluscipoxvirus*, and HIV), parasites (eg, *Sarcoptes* mites)

Foreign agents

Tattoo dyes, injected vaccination, or allergen extracts for hyposensitization, piercing)

Other

Insect bites, drugs, and photosensitivity

---

2. Pseudo–mycosis fungoides (pseudo-MF): mimics mycosis fungoides predominately on histologic grounds
3. Other PSLs: distinct clinical entities, for example, acral papular angiokeratoma of childhood
4. Intravascular PSL

In addition, there are numerous infectious and noninfectious conditions characterized by a lymphocyte-rich infiltrate, which, therefore, are prone to be misinterpreted as cutaneous lymphoma primarily on histologic grounds.

## DIAGNOSTIC APPROACH

The clinical presentation of cutaneous PSL ranges from solitary nodule, clustered, or disseminated papules to erythroderma.[2,4] The histologic analysis plays a crucial role in the diagnostic approach to cutaneous PSL. Different infiltrate patterns (nodular vs epidermotropic infiltrates), the size of the lymphocytes (mostly small, occasionally medium-sized and large cells), immunophenotype (T cell vs B cell, CD4 vs CD8, and CD30) can be distinguished. Molecular studies for clonality and infectious agents, especially *Borrelia burgdorferi*, are adjunctive diagnostic tools. It is important to emphasize that the detection of a clonal T-cell or B-cell population per se does not indicate the presence of malignant lymphoma. Moreover, some PSL cases have been reported to harbor clonal T cells or B cells.[5–8] Thus, the histologic as well as the molecular findings always need to be interpreted in synopsis with the clinical context, that is, the clinicopathologic correlation is essential to achieve the final diagnosis.

The diagnostic work-up includes the medical history (in particular, exposure to arthropods, allergens, and exogenic material and drugs) and physical examination, including palpation of lymph nodes. Moreover, examination of peripheral blood

(differential blood count and serology for infectious agents, especially *Borrelia burgdorferi*, syphilis, and HIV – depending on the infiltrate type) is recommended. Because PSLs represent benign lymphocytic proliferations without the potential for extracutaneous spread, staging examination generally seems to be not indicated. Nevertheless, a clear allocation to cutaneous PSL and a safe exclusion of lymphoma (primary or secondary cutaneous) is often only possible in knowledge of the clinical behavior. Therefore, staging procedures (CT or PET-CT) should be considered, especially in cases of unusual manifestation (eg, multiple nodular lesions, monotypic expression of immunoglobulin (Ig) light chains, detection of T-cell or B-cell clonality, or other inconsistent or unexpected histologic, phenotypic, or genotypic findings).

## CLINICAL COURSE AND TREATMENT

The course of cutaneous PSL is variable. Some lesions show regression after biopsy, but many persist over several months or even years. Recurrences can be observed particularly after re-exposure to the inducing agent in cases induced by drugs or allergens. Progression of PSL has been reported but is a rare event, if it exists at all.[9]

If a causing agent has been identified, it should be removed, if possible. In general, solitary lesions can be treated by complete surgical excision. Alternative treatment options are topical or intralesional corticosteroids and cryotherapy. Especially in tattoo-induced PSL, laser treatment has been reported effective.[10] If those therapeutic approaches are not possible or successful, radiation therapy may be considered. In patients with multiple PSL lesions, in particular those with idiopathic multifocal PSL, systemic corticosteroids or intralesional or systemic interferon alpha[11] or oral hydroxychloroquine can be used.[12] Avoidance of re-exposure to the inducing agent (ie, vaccines, allergen injection, other drugs, *Hirudo medicinalis* treatment, acupuncture, and tattoo) is the most important step to preventing persistence and recurrence of PSL.

## NODULAR PSEUDOLYMPHOMA

Nodular PSL represents one of the most common forms of PSL. It is characterized by solitary or multiple nodules, simulating cutaneous T-cell or B-cell lymphomas on clinical and histologic grounds. Based on histology, nodular PSL can be classified according to the predominant lymphocytic subset into B-cell, T-cell, and mixed (T-cell/B-cell) PSL.[2,4]

This classification is somewhat artificial because B-PSL always contains T-cells and vice versa.

## CUTANEOUS B-CELL PSEUDOLYMPHOMA

B-PSL is often also referred as lymphocytoma cutis or cutaneous lymphoid hyperplasia.

### Clinical Findings

The localized form of B-PSL presents with a solitary nodule, measuring up to 4 cm in most of the cases. One-third of the patients develop multiple lesions (generalized form) either aggregated in clusters (agminated form) or as disseminated papules (miliarial form).

The face, especially the nose and the cheeks; the upper trunk; and the arms are the most commonly involved sites (Fig. 1A). A male-to-female ratio of 3:1 has been described.[13] Approximately two-thirds of patients with B-PSL are under the age of 40 years and less than 10% are children and adolescents[14] (Table 1).

### Histology

Nodular B-PSL is characterized by a dense nodular infiltrate, predominantly located in the reticular dermis and occasionally extending into the superficial parts of the subcutis (see Fig. 1B). The infiltrate is mostly composed of small lymphocytes with chromatin dense nuclei and reactive germinal centers (see Fig. 1C) containing tingible body macrophages. The lymphocytes do not show significant nuclear atypia. There is an admixture of diffusely scattered plasma cells. Sometimes admixed eosinophils and a granulomatous component can be observed. In a majority of B-PSL plasmacytoid dendritic cells (CD123+) are found, arranged in clusters with close vicinity to T cells and plasma cells.[15,16] There is an admixture of a variable number of T cells, which usually account for less than 30% of the infiltrate (see Table 1).

### Immunohistochemistry and Molecular Diagnostics

The majority of the infiltrate is represented by CD19+, CD20+, CD79a+, and PAX-5+ B cells. The cells in the reactive follicles express bcl-6 (see Fig. 1D) and are negative for bcl-2 (see Fig. 1E). The small B cells in the interfollicular area express bcl-2 but are negative for bcl-6. The networks of CD21+ follicular dendritic cells (FDCs) are sharply demarcated and regularly structured (see Fig. 1F). In Ki-67 or MIB-1 stain, the proliferative activity is elevated and mainly confined to the germinal centers. With a few exceptions, the expression of Ig light chains kappa and lambda by plasma cells are polytypic (immunohistochemistry or in situ hybridization) and no monoclonal rearrangement of Ig heavy chain genes by polymerase chain reaction (PCR) or Southern blot (see Table 1) is found.

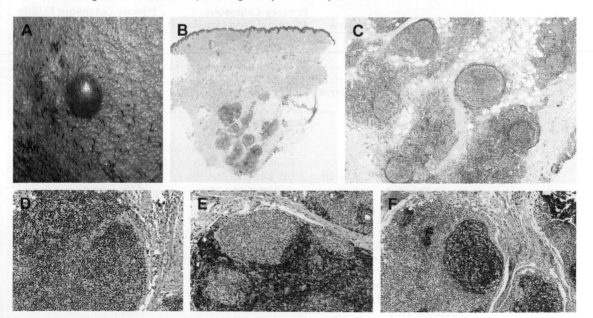

Fig. 1. B-PSL. (A) Erythematous nodule on the cheek. (B) Dense nodular infiltrate encompassing the deep dermis and superficial parts of the subcutis (hematoxylin-eosin, ×20). (C) Reactive germinal centers of different size (hematoxylin-eosin, ×100). The cells in reactive follicles express bcl-6 (D) (×200) and are negative for bcl-2 (E) (×200). (F) The networks of CD21+ FDCs are sharply restricted to the germinal centers (×200).

*Table 1*
**Clinical and histologic characteristics of B-cell pseudolymphoma**

| Clinical Characteristics | Histologic Characteristics | Immunohistochemistry |
|---|---|---|
| Male:female ratio 3:1 | Nodular infiltrate in the dermis and superficial parts of subcutis | |
| 75% <40 y | Small B cells, no nuclear atypia | CD5$^-$, CD20$^+$, CD23$^-$, CD43$^-$ |
| Face (especially nose and cheeks), upper trunk, arms | Reactive germinal centers | Follicle centers: bcl2$^-$, bcl6$^+$, well defined and regular structured networks of CD21$^+$ FDCs, elevated Ki-67 rate mostly confined to the germinal centers |
| | Tingible body macrophages | CD68$^+$ |
| | Scattered plasma cells | CD79a$^+$, CD138$^+$, no light chain restriction (kappa, lambda) |
| | Sometimes eosinophils | |
| | Admixed T cells at variable degree (commonly <30%) | CD3$^+$, CD4$^+$, and CD8$^+$ |
| | Small clusters of plasmacytoid dendritic cells | CD123$^+$ |

## Differential Diagnoses

The differential diagnosis of B-PSL primarily includes primary cutaneous marginal zone lymphoma (PCMZL) and primary cutaneous follicle center lymphoma (PCFCL) or their nodal or other extranodal counterparts presenting with secondary cutaneous infiltrates (Table 2).

PCMZL presents with nodular infiltrates in the reticular dermis and superficial subcutis.[17] In comparison with B-PSL, the plasma cells in PCMZL are

*Table 2*
**Differential diagnosis of B-cell pseudolymphoma**

| | B-Cell Pseudolymphoma | Primary Cutaneous Marginal Zone Lymphoma | Primary Cutaneous Follicle Center Lymphoma |
|---|---|---|---|
| Gender (female:male) | 3:1 | 1:2 | 1:1.5 |
| Age (y) | 75% < 40 | 55 | 51 |
| Localization | Face > upper trunk > arms | Upper trunk > upper arms > face/head | Head/face > upper trunk |
| Histology | Dermal/superficial subcutis, reactive germinal centers, tingible body macrophages, scattered plasma cells | Dermal/superficial subcutis, reactive germinal centers can be found, plasma cells in the periphery of the infiltates and near by the epidermis | Dermal/superficial subcutis, neoplastic irregular germinal centers of different size (CAVEAT: not found in diffuse type) |
| Immuno-histochemistry | CD20$^+$; reactive germinal centers (bcl-2$^-$, bcl-6$^+$); high proliferative activity in geminal centers (Ki-67 $^+$ or MIB-1$^+$), sharply restricted networks of FDCs (CD21$^+$) | Tumor cells: CD20$^+$ bcl-2$^+$; bcl-6$^-$, CD5$^-$, CD10$^-$, CD43$^-$; reactive germinal centers (bcl-2$^-$, bcl-6$^+$) | Tumor cells: CD20$^+$, bcl-6$^+$; bcl-2$^-$ (90%); neoplastic germinal centers (bcl-2$^-$, bcl-6$^+$); proliferating cells (Ki-67$^+$ or MIB-1$^+$) are scattered; irregular networks of FDCs (CD21$^+$) |
| Molecular diagnostics | Polytypic light chains, polyclonal IgH | Monoclonal IgH (up to 90%) | Monotypic light chain (85%) monoclonal IgH (60%–70%) |

usually more prominent and found in sheets, particularly at the periphery of the infiltrates and near by the epidermis.[18] The most important histopathologic diagnostic finding is the monotypic expression of Ig light chains (lambda or kappa) in PCMZL with a ratio of at least 5:1 or 10:1. The presence and number of eosinophils are not useful findings for discrimination between both entities. In 50% to 70% of PCMZL a clonal B-cell population can be detected and used as an additional diagnostic hint.

PCFCL is characterized by the predominance of centrocyte-like differentiated tumor cells arranged in large neoplastic follicles. Tingible body macrophages are only found in small minority of PCFCL.[19] Furthermore, a low proliferative activity in the neoplastic follicles of PCFCL is a characteristic finding, which contrasts with the high proliferative activity in the reactive germinal centers of B-PSL. The networks of CD21[+] FDCs in PCFCL are irregular and disrupted in contrast to the sharply demarcated and regularly structured networks in B-PSL. A clonal B-cell population is detectable in the majority of PCFCL by PCR or Southern blot. A vast majority of PCFCLs do not show expression of bcl-2 by the neoplastic centrocyte-like differentiated cells. Therefore, the expression of bcl-2 is not of diagnostic value for the discrimination of PCFCL from B-PSL. In cases of expression of bcl-2 by the centrocyte-like tumor cells, secondary cutaneous infiltration by a nodal FCL has to be considered because nodal FCL exhibits expression of bcl-2 by the neoplastic cells due to underlying t(14;18) translocation in a majority of the cases.

Other differential diagnoses include cutaneous infiltrates of B-cell chronic lymphocytic leukemia (CD5[+], CD23[+], and CD43[+]) or small cell lymphocytic lymphoma, although the latter one do usually not show reactive germinal centers.[20,21]

Clonality studies in B-PSL are of limited value in the distinction from cutaneous B-cell lymphomas because approximately 10% to 20% of PSL harbor a clonal B-population.[6,22] In some studies, even a higher percentage of cases of clonal B cells was detected in nodular PSL.[23] In lesions with subtle infiltrates, pseudoclonality should always be ruled out because it represents a diagnostic pitfall.[24]

## BORRELIA-ASSOCIATED B-CELL PSEUDOLYMPHOMA

Lymphocytoma cutis and lymphadenosis cutis benigna often are synonymously used. The diagnosis is based on histology, the clinical context (history of tick bite and localization at predilection site), serologic findings, and/or detection of Borrelia burgdorferi species DNA in the tissue by PCR.

### Clinical Findings

Approximately 1% of clinically apparent Borrelia species infections manifest as B-PSL. A slight female preponderance is observed in some but not all studies.[8] This form of B-PSL has more often been reported in white than in African Americans. Borrelia-associated B-PSL affects typically children and occurs in early adulthood but may be seen in all age groups.[14]

Usually Borrelia-associated B-PSL presents with a solitary red to violaceous nodule. In 10% to 15% of the patients, multifocal skin lesions can be observed. The earlobes (**Fig. 2**A), nipples, and scrotum are the predilection sites, but the trunk and extremities may also be involved.[8]

### Histology

A dense dermal nodular infiltrate of small B cells and reactive germinal centers is found[8] (see **Fig. 2**B). In Borrelia-associated B-PSL, the germinal centers tend to be larger and confluent with only a small or completely lost mantle zone[8] (see **Fig. 2**B). A lack of polarization is found in up to 20% of the cases.[8,22] Due to the confluence of the large germinal centers, the lesions resemble the neoplastic follicles in PCFCL (follicular growth pattern).[22] Tingible body macrophages are found in all cases (see **Fig. 2**C). Plasma cells are almost always present and found particularly at the periphery of the infiltrates. Eosinophils are often admixed. Colli and colleagues[8] provide an overview of histologic findings in Borrelia-associated PSL, summarized in **Box 2**.

In rare cases of so-called large cell lymphocytoma associated with Borrelia infection, a predominance of large blasts, resembling centroblasts and immunoblasts, are found simulating the findings in large B-cell lymphoma.[25] Therefore, those cases are prone to be misdiagnosed as diffuse large B-cell lymphoma.

### Immunohistochemistry and Molecular Diagnostics

Immunohistochemically, the typical findings of B-PSL are found (discussed previously). Molecular studies for the detection of Borrelia burgdorferi species DNA by PCR are a helpful adjunctive diagnostic tool with a sensitivity of approximately 70%.[26] In a vast majority of the cases of Borrelia-associated B-PSL, molecular studies show a polyclonal rearrangement of IgH genes, but detection of monoclonal B cells has been observed and, therefore, does not exclude this diagnosis.[8] The

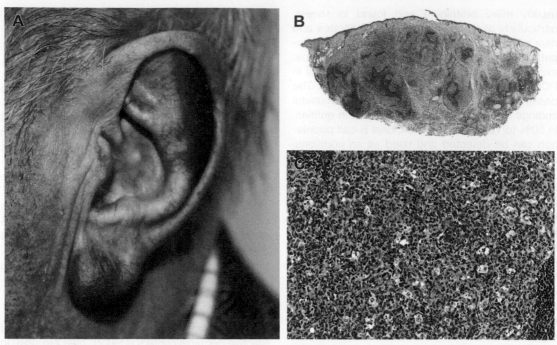

**Fig. 2.** *Borrelia*-associated B-PSL. (*A*) Blue nodule at the earlobe. (*B*) Dense dermal nodular infiltrate with reactive germinal centers with small or completely lost mantle zones (hematoxylin-eosin, ×20). (*C*) Germinal centers with multiple tingible body macrophages (hematoxylin-eosin, ×200).

light chains are predominately polyclonal, but a few cases of monoclonal Ig light chains have been reported.[27]

## Laboratory Tests

Serology shows antibodies against *Borrelia burgdorferi* species with variable pattern, that is, IgG and/or IgM may be elevated. Nevertheless, cases of negative serologic findings can be seen[8] so that negative serology does not exclude *Borrelia*-induced B-PSL.

---

**Box 2**
**Histologic findings in *Borrelia*-associated B-cell pseudolymphoma**

Mostly the entire dermis is involved

Grenz zone, epidermal component in approximately 10%

High number of admixed T cells

Germinal centers (77%), often large and confluent

Absence of mantle zone (88%)

Tingible body macrophages (100%)

Plasma cells (99%)

Eosinophils (84%)

---

## PSEUDOLYMPHOMA T-CELL AND MIXED PSEUDOLYMPHOMA

Nodular T-PSL is characterized by a dense dermal T-cell–rich nodular infiltrate, which is accompanied by variable number of B cells, which can reach up to 30% of the entire infiltrate.[28] Mixed forms of PSL contain an equal number of T cells and B cells. All causes identified in B-PSL can also be found as underlying stimuli in T-PSL and mixed PSL. Most cases, however, are without known cause and, therefore, are referred to as idiopathic T-PSL or mixed PSL.

## Clinical Findings

T-PSL and mixed PSL usually present with a solitary or multiple red to violaceous nodules similar to B-PSL (**Fig. 3**A). There are no detailed epidemiologic data on the prevalence of T-PSL or mixed PSL. They affect patients of both genders and all age and ethnic groups.

## Histology

In most cases, a dense nodular infiltrate in the entire dermis and in the superficial parts of the subcutis is found (see **Fig. 3**B). The infiltrate is predominantly composed of small lymphocytes with chromatin dense nuclei. A variable number of slightly enlarged lymphocytes with chromatin

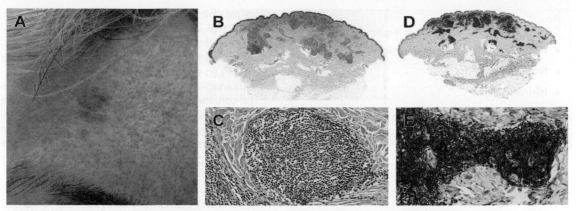

**Fig. 3.** Nodular T-PSL. (*A*) Solitary red flat nodule on the forehead. (*B*) Dense nodular wedge shaped infiltrate in the entire dermis (hematoxylin-eosin, ×20). (*C*) Variable number of slightly enlarged lymphocytes with chromatin dense nuclei (hematoxylin-eosin, ×200). (*D*) CD4⁺ expression in a majority of the small lymphocytes (hematoxylin-eosin, ×20); (*E*) detail (hematoxylin-eosin, ×200).

dense nuclei can be seen (see **Fig. 3**C). There is an admixture of a variable number of eosinophils, histiocytes, and plasma cells. The B cells can be arranged in small aggregates, but germinal centers are only rarely found. Granuloma formation can be observed. There may be exocytosis of T-lymphocytes into the epithelia of the hair follicles, but usually there is no significant exocytosis of lymphocytes into the overlying interfollicular epidermis.

## Immunohistochemistry and Molecular Diagnostics

A majority of the small lymphocytes belongs to CD4⁺ CD30⁻ T cells in most cases (see **Fig. 3**D, E). A few activated CD30⁺ lymphocytes can be admixed. The number of admixed B-lymphocytes is variable.

Clonality studies reveal a polyclonal infiltrate in a majority of T-PSL, but PSL with clonal T-cells have been reported and referred to as so-called clonal PSL. Some of those cases may progress to overt lymphoma and may present very early stages of lymphoma genesis rather than genuine PSLs.

## Differential Diagnosis

Differential diagnosis of nodular T-PSL and mixed PSL includes cutaneous CD4⁺ small/medium-sized T-cell lymphoma/lymphoproliferative disorder (LPD) (World Health Organization [WHO] classification 2008/2016), which shows overlapping histologic and immunophenotypic features.[29,30] The latter also presents usually with a solitary lesion located mostly on the head and neck area and shows an indolent course. Because nodular T-PSL and cutaneous CD4⁺ small/medium-sized T-cell lymphoma/LPD cannot be

distinguished with certainty either on clinical nor on histopathologic or phenotypic features, some investigators consider them to represent the same process. Therefore, the encompassing term, cutaneous CD4⁺ small/medium sized T-cell LPD, has been introduced in the updated WHO classification 2016 to emphasize the indolent nature of this process. The expression of PD-1 originally thought to be a discriminative marker is not of diagnostic value in this setting.

Nodular T-PSL should be differentiated from MF in tumor stage. MF in tumor stage presents more often with medium-sized T-cells with atypia. Eosinophils are often admixed and, therefore, are not helpful to differentiate it from T-PSL. A monoclonal T-cell receptor (TCR) rearrangement is a common finding in tumor stage MF. Nevertheless, the most important distinction criterion is the clinical presentation with patches and plaques preceding the tumors in MF. The differential diagnosis further includes secondary cutaneous infiltrates, for example, of angioimmunoblastic T-cell lymphoma (AITL). In AITL, small CD4⁺ and PD-1⁺ T cells are accompanied by a significant number of B cells. The clinical context with B symptoms, serologic findings, the nodal involvement shown by radiologic staging examinations, a high proliferation rate in AITL infiltrates, and the association with Epstein-Barr virus in some of the cases of AITL are useful findings for the distinction of AITL from nodular T-PSL. In the authors' experience, sometimes primary cutaneous marginal zone lymphoma with an unusual high number of admixed T cells (>50%) can be observed, which are challenging to differentiate from T-PSL.

Among inflammatory skin disorders, lupus erythematosus (in particular the tumid type) has to be considered, which also can present with dense dermal lymphocytic infiltrates. Mucin deposits might be helpful in this context. Vacuolization at the interface of the epidermis and the hair follicle epithelium is not found in tumid type of lupus erythematosus.

## CD30⁺ T-CELL PSEUDOLYMPHOMA

CD30⁺ PSL represent a histologic subtype of T-cell PSL of the skin, which is characterized by the presence of medium-sized to large atypical CD30⁺ T cells.[31,32] This has been reported in the context various infections and other diseases (**Box 3**).[31,33,34]

In CD30⁺ PSL, immunohistochemistry shows medium-sized to large CD30⁺ blastlike cells usually found as single units scattered throughout the infiltrate (**Fig. 4**). The infiltrate is otherwise dominated by small T cells. In some cases, the underlying disease (eg, molluscum contagiosum) could be identified. A significant number of B cells

and plasma cells argue for a reactive process. CD30⁺ PSL does not harbor a clonal T-cell population in most of the cases.

As differential diagnosis, lymphomatoid papulosis (LYP) (in particular histologic type A) and cutaneous anaplastic large cell lymphoma (ALCL) have to be considered. In contrast to LYP and ALCL, the CD30⁺ cells in CD30⁺ PSL are usually not arranged in aggregates as in LYP and ALCL. Helpful histologic criteria to differentiate CD30⁺ PSL from CD30⁺ lymphoproliferative disease are given in **Table 3**.

## PSEUDO-MYCOSIS FUNGOIDES—HISTOLOGIC SIMULATORS OF MYCOSIS FUNGOIDES

The term pseudo-MF describes a group of disorders of different etiology, which histologically mimic MF. The clinicopathologic correlation is crucial to avoid misinterpretation.

### HISTOLOGY

Pseudo-MF is characterized by a bandlike (**Fig. 5**) or perivascular infiltrate of mostly small lymphocytes, which show exocytosis into the epidermis (see **Fig. 5**) and may exhibit subtle nuclear atypia thereby simulating epidermotropic cutaneous T-cell lymphoma.

### IMMUNOHISTOCHEMISTRY

A Predominance of CD4⁺ or CD8⁺ cells can be found. In addition, a variable expression of CD30 can be seen in some cases of pseudo-MF. As in other forms of PSL, the lymphocytes are polyclonal in a majority of cases. In some diseases, such as

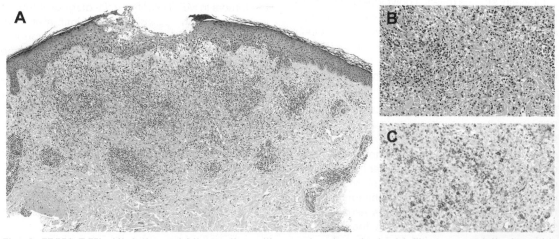

**Fig. 4.** CD30⁺ T-PSL. (*A*) Arthropod bite reaction with a wedge shaped mixed infiltrate, spongiotic dermatitis, and papillary edema (hematoxylin-eosin, ×40). (*B*) The infiltrate consists of lymphocytes, histiocytes, and eosinophils. A few (immuno-) blastlike cells are admixed (hematoxylin-eosin, ×200). (*C*) These cells were positive for CD30 (×200).

**Table 3**
**Histologic criteria to differentiate a neoplastic and reactive CD30$^+$ infiltrate**

|  | Neoplastic | Reactive |
|---|---|---|
| Number of CD30$^+$ cells | Often higher number | Lower number |
| Arrangement | Little clusters or sheets | More scattered distribution as single units |
| CD30 staining intensity | Often more intensive | Often weak |
| Composition of the infiltrate | Depending on the type of CD30$^+$ LPD (eg, in LYP type A: mixed infiltrate with many histiocytes, ALCL: predominantly CD30$^+$ cells arranged in sheets) | Higher number of admixed B cells and plasma cells |

pityriasis lichenoides et varioliformis acuta, clonal T cells are found in a significant percentage but do not indicate malignancy or a risk for progression to lymphoma.

## DIFFERENTIAL DIAGNOSES

Most important differential diagnoses include MF and Sézary syndrome. In cases of predominantly CD8$^+$ infiltrate, CD8$^+$ MF, cutaneous CD8$^+$ aggressive epidermotropic cytotoxic T-cell lymphoma, and primary cutaneous LYP (types D and E) should be considered. Profound nuclear atypia, predominance of medium-sized to large cells, loss of pan T-cell markers, and monoclonal rearrangement of TCR genes, are findings in favor of cutaneous T-cell lymphoma. The diagnosis of Sézary syndrome can be excluded by blood analysis.

### Lymphomatoid Contact Dermatitis

Lymphomatoid contact dermatitis (LCD) is a chronic contact dermatitis, which histologically simulates MF.[35]

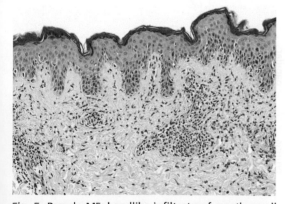

*Fig. 5.* Pseudo-MF: bandlike infiltrate of mostly small lymphocytes with exocytosis into the epidermis. Many admixed eosinophils in the upper dermis (H&E, original magnification ×100).

Clinically, LCD presents with eczematous and pruritic papules, patches or plaques. In rare cases, erythroderma can be found. LCD occurs mostly in adults and affects both genders.

Histologically, there is a superficial bandlike infiltrate with variable exocytosis of lymphocytes into the spongiotic epidermis. Intra-epidermal accumulations of Langerhans cells (so called pseudo-Pautrier collections) can be found. A mild atypia of the lymphocytes has been described. Eosinophils are generally admixed. The ratio of CD4$^+$ to CD8$^+$ lymphocytes is balanced. An admixture of slightly enlarged activated CD30$^+$ cells may be observed. For differential diagnoses, see **Table 4**.

### Lymphomatoid Drug Reaction

Apart from its nodular form, drug-related PSL clinically more commonly presents with macular or papular eruptions.[2,36]

Histologically, in lymphomatoid drug reaction, a bandlike infiltrate in the upper dermis with variable degree of exocytosis of lymphocytes is found.[37] Vacuolar alteration at the dermoepidermal junction and apoptotic keratinocytes may be present. Eosinophils are commonly found but also may be absent. Immunohistochemistry reveals either a predominance of CD4$^+$ or CD8$^+$ lymphocytes and admixture of a variable number of CD30$^+$ lymphocytes.[38] Loss of pan T-cell markers is not observed. The differential diagnoses are given in **Table 4**.

### Actinic Reticuloid

Actinic reticuloid is a chronic multifactorial dermatitis with severe photosensitivity, which histologically mimics epidermotropic cutaneous T-cell lymphoma.[39]

Clinically, actinic reticuloid affects mostly middle-aged and older men.[40] It presents with persistent erythematous lichenoid papules and plaques on light-exposed skin areas, particularly

*Table 4*
Clinical and histologic characteristics of T-cell pseudolymphoma and their differential diagnoses

| | Lymphomatoid Contact Dermatitis | Lymphomatoid Drug Reaction | Actinic Reticuloid | CD8+ T-cell Pseudolymphoma in Immunodefiency | Borrelia-Associated T-cell Pseudolymphoma | Papuloerythroderma of Ofuji | Mycosis Fungoides | Sézary Syndrome |
|---|---|---|---|---|---|---|---|---|
| Mean age | Adults | Adults | Middle and older age | NA | 60 | 70 | 55–60 | Adults |
| Gender | Male = female | NA | Male >> female | NA | Male = female | Male > female | Male > female | Male > female |
| Prediliction sites | Areas exposed to the allergen(s) | Variable, generalized | Face, neck | Generalized | Lower limb > trunk | Generalized, especially trunk and limbs | Initial skin lesions: buttocks and other sun-protected areas | Generalized |
| Clinical picture | Eczematous and pruritic papules, patches or plaques | Rush, macular-papular eruptions | In sun exposed areas: persistent erythematous lichenoid papules and plaques, facies leonina | Variable: plaques -> erythroderma, palmoplantar hyperkeratosis, lymphadenopathie | Variable: erythema chronicum migrans, acrodermatitis chronica atrophicans, MF-like, lichenoid aspect | Itchy flat topped red to brownisch papules, erythoderma with (deck chair sign), palmoplantar hyperkeratosis, lymphadenopathy | Patch, plaques and tumors (depending on the stage) | Erythroderma, palmoplantar hyperkeratosis, enlarged lymph nodes |
| Histology | Superficial bandlike infiltrate, spongiosis, pseudo-Pautrier collections, eosinophils | Superficial, bandlike, eosinohils | Psoriasiform hyperplasia, mild spongiosis, eosinophils, coarsed and vertically arranged collagen bundles in the papillary dermis | Superficial and mid-dermal infiltrate, no atypia | Bandlike or deep, lichenoid aspect, lymphocytes, histiocytes (pseudorosettes), variable number of plasma cells | Pattern of chronic dermatitis with a variable epidermal hyperplasia with mild spongiosis and a mixed inflammatory infiltrate, predominately consist of lymphocytes, histiocytes and eosinophils | Lining up, Pautrier collections, atypia, eosinophils are uncommon in patch MF | Often unspecific, epiderotropism may be absent, often only mild atypia |

|  |  |  |  |  |  |  |  |  |
|---|---|---|---|---|---|---|---|---|
| Immunohistochemistry | CD4 = CD8, sometimes admixed larger CD30+ cells | CD4 or CD8 predominance, admixed CD30+ cells. Caveat: loss pf pan-T-cell markers is possible | CD8+ | CD8+, TIA-1, granzyme B | CD4+ | CD4 = CD8 | CD4+ or CD8+ or CD4−/CD8−, loss of pan T-cell markers, admixed CD30+ cells possible | CD4+, PD-1+, TOX+ |
| Molecular diagnostics (tissue) | TCR mostly polyclonal | TCR mostly polyclonal | TCR mostly polyclonal | TCR mostly polyclonal | TCR mostly polyclonal | TCR mostly polyclonal | TCR monoclonal up to 90% | Blood involvement |
| Additional findings | Identification of allergen (patch test) |  | Increased number of circulating CD8+ cells in the peripheral blood, photosensitivity | HIV with deep immunosuppression, other type of immunosuppression, often monoclonal cells in peripheral blood | Detection of Borrelia burgdorferi PCR, serology | Blood eosinophilia | Blood involvement (see criteria of International Society for Cutaneous Lymphomas) |  |

*Abbreviation:* NA, not available.

on the face and neck, in some patients with a facies leonina–like aspect. Progression into erythroderma can be observed. Lichenification and erosions usually occur over time. The skin lesions are accompanied by intense pruritus.

Histologically, actinic reticuloid shows a psoriasiform hyperplasia of the epidermis with slight spongiosis. The cornified layer is compact orthokeratotic with focal parakeratosis. In the dermis, a predominating superficial perivascular infiltrate composed of small lymphocytes, eosinophils, and plasma cells is found. Coarse bundles of collagen arranged in vertical streaks are found in the papillary dermis. Multinucleated fibroblasts may be present. The lymphocytes may show slightly atypical nuclei and exocytosis into the overlying epidermis. Immunohistochemistry reveals a predominance of CD8+ T cells.[41]

In the peripheral blood, an increased number of CD8+ T cells (reversed CD4:CD8 ratio) is characteristic for actinic reticuloid, particularly in erythrodermic patients.[40] The atypical circulating lymphocytes show indented nuclei. For differential diagnosis, see **Table 4**.

## CD8+ T-Cell Pseudolymphoma in Immunodeficiency

In patients with immunodeficiency, in particular HIV infections, infiltrates of CD8+ lymphocytes mimicking MF or Sézary syndrome may rarely develop. In HIV, most of the patients are deeply immunosuppressed (CD4+ count <50/mm$^3$) and have a high HIV-RNA load.[42] This condition seems not to be exclusively limited to patients with HIV infection, because similar features were recently described in a renal transplant recipient.[43]

Clinically, a variety of clinical presentations were described. Often erythematous, infiltrated cutaneous plaques with progression to erythroderma have been observed[44–46]; in addition, palmoplantar hyperkeratosis could be found with generalized lympadenopathy. These

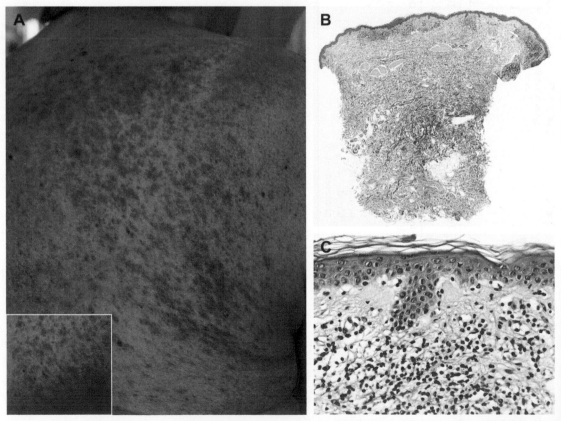

**Fig. 6.** *Borrelia*-associated T-PSL. (*A*) Multiple lichenoid red-brownish maculae and flat papules on the back, detail (*inset*). (*B*) Superficial bandlike lymphocytic infiltrate (hematoxylin-eosin, ×20). (*C*) The infiltrate predominately consists about T-lymphocytes with a few admixed plasma cells. Vacular alteration of the junctional zone (hematoxylin-eosin, ×200).

eruptions can, therefore, clinically mimic Sézary syndrome. Some investigators reported a worsening of skin symptoms after ultraviolet light exposure.

Histologically, a superficial and sometimes mid-dermal infiltrate is found, consisting of small lymphocytes without nuclear atypia. Eosinophils are admixed. Immunophenotyping shows a predominance of CD3+ and CD8+ lymphocytes, with expression of cytotoxic markers (granzyme B and T-cell–restricted intracellular antigen [TIA-1]). Molecular studies revealed the polyclonal skin infiltrate but often monoclonal cells in the peripheral blood.[42] The differential diagnosis is given in **Table 4**.

### Borrelia-Associated T-Cell Pseudolymphoma

Recently *Borrelia burgdorferi* species infection with T cell–rich pseudolymphomatous infiltrates has been reported.[47]

Clinically, *Borrelia*-associated T-PSL can resemble MF, sometimes a lichenoid aspect is evident (**Fig. 6**A). Other clinical presentations included the typical findings of erythema migrans or acrodermatitis chronica atrophicans. *Borrelia*-serology and detection of *Borrelia* in the skin infiltrate by PCR are necessary to confirm the diagnosis.

Histologically, the dermal T-cell infiltrate is either bandlike (sometimes with vacuolar interface

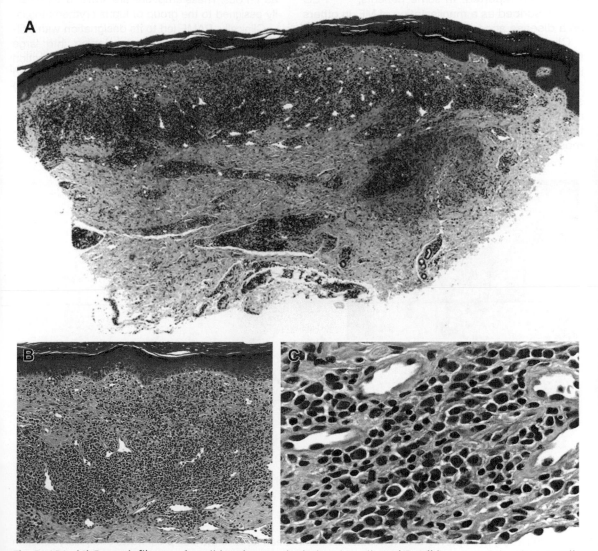

*Fig. 7.* APA. (*A*) Dense infiltrate of small lymphocytes (polyclonal T cells and B cells), eosinophils, plasma cells, and histiocytes, and sometime histiocytic giant cells is found (hematoxylin-eosin, ×20). (*B, C*) Thick-walled vessels lined by plump endothelia, surrounded by plasma cells (hematoxylin-eosin, ×100; detail: hematoxylin-eosin, ×200).

dermatitis) (see **Fig. 6**B) or diffuse. The infiltrate displays focal epidermotropism with lining up of lymphocytes along the junctional zone (see **Fig. 6**C). In addition, a minor interstitial histiocytic component of the infiltrate can be observed. Sometimes histiocytic pseudorosettes are found. The number of admixed plasma cells is variable.[47] For differential diagnosis, see **Table 4**.

### Papuloerythroderma Ofuji

Papuloerythroderma of Ofuji (PEO) is a rare pruritic erythrodermic dermatosis, which clinically may simulate cutaneous T-cell lymphoma.[48] Association with drugs, Hodgkin lymphoma, visceral malignancies, and immunodeficiency syndromes have been reported. In some patients,[49,50] PEO was described as a manifestation of MF, in others as a disease accompanying MF.[51]

Clinically, PEO manifests with generalized itchy flat topped red to brownish papules. The axillae, inguinal regions, antecubital and popliteal fossae, and big furrows on the abdomen are typically spared (so-called deck chair sign).[52] The median age is 70 years. It occurs more frequently in men than in women. Blood eosinophilia is detected in most of the patients.

Histologically, PEO resembles chronic dermatitis, with a variable epidermal hyperplasia with mild spongiosis and a mixed inflammatory infiltrate, predominately consisting of lymphocytes, histiocytes and eosinophils.[53] In approximately 10%, plasma cells are admixed.[50] Immunohistochemistry shows numerous dendritic cells and mature CD4[+] T cells in the dermis. For differential diagnosis, see **Table 4**.

### Lymphocytic Infiltration of the Skin and Palpable Arciforme Migratory Erythema

Jessner-Kanof lymphocytic infiltration of the skin (LIS) and palpable arciform migratory erythema (PAME) have been regarded by some investigators as T-PSLs. These eruptions are nowadays primarily assigned to the group of lupus erythematosus.

Clinically, PAME led to its designation with infiltrated annular erythema developing into large migrating lesions.[54] The trunk is the predilection site. LIS is characterized by sharply demarked often symmetric infiltrated plaques, which typically occur on the face.[55]

Histologically, the findings are similar in PAME and LIS. Both shows dense perivascular and periadnexal predominantly lymphocytic infiltrate.[56]

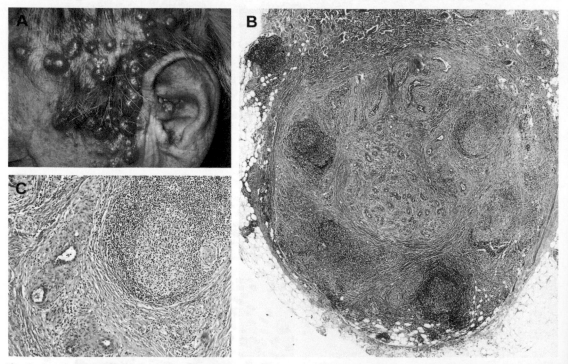

*Fig. 8.* ALHE. (*A*) Multiple red-brown nodules around the ear. (*B*) Circumscribed proliferates of capillary vessels in the deep dermis and superficial subcutis. These vessels are surrounded by a dense lymphocytic infiltrate with reactive germinal centers (hematoxylin-eosin, ×40). (*C*) The vessels show prominent endothelia with typical vacuolization. The vessels are surrounded by a dense lymphocytic infiltrate, consisting eosinophils and plasma cell. Reactive germinal centers (hematoxylin-eosin, ×200).

Many investigators reported that interstitial mucin deposits are absent. Immunohistochemistry reveals an infiltrate dominated by T cells with admixture of B cells and histiocytes. The lymphocytes are polyclonal. Phenotypically, the infiltrate in LIS is mostly composed of CD8+ lymphocytes.[57]

## Infections as Simulators of Lymphomas

Various infections, in particular those caused by viruses and parasites, may show dense lymphocyte-rich infiltrates and thereby simulating a lymphoma.

Cutaneous leishmaniasis can histologically simulates lymphoma and, therefore, can be difficult to diagnose, especially in cases of a low number of parasites. The infiltrate is composed of numerous lymphocytes, histiocytes, and plasma cells.[58] The detection of the agents is essential to making a correct diagnosis. Molecular studies demonstrate that a PCR diagnostic is helpful to identify the agent if it cannot be identified by conventional histology or special stains, for example, in Giemsa stain alone.[59]

In infections with herpes simplex virus and varicella zoster virus, occasionally lymphocyte-rich infiltrates without the pathognomonic epithelial changes can be observed and have been referred to as herpes incognito.[60] Lymphocytes with slightly enlarged and atypical-appearing chromatin dense nuclei as well as enlarged CD30+ lymphocytes may be found. Those infiltrates are prone to be misinterpreted as lymphoma. Detection of viral antigens by immunohistochemistry and/or detection of viral DNA by PCR allow identifying those infiltrates as herpesvirus-related T-cell reactions.[60]

Parapoxvirus infections may induce cytomorphological changes and expression of CD30 by

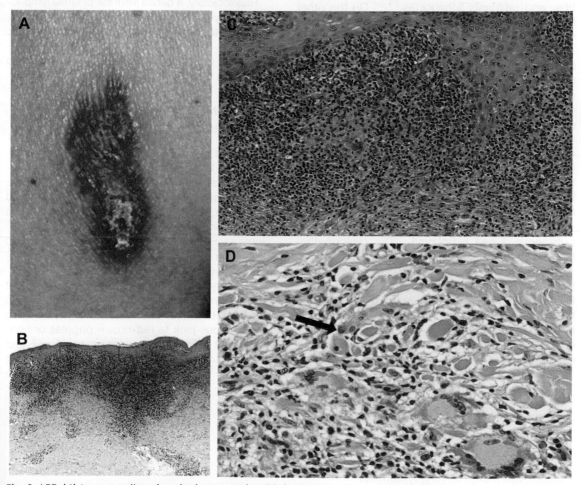

*Fig. 9.* LPP. (*A*) Longstanding sharply demarcated reddish plaque with scaling. (*B*) Epidermal hyperplasia with a bandlike and superficial perivascular infiltrate (hematoxylin-eosin, ×100). (*C*) The infiltrate consists of lymphocytes, histiocytes, and plasma cells (hematoxylin-eosin, ×200). (*D*) Interstitial histiocytic granulomas around sclerotic collagen bundles (so-called pseudorosettes [*arrow*]) (hematoxylin-eosin, ×400).

the infiltrating T cells, which make distinction from pleomorphic lymphocytes in the context of CD30-LPDs challenging.[31,32] The presence of epithelial changes with inclusion bodies typical for parapox-virus infection, absence of loss of T-cell markers, and lack of monoclonal rearrangement of TCR gamma genes are diagnostic hints to distinguish those infiltrates from cutaneous T-cell lymphoma, in particular CD30[+] LPDs. The diagnosis is based on the detection of the virus by immunohistochem-istry, electron microscopy or PCR.

## Inflammatory Disorders as Simulators of T-Cell Lymphoma

Various disorders, especially diseases with inter-face dermatitis, are prone to be misinterpreted as epidermotropic cutaneous T-cell lymphoma. These disorders include lichen planus, lichen scle-rosus et atrophicus, pigmented purpuric derma-titis, and pityriasis lichenoides.[61–64] On the other hand, MF can sometimes present with an interface dermatitis.

Clonal T-cell populations have been found in some cases in the inflammatory skin conditions (discussed previously), for example, in lichen pla-nus and lichen sclerosus et atrophicans, in which clonal T cells were found in 6% and 13% of the cases, respectively. Remarkably, a monoclonal rearrangement of TCR genes is commonly found in pityriasis lichenoides harboring clonal T cells in up to 60% of the cases.[62,65] The significance of these T cell clones is unclear. As a consequence, for the diagnostic work-up of lymphocyte-rich infil-trates, detection of a clonal T-cell population cannot be used as a sufficient finding to diagnose cutaneous T-cell lymphoma.[7] The clinicopatho-logic correlation is essential.

Furthermore, inflammatory diseases with lymphocyte-rich dermal and/or subcutaneous in-filtrates, such as lupus erythematosus, in particular the tumid type and lupus panniculitis, have to be differentiated from cutaneous T-cell lymphoma, in particular subcutaneous panniculitis-like T-cell lymphoma.

## OTHER PSEUDOLYMPHOMA (ALPHABETICAL ORDER)

### ACRAL PSEUDOLYMPHOMATOUS ANGIOKERATOMA

Acral pseudolymphomatous angiokeratoma (APA) has originally been described as occurring in children (original name, APA of childhood [APACHE]), but it has been shown to also affect adults.[66–68] Some investigators consider the le-sions to represent persistent arthropod bite re-actions, whereas others categorize APA a benign vascular process with a prominent lym-phocytic infiltrate, that is, a form of cutaneous PSL.[66,68]

Clinically, APA manifests as a unilateral eruption of clustered red to violaceous angiomatous pap-ules (diameter 1–5 mm) on acral sites, that is, hands and feet[66] (Fig. 7A).

Histologically, a dense infiltrate of small lympho-cytes (polyclonal T cells and B cells), eosinophils, plasma cells, histiocytes, and sometime histiocytic giant cells is found (see Fig. 7B). Within the infil-trate there are thick-walled vessels lined by plump endothelia (see Fig. 7C).

### ANGIOLYMPHOID HYPERPLASIA WITH EOSINOPHILIA

Nowadays angiolymphoid hyperplasia with eosin-ophilia (ALHE) is commonly as an angioprolifera-tive process due to the presence of prominent, bizarrely shaped blood vessels and epithelioid endothelia, leading to its alternative synonymous designation as epithelioid hemangioma.[69,70] Some investigators consider ALHE a hyperplastic process in response to tissue damage and forma-tion of vascular shunts.

Clinically, ALHE affect both genders without gender predominance.[70] Most patients are in the third or fourth decade. ALHE presents as angiomatous pink to red-brown papules or nod-ules most commonly found on the head and neck, especially on the face and ears (Fig. 8A)

---

**Box 4**
**Differential diagnosis of lymphoplasmacytoid plaque**

Cutaneous plasmocytosis

Lymphocytoma cutis

Cutaneous marginal zone lymphoma

Primary and secondary cutaneous plasmacytoma

Infections (eg, fungal, mycobacterial, and spirochetal)

but also occurring at the extremities and genital area.

Histologically, there are dermal proliferates of capillary vessels with prominent endothelia (see Fig. 8B), which presented typical cytoplasmic vacuoles (see Fig. 8C). These vessels are surrounded by a dense lymphocytic infiltrate with reactive germinal centers (see Fig. 8B) and eosinophils (see Fig. 8C).[71] By immunohistochemistry the endothelial cells were positive for CD31 and ERG but negative for podoplanin/D2-40. A majority of lymphocytes are of T-cell lineage. Admixed B cells may form lymphoid follicles. Clonal T cells have been detected.[72,73]

## CUTANEOUS PLASMOCYTOSIS

Cutaneous plasmocytosis is a rare disease, which has been reported in Asian countries, especially Japan. It mostly affects adults.[74,75] It is characterized by multiple brownish small plaques and nodules occurring all over the body. Histology shows dermal infiltrates composed predominantly of mature polyclonal plasma cells.[74,75] In some patients signs of a systemic involvement (eg, lymphadenopathy, hepatospenomegaly, hypergammaglobulinemia, increased levels of interleukin 6 in the serum, and elevated erythrocyte sedimentation rate) can be present.

## LYMPHOPLASMACYTIC PLAQUE

Lymphoplasmacytic plaque (LPP) is a recently described rare skin disease, which is considered a form of PSL of unknown etiology. The diagnosis is based on clinicopathologic correlation. Originally, it was reported in children with the pretibial region as predilection site.[76,77] A recent study indicates that LPP can also affect adults and involve the trunk and arms.[78] A female preponderance can be observed.

Clinically, LPP shows a distinct presentation characterized by a longstanding plaque or circumscribed, often linear arranged reddish and brownish papules and plaques (Fig. 9A).[78,79]

Histology reveals a superficial, bandlike (see Fig. 9B), or deep nodular and interstitial infiltrate, often accentuated around adnexal structures or blood vessels. An epidermal hyperplasia is common (see Fig. 9B). The infiltrate consists of lymphocytes and histiocytes with numerous polyclonal plasma cells accounting for up to 25% of the entire infiltrate (see Fig. 9C). The interstitial histiocytes may form granulomas around sclerotic collagen bundles (so-called pseudorosettes) (see Fig. 9D). Histiocytic giant cells and an increased number of vessels can be seen.[78]

LPPs have been differentiated from other conditions containing plasma cells and histiocytes (Box 4). LPP and APA show overlapping clinical and histologic features. Thus it has been postulated

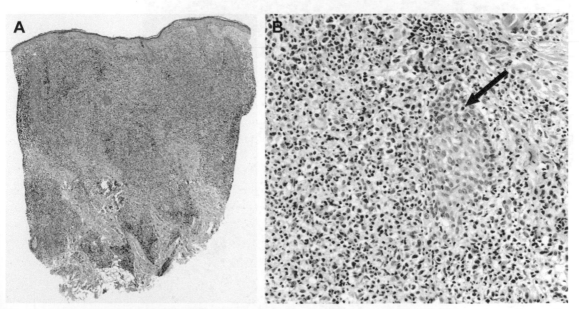

Fig. 10. Pseudolymphomatous folliculitis. (A) The lymphocytic infiltrates are located throughout the entire dermis and may extend into the subcutis (hematoxylin-eosin, ×20). (B) Exocytosis of lymphocytes (arrow) into the hair follicles (hematoxylin-eosin, ×200).

that both entities belong to the same spectrum of diseases and represent a plasma cell–rich PSL with a prominent vascular component.[78]

### Pseudolymphomatous Folliculitis

The pseudolymphomatous folliculitis was first described in 1988 by Kibbi and colleagues.[80] It presents with a solitary nodule preferentially located on the face.[81,82] Histologically, T-cell predominance is more often found than predominating B cells; in some cases, these cell types were equally distributed.[82] Admixed epithelioid histiocytes and granulomas are found. The lymphocytic infiltrates are located throughout the entire dermis and may extend into the subcutis (Fig. 10A). The epidermis is spared. There is exocytosis of lymphocytes into

the hair follicles often showing broadened epithelia[83] (see Fig. 10B). A hyperplasia of eccrine and apocrine ducts is often observed. An admixture of numerous dendritic cells with expression of CD1a and S-100 was identified in all cases.[81] Kazakov and colleagues[82] reported an unusual high number (approximately 50% of the cases) of clonal T cells and less often about a monoclonal IgH rearrangement in this entity. These cases have to be carefully differentiated from T-cell or B-cell lymphoma, which can also show follicular involvement.

## INTRAVASCULAR PSEUDOLYMPHOMA

Recently, benign intravascular proliferation of blasts with or without expression of CD30

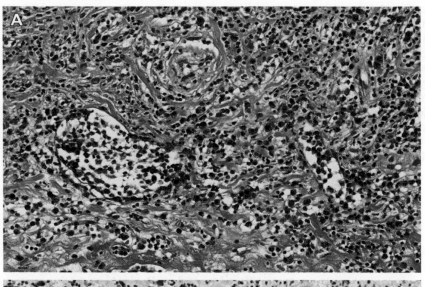

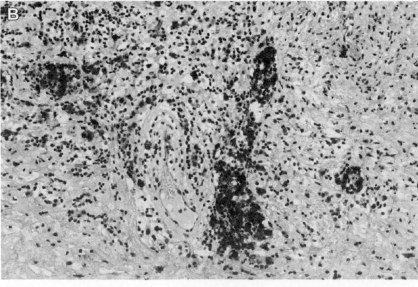

Fig. 11. Benign intravascular CD30+ lymphoproliferation. (A) The vessels are filled with activated large lymphocytes (hematoxylin-eosin, ×200). (B) The intravascular lymphocytes are positive for CD30 (×200).

have been reported. This condition arises in areas with inflammatory skin diseases or trauma of the skin.[84–86] Pathogenetically, obstruction of lymphatic vessels due to inflammation with disrupted immune cell trafficking may result in the accumulation of activated CD30[+] lymphocytes (Fig. 11A, B). The lymphocytes are large and have a blastlike morphology. They express T-cell markers (CD3 and CD4) and in some cases CD30. There is no association with Epstein-Barr virus infection. Clonality studies reveal the polyclonal nature of the process. Intravascular lymphoma is the most important differential diagnosis because it is an aggressive lymphoma with various phenotypic forms (B cell, T cell, or natural killer cell/T cell). In addition, benign intravascular proliferation of lymphoid cells needs to be distinguished from intralymphatic histiocytosis representing a reactive proliferation of histiocytes in the lumina of lymphatics in patients with rheumatoid arthritis or orthopedic metal implants.

## REFERENCES

1. Rijlaarsdam JU, Willemze R. Cutaneous pseudolymphomas: classification and differential diagnosis. Semin Dermatol 1994;13:187–96.
2. Ploysangam T, Breneman DL, Mutasim DF. Cutaneous pseudolymphomas. J Am Acad Dermatol 1998;38:877–95.
3. Gilliam AC, Wood GS. Cutaneous lymphoid hyperplasias. Semin Cutan Med Surg 2000;19:133–41.
4. van Vloten WA, Willemze R. The many faces of lymphocytoma cutis. J Eur Acad Dermatol Venereol 2003;17:3–6.
5. Hammer E, Sangueza O, Suwanjindar P, et al. Immunophenotypic and genotypic analysis in cutaneous lymphoid hyperplasias. J Am Acad Dermatol 1993;28:426–33.
6. Bouloc A, Delfau-Larue MH, Lenormand B, et al. Polymerase chain reaction analysis of immunoglobulin gene rearrangement in cutaneous lymphoid hyperplasias. French Study Group for cutaneous lymphomas. Arch Dermatol 1999;135:168–72.
7. Holm N, Flaig MJ, Yazdi AS, et al. The value of molecular analysis by PCR in the diagnosis of cutaneous lymphocytic infiltrates. J Cutan Pathol 2002;29:447–52.
8. Colli C, Leinweber B, Mullegger R, et al. Borrelia burgdorferi-associated lymphocytoma cutis: clinicopathologic, immunophenotypic, and molecular study of 106 cases. J Cutan Pathol 2004;31:232–40.
9. Goodlad JR, Davidson MM, Hollowood K, et al. Borrelia burgdorferi-associated cutaneous marginal zone lymphoma: a clinicopathological study of two cases illustrating the temporal progression of B.

burgdorferi-associated B-cell proliferation in the skin. Histopathology 2000;37:501–8.
10. Tan LS, Oon HH, Lee JS, et al. Successful treatment of tattoo-induced pseudolymphoma with sequential ablative fractional resurfacing followed by Q-Switched Nd: YAG 532 nm laser. J Cutan Aesthet Surg 2013;6:226–8.
11. Singletary HL, Selim MA, Olsen E. Subcutaneous interferon alfa for the treatment of cutaneous pseudolymphoma. Arch Dermatol 2012;148:572–4.
12. Moulonguet I, Ghnassia M, Molina T, et al. Miliarial-type perifollicular B-cell pseudolymphoma (lymphocytoma cutis): a misleading eruption in two women. J Cutan Pathol 2012;39:1016–21.
13. Brodell RT, Santa Cruz DJ. Cutaneous pseudolymphomas. Dermatol Clin 1985;3:719–34.
14. Caro WA, Helwig HB. Cutaneous lymphoid hyperplasia. Cancer 1969;24:487–502.
15. Kempf W, Kerl H, Kutzner H. CD123-positive plasmacytoid dendritic cells in primary cutaneous marginal zone B-cell lymphoma: a crucial role and a new lymphoma paradigm. Am J Dermatopathol 2009;32:194–6.
16. Kutzner H, Kerl H, Pfaltz MC, et al. CD123-positive plasmacytoid dendritic cells in primary cutaneous marginal zone B-cell lymphoma: diagnostic and pathogenetic implications. Am J Surg Pathol 2009;33:1307–13.
17. Baldassano MF, Bailey EM, Ferry JA, et al. Cutaneous lymphoid hyperplasia and cutaneous marginal zone lymphoma: comparison of morphologic and immunophenotypic features. Am J Surg Pathol 1999;23:88–96.
18. Kempf W, Mitteldorf C. Pathologic diagnosis of cutaneous lymphomas. Dermatol Clin 2015;33:655–81.
19. Leinweber B, Colli C, Chott A, et al. Differential diagnosis of cutaneous infiltrates of B lymphocytes with follicular growth pattern. Am J Dermatopathol 2004;26:4–13.
20. Kash N, Fink-Puches R, Cerroni L. Cutaneous manifestations of B-cell chronic lymphocytic leukemia associated with Borrelia burgdorferi infection showing a marginal zone B-cell lymphoma-like infiltrate. Am J Dermatopathol 2011;33:712–5.
21. Levin C, Mirzamani N, Zwerner J, et al. A comparative analysis of cutaneous marginal zone lymphoma and cutaneous chronic lymphocytic leukemia. Am J Dermatopathol 2012;34:18–23.
22. Boudova L, Kazakov DV, Sima R, et al. Cutaneous lymphoid hyperplasia and other lymphoid infiltrates of the breast nipple: a retrospective clinicopathologic study of fifty-six patients. Am J Dermatopathol 2005;27:375–86.
23. Nihal M, Mikkola D, Horvath N, et al. Cutaneous lymphoid hyperplasia: a lymphoproliferative continuum with lymphomatous potential. Hum Pathol 2003;34:617–22.

24. Boer A, Tirumalae R, Bresch M, et al. Pseudoclonality in cutaneous pseudolymphomas: a pitfall in interpretation of rearrangement studies. Br J Dermatol 2008;159:394–402.

25. Grange F, Wechsler J, Guillaume JC, et al. Borrelia burgdorferi-associated lymphocytoma cutis simulating a primary cutaneous large B-cell lymphoma. J Am Acad Dermatol 2002;47:530–4.

26. Kempf W, Flaig MJ, Kutzner H. Molecular diagnostics in infectious skin diseases. J Dtsch Dermatol Ges 2013;11(Suppl 4):50–8.

27. Bertolotti A, Pham-Ledard A, Petrot D, et al. Two cases of proliferation of monoclonal and monotypic lymphocytes and plasma cells corresponding to acrodermatitis chronica atrophicans. Ann Dermatol Venereol 2014;141:452–7, [in French].

28. Rijlaarsdam JU, Scheffer E, Meijer CJ, et al. Cutaneous pseudo-T-cell lymphomas. A clinicopathologic study of 20 patients. Cancer 1992;69:717–24.

29. Bergman R, Khamaysi Z, Sahar D, et al. Cutaneous lymphoid hyperplasia presenting as a solitary facial nodule: clinical, histopathological, immunophenotypical, and molecular studies. Arch Dermatol 2006;142:1561–6.

30. Leinweber B, Beltraminelli H, Kerl H, et al. Solitary small- to medium-sized pleomorphic T-cell nodules of undetermined significance: clinical, histopathological, immunohistochemical and molecular analysis of 26 cases. Dermatology 2009;219:42–7.

31. Kempf W. CD30+ lymphoproliferative disorders: histopathology, differential diagnosis, new variants, and simulators. J Cutan Pathol 2006;33(Suppl 1):58–70.

32. Werner B, Massone C, Kerl H, et al. Large CD30-positive cells in benign, atypical lymphoid infiltrates of the skin. J Cutan Pathol 2008;35:1100–7.

33. Gonzalez LC, Murua MA, Perez RG, et al. CD30+ lymphoma simulating orf. Int J Dermatol 2010;49: 690–2.

34. Fukamachi S, Sugita K, Sawada Y, et al. Drug-induced CD30+ T cell pseudolymphoma. Eur J Dermatol 2009;19:292–4.

35. Gomez-Orbaneja J, Diez LI, Lozano JL, et al. Lymphomatoid contact dermatitis: a syndrome produced by epicutaneous hypersensitivity with clinical features and a histopathologic picture similar to that of mycosis fungoides. Contact Dermatitis 1976;2:139–43.

36. Wolf IH, Cerroni L, Fink-Puches R, et al. [The morphologic spectrum of cutaneous pseudolymphomas]. J Dtsch Dermatol Ges 2005;3:710–20, [quiz: 721].

37. Souteyrand P, d'Incan M. Drug-induced mycosis fungoides-like lesions. Curr Probl Dermatol 1990; 19:176–82.

38. Pulitzer MP, Nolan KA, Oshman RG, et al. CD30+ lymphomatoid drug reactions. Am J Dermatopathol 2013;35:343–50.

39. Ive FA, Magnus IA, Warin RP, et al. "Actinic reticuloid"; a chronic dermatosis associated with severe photosensitivity and the histological resemblance to lymphoma. Br J Dermatol 1969;81:469–85.

40. Toonstra J, Henquet CJ, van Weelden H, et al. Actinic reticuloid. A clinical photobiologic, histopathologic, and follow-u study of 16 patients. J Am Acad Dermatol 1989;21:205–14.

41. Toonstra J. Actinic reticuloid. Semin Diagn Pathol 1991;8:109–16.

42. Sbidian E, Battistella M, Rivet J, et al. Remission of severe CD8(+) cytotoxic T cell skin infiltrative disease in human immunodeficiency virus-infected patients receiving highly active antiretroviral therapy. Clin Infect Dis 2010;51:741–8.

43. Bayal C, Büyükbani N, Seckin D, et al. Cutaneous atypical papular CD8+ lymphoproliferative disorder at acral sites in a renal transplant patient. Clin Exp Dermatol, in press.

44. Ingen-Housz-Oro S, Sbidian E, Ortonne N, et al. HIV-related CD8+ cutaneous pseudolymphoma: efficacy of methotrexate. Dermatology 2013;226:15–8.

45. Longacre TA, Foucar K, Koster F, et al. Atypical cutaneous lymphoproliferative disorder resembling mycosis fungoides in AIDS. Report of a case with concurrent Kaposi's sarcoma. Am J Dermatopathol 1989;11:451–6.

46. Egbers RG, Do TT, Su L, et al. Rapid clinical change in lesions of atypical cutaneous lymphoproliferative disorder in an HIV patient: a case report and review of the literature. Dermatol Online J 2011;17:4.

47. Kempf W, Kazakov DV, Hubscher E, et al. Cutaneous Borreliosis With a T-Cell-Rich Infiltrate and Simultaneous Involvement by B-Cell Chronic Lymphocytic Leukemia With t(14;18)(q32;q21). Am J Dermatopathol 2015;37:715–8.

48. Ofuji S, Furukawa F, Miyachi Y, et al. Papuloerythroderma. Dermatologica 1984;169:125–30.

49. Sugita K, Kabashima K, Nakamura M, et al. Drug-induced papuloerythroderma: analysis of T-cell populations and a literature review. Acta Derm Venereol 2009;89:618–22.

50. Torchia D, Miteva M, Hu S, et al. Papuloerythroderma 2009: two new cases and systematic review of the worldwide literature 25 years after its identification by Ofuji, et al. Dermatology 2010;220: 311–20.

51. Shah M, Reid WA, Layton AM. Cutaneous T-cell lymphoma presenting as papuloerythroderma–a case and review of the literature. Clin Exp Dermatol 1995;20:161–3.

52. Aste N, Fumo G, Conti B, et al. Ofuji papuloerythroderma. J Eur Acad Dermatol Venereol 2000; 14:55–7.

53. Bech-Thomsen N, Thomsen K. Ofuji's papuloerythroderma: a study of 17 cases. Clin Exp Dermatol 1998;23:79–83.

54. Abeck D, Ollert MW, Eckert F, et al. Palpable migratory arciform erythema. Clinical morphology, histopathology, immunohistochemistry, and response to treatment. Arch Dermatol 1997;133:763–6.

55. Remy-Leroux V, Leonard F, Lambert D, et al. Comparison of histopathologic-clinical characteristics of Jessner's lymphocytic infiltration of the skin and lupus erythematosus tumidus: Multicenter study of 46 cases. J Am Acad Dermatol 2008;58:217–23.

56. Wagner G, Bartsch S, Rose C, et al. Palpable arciforme migratory erythema. Hautarzt 2012;63: 965–8, [in German].

57. Poenitz N, Dippel E, Klemke CD, et al. Jessner's lymphocytic infiltration of the skin: a CD8+ polyclonal reactive skin condition. Dermatology 2003;207: 276–84.

58. Mitteldorf C, Tronnier M. Histologic features of granulomatous skin diseases. J Dtsch Dermatol Ges 2016;14:378–88.

59. Boer A, Blodorn-Schlicht N, Wiebels D, et al. Unusual histopathological features of cutaneous leishmaniasis identified by polymerase chain reaction specific for Leishmania on paraffin-embedded skin biopsies. Br J Dermatol 2006;155:815–9.

60. Boer A, Herder N, Blodorn-Schlicht N, et al. Herpes incognito most commonly is herpes zoster and its histopathologic pattern is distinctive! Am J Dermatopathol 2006;28:181–6.

61. Toro JR, Sander CA, LeBoit PE. Persistent pigmented purpuric dermatitis and mycosis fungoides: simulant, precursor, or both? A study by light microscopy and molecular methods. Am J Dermatopathol 1997;19:108–18.

62. Magro C, Crowson AN, Kovatich A, et al. Pityriasis lichenoides: a clonal T-cell lymphoproliferative disorder. Hum Pathol 2002;33:788–95.

63. Citarella L, Massone C, Kerl H, et al. Lichen sclerosus with histopathologic features simulating early mycosis fungoides. Am J Dermatopathol 2003;25: 463–5.

64. Kempf W, Kazakov DV, Palmedo G, et al. Pityriasis lichenoides et varioliformis acuta with numerous CD30+ cells: a variant mimicking lymphomatoid papulosis and other cutaneous lymphomas. A clinicopathologic, immunohistochemical, and molecular biological study of 13 cases. Am J Surg Pathol 2012;36:1021–9.

65. Dereure O, Levi E, Kadin ME. T-Cell clonality in pityriasis lichenoides et varioliformis acuta: a heteroduplex analysis of 20 cases. Arch Dermatol 2000;136: 1483–6.

66. Kaddu S, Cerroni L, Pilatti A, et al. Acral pseudolymphomatous angiokeratoma. A variant of the cutaneous pseudolymphomas. Am J Dermatopathol 1994;16:130–3.

67. Okada M, Funayama M, Tanita M, et al. Acral angiokeratoma-like pseudolymphoma: one adolescent and two adults. J Am Acad Dermatol 2001;45:S209–11.

68. Wagner G, Rose C, Sachse MM. Papular pseudolymphoma of adults as a variant of acral pseudolymphomatous angiokeratoma of children (APACHE). J Dtsch Dermatol Ges 2014;12:423–4.

69. Requena L, Sangueza OP. Cutaneous vascular proliferation. Part II. Hyperplasias and benign neoplasms. J Am Acad Dermatol 1997;37:887–919, [quiz: 920–2].

70. Adler BL, Krausz AE, Minuti A, et al. Epidemiology and treatment of angiolymphoid hyperplasia with eosinophilia (ALHE): A systematic review. J Am Acad Dermatol 2016;74:506–512 e511.

71. Olsen TG, Helwig EB. Angiolymphoid hyperplasia with eosinophilia. A clinicopathologic study of 116 patients. J Am Acad Dermatol 1985;12:781–96.

72. Chim CS, Fung A, Shek TW, et al. Analysis of clonality in kimura's disease. Am J Surg Pathol 2002;26: 1083–6.

73. Kempf W, Haeffner AC, Zepter K, et al. Angiolymphoid hyperplasia with eosinophilia: evidence for a T-cell lymphoproliferative origin. Hum Pathol 2002; 33:1023–9.

74. Uhara H, Saida T, Ikegawa S, et al. Primary cutaneous plasmacytosis: report of three cases and review of the literature. Dermatology 1994;189:251–5.

75. Honda R, Cerroni L, Tanikawa A, et al. Cutaneous plasmacytosis: report of 6 cases with or without systemic involvement. J Am Acad Dermatol 2013;68: 978–85.

76. Gilliam AC, Mullen RH, Oviedo G, et al. Isolated benign primary cutaneous plasmacytosis in children: two illustrative cases. Arch Dermatol 2009; 145:299–302.

77. Fried I, Wiesner T, Cerroni L. Pretibial lymphoplasmacytic plaque in children. Arch Dermatol 2010; 146:95–6.

78. Mitteldorf C, Palmedo G, Kutzner H, et al. Diagnostic approach in lymphoplasmacytic plaque. J Eur Acad Dermatol Venereol 2015;29:2206–15.

79. Moulonguet I, Hadj-Rabia S, Gounod N, et al. Tibial lymphoplasmacytic plaque: a new, illustrative case of a recently and poorly recognized benign lesion in children. Dermatology 2012;225:27–30.

80. Kibbi AG, Scrimenti RJ, Koenig RR, et al. A solitary nodule of the left cheek. Pseudolymphomatous folliculitis. Arch Dermatol 1988;124: 1272–3, 1276.

81. Arai E, Okubo H, Tsuchida T, et al. Pseudolymphomatous folliculitis: a clinicopathologic study of 15 cases of cutaneous pseudolymphoma with follicular invasion. Am J Surg Pathol 1999;23:1313–9.

82. Kazakov DV, Belousova IE, Kacerovska D, et al. Hyperplasia of hair follicles and other adnexal structures in cutaneous lymphoproliferative disorders: a study of 53 cases, including so-called

pseudolymphomatous folliculitis and overt lymphomas. Am J Surg Pathol 2008;32:1468–78.

83. Petersson F. Pseudolymphomatous folliculitis with marked lymphocytic folliculo- and focal epidermotropism–expanding the morphologic spectrum. Am J Dermatopathol 2011;33:323–5.

84. Riveiro-Falkenbach E, Fernandez-Figueras MT, Rodriguez-Peralto JL. Benign atypical intravascular CD30(+) T-cell proliferation: a reactive condition mimicking intravascular lymphoma. Am J Dermatopathol 2013;35:143–50.

85. Kempf W, Keller K, John H, et al. Benign atypical intravascular CD30+ T-cell proliferation: a recently described reactive lymphoproliferative process and simulator of intravascular lymphoma: report of a case associated with lichen sclerosus and review of the literature. Am J Clin Pathol 2014;142: 694–9.

86. Calamaro P, Cerroni L. Intralymphatic proliferation of T-cell lymphoid blasts in the setting of hidradenitis suppurativa. Am J Dermatopathol 2016;38: 536–40.

# Histopathologic Spectrum of Connective Tissue Diseases Commonly Affecting the Skin

Alvaro C. Laga, MD, MMSc[a],*, Allison Larson, MD[b],
Scott R. Granter, MD[a]

## KEYWORDS

- Histopathology • Connective • Lupus • Scleroderma • Dermatomyositis • Patterns • Neutrophilic

## Key Points

- Connective tissue diseases affecting the skin may show the following histologic patterns: interface alteration, vasculitis, vasculopathy, neutrophilic dermatosis, and dermal sclerosis.
- The main role of histopathology in the diagnosis of connective tissue disorders is to confirm, exclude, or alert clinicians of connective tissue disease as a diagnostic category rather than specific entities.
- Clinical and serologic correlation is needed to arrive at the correct diagnosis.
- Neutrophilic dermatosis may be the initial (presenting) manifestation of connective tissue disease.

## ABSTRACT

Connective tissue disorders (CTDs), also known as collagen vascular diseases, are a heterogeneous group of diseases with a common pathogenic mechanism: autoimmunity. Precise classification of CTDs requires clinical, serologic, and pathologic correlation and may be difficult because of overlapping clinical and histologic features. The main contribution of histopathology in the diagnosis of these disorders is to confirm, rule out, or alert clinicians to the possibility of CTD as a disease category, rather than producing definitive diagnoses of specific entities. This article discusses the histopathologic spectrum of 3 common rheumatologic skin disorders: lupus erythematosus, dermatomyositis, and morphea (localized scleroderma).

## OVERVIEW

Connective tissue disorders (CTDs), also known as collagen vascular diseases, are a heterogeneous group of diseases with a common pathogenic mechanism: the loss of self-tolerance and development of so-called autoimmunity. Although the exact cause is unknown, it is generally accepted that genetic predisposition and environmental factors such as infection play an important role in unmasking self-antigens that are then recognized by autoreactive clones with consequent target cell/organ injury.[1] Autoimmune disorders can be broadly categorized into organ-specific disorders (eg, diabetes mellitus [DM] type 1, Hashimoto thyroiditis, localized scleroderma, chronic cutaneous lupus erythematosus) and systemic disorders (eg, systemic lupus erythematosus [SLE], dermatomyositis, systemic

Disclosure: The authors have nothing to disclose.
[a] Department of Pathology, Brigham and Women's Hospital, Harvard Medical School, Amory-3, 75 Francis Street, Boston, MA 02115, USA; [b] Department of Dermatology, Boston University School of Medicine, 609 Albany Street, J202, Boston, MA 02118, USA
* Corresponding author.
E-mail address: alaga@partners.org

Surgical Pathology 10 (2017) 477–503
http://dx.doi.org/10.1016/j.path.2017.01.012

sclerosis).[2,3] Precise classification of CTDs requires clinical, serologic, and pathologic correlation and may be difficult at times because of overlapping clinical and histologic features. Although there are classic or characteristic histopathologic changes of CTD, the main contribution of histopathology in the diagnosis of these disorders is perhaps to confirm, rule out, or alert clinicians to the possibility of CTD as a disease category, rather than producing definitive diagnoses of specific entities. Although some histologic patterns (eg, vacuolar interface alteration) are readily associated with CTD by pathologists, there are other patterns (eg, neutrophilic dermatosis) that, despite having characteristic histopathologic features, only recently have emerged as distinctive manifestations of CTD.[4–7] This article discusses the histopathologic spectrum of 3 common rheumatologic disorders involving the skin: lupus erythematosus, dermatomyositis, and morphea (localized scleroderma).

## LUPUS ERYTHEMATOSUS

### CLINICAL FEATURES

Lupus erythematosus is an inflammatory disease with a protracted clinical course and potential for multiorgan disorder. Skin involvement is seen in more than 80% of patients.[3] Although severity and clinical manifestations vary from patient to patient, multiple clinical and pathologic patterns of skin disease may be encountered and should alert clinicians and pathologists to this diagnosis.

Lupus erythematosus is predominantly observed in young women, but can occasionally affect men and may occur at any age. Cutaneous manifestations of lupus can be divided into acute, subacute, and chronic cutaneous lupus. Chronic cutaneous lupus, in turn, can be subdivided into discoid lupus (the most common form), lupus panniculitis, chilblain lupus (lupus perniosis), and tumid lupus, this last form being controversial.[8–10]

Acute cutaneous lupus erythematosus (ACLE) is a manifestation of SLE and presents with the classic malar erythema (butterfly rash) spreading over the cheeks and bridge of the nose, with sparing of the nasolabial folds, which are relatively sun protected. ACLE manifests in up to 50% of patients with SLE after sun exposure and can be confused with sunburn. Subacute cutaneous lupus erythematosus (SCLE) is characterized by annular, polycyclic, or psoriasiform scaly papules and plaques on photosensitive areas of the chest, upper back, and arms. The central face is typically spared and most patients

have anti-Ro (SSA) antibodies. SCLE is frequently induced by medications but can be idiopathic; both forms are indistinguishable clinically, serologically, and by histopathology. Permanent pigmentary changes and scarring do not occur. Discoid lupus erythematosus (DLE) presents with indurated pink, violaceous, or hyperpigmented plaques that may develop central hypopigmentation and scarring. Scale is frequently seen, and follicular plugging may be evident. Involvement of the scalp is common and results in scarring alopecia. The head and neck are most frequently involved. There is minimal risk of systemic involvement. Long-standing DLE lesions are at increased risk for squamous cell carcinoma formation, and these squamous cell carcinomas confer a higher rate of recurrence, metastasis, and death. Lupus panniculitis presents with indurated nodules, most frequently on the head, neck, and arms, and heals with depressed scars. Lupus panniculitis may represent purely cutaneous disease or may be a manifestation of SLE. Bullous lupus erythematosus occurs in patients with SLE and presents with tense vesicles and bullae on both sun-exposed and sun-protected sites.[8–13]

### MICROSCOPIC FEATURES

The key features of histologic patterns encountered in lupus erythematosus, dermatomyositis, and morphea are summarized in **Box 1**.

### HISTOLOGIC PATTERNS SEEN IN LUPUS ERYTHEMATOSUS

### INTERFACE DERMATITIS

Vacuolar interface alteration, consisting of vacuolar or hydropic degeneration of the epidermal basal cell layer, is the most common histologic pattern in lupus erythematosus and can be seen in the acute, subacute, and chronic forms of cutaneous lupus. Early lesions of ACLE may show subtle, nonspecific findings such as dermal edema and sparse mononuclear inflammation. Well-developed lesions show vacuolar interface alteration, indistinguishable histologically from SCLE (**Fig. 1**A). In SCLE, there is vacuolar interface dermatitis, sometimes associated with colloid bodies in the papillary dermis and edema. There is a lymphocytic inflammatory infiltrate, but it tends to be less conspicuous than in DLE (**Fig. 1**B). SCLE is also the most frequent pattern seen in neonatal lupus erythematosus. In DLE, there is interface dermatitis and prominent mononuclear inflammatory infiltrates near the dermal-epidermal

---

**Box 1**
**Key features of histopathologic patterns in connective tissue diseases**

*Interface dermatitis*

- Characterized by hydropic (also termed granulovacuolar) degeneration of basal keratinocytes.

- May be pauci-inflammatory (vacuolar type) or show bandlike infiltrate of lymphocytes obscuring the dermal-epidermal junction (lichenoid type).

- The presence of dermal mucin, perivascular (superficial and deep), and periadnexal lymphocytic infiltrates associated with interface alteration is characteristic of connective tissue disease.

- Eosinophils, particularly when numerous, should raise consideration of a hypersensitivity reaction (eg, drug eruption).

- Precise classification of CTDs requires clinical and serologic correlation.

*Vasculitis*

- Leukocytoclastic vasculitis is a histologic pattern that may be seen in connective tissue disease, but it is nonspecific.

- Medium-vessel vasculitis may present in association with CTD (eg, SLE).

- Immunofluorescence studies are of limited value in ascribing an cause to vasculitis and should be used judiciously.

- A vasculitis work-up may be necessary to determine the cause.

- So-called lymphocytic vasculitis in acral skin is characteristic of perniosis (chilblains), which may be a manifestation of CTD (ie, SLE).

*Vasculopathy*

- The presence of fibrin thrombi within dermal vessels (thrombotic vasculopathy) is a histologic pattern that includes CTD as a possible cause in the differential diagnosis.

- The main role of histopathology is distinction from vasculitis, which sometimes is difficult.

- A coagulopathy work-up may be necessary to establish the cause.

*Neutrophilic dermatosis*

- Neutrophilic dermatosis may be the presenting manifestation of CTD.

- Hypercellular (Sweet syndrome–like), moderately cellular, and paucicellular (urticarial) patterns may be seen.

- The diagnosis of neutrophilic dermatosis requires exclusion of infection.

- Lupus erythematosus, dermatomyositis, rheumatoid arthritis, Sjögren syndrome, and many other CTDs have been associated with neutrophilic dermatosis.

*Dermal sclerosis*

- Characterized by prominent deposition of collagen in the dermis and subcutis, with distortion of the normal architecture (entrapping and/or loss of adnexal structures).

- May be a manifestation of localized scleroderma (morphea) or systemic sclerosis.

- The differential diagnosis includes radiation dermatitis, eosinophilic fasciitis, chronic graft-versus-host disease, and other scarring processes.

- Papillary dermal sclerosis (hyalinization) may coexist (overlap lichen sclerosus/morphea syndrome).

---

junction and around vessels and hair follicles. Hyperkeratosis of the follicular ostia (follicular plugging) and thickening of the basement membrane are characteristic (**Fig.** 1C). Mucin deposition is seen as a faint bluish substance between dermal collagen fibers. Pigment incontinence is frequently observed.[2,14]

Lichenoid interface dermatitis and reactive epidermal hyperplasia may be seen in a minority of patients (~2%) with hypertrophic or verrucous

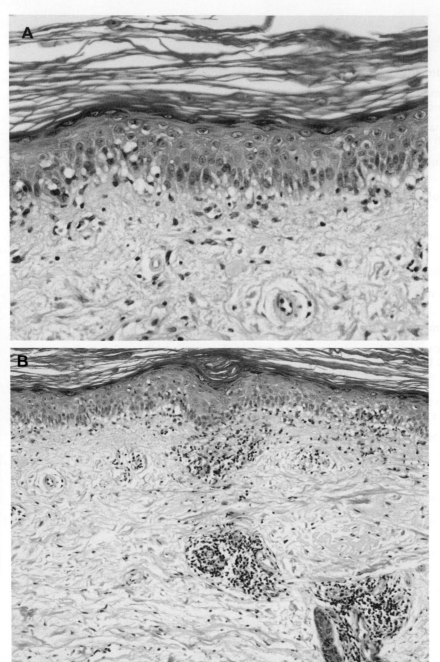

*Fig. 1.* Lupus erythematosus. (*A*) Vacuolar interface alteration in acute lupus; note the prominent vacuolization of the basal cell layer and low level of inflammatory infiltrate (hematoxylin-eosin [H&E], original magnification ×400). (*B*) Interface alteration with subtle perivascular and periadnexal lymphocytic infiltrates is characteristic of SCLE (H&E, original magnification ×200).

lupus erythematosus. There is a brisk lichenoid mononuclear infiltrate and a proliferative epidermal response resembling lichen planus (**Fig.** 1D). The squamous hyperplasia of hypertrophic lupus erythematosus can show significant atypia and may be confused with well-differentiated squamous cell carcinoma by the unwary.[15]

## PANNICULITIS

Lupus panniculitis, also known as lupus profundus, is a rare manifestation occurring in 1% to 3% of patients with cutaneous or systemic lupus.[16,17] Approximately 67% of patients with lupus panniculitis have prototypic discoid plaques either overlying the area of panniculitis or distant

*Fig. 1. (continued).* (*C*) Prominent perivascular and periadnexal lymphocytic inflammation and hyperkeratosis of follicular ostia (follicular plugging) are characteristic of DLE (H&E, original magnification ×100). (*D*) A bandlike lymphocytic infiltrate with squamatization and sawtoothing of the basal cell layer are seen in hypertrophic lupus erythematosus. These findings mimic lichen planus.

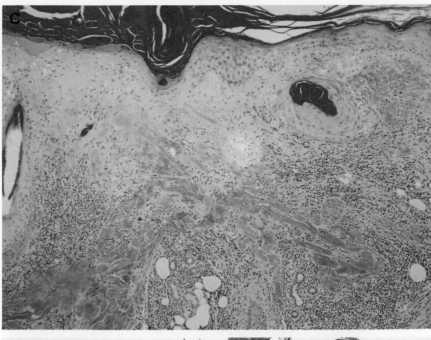

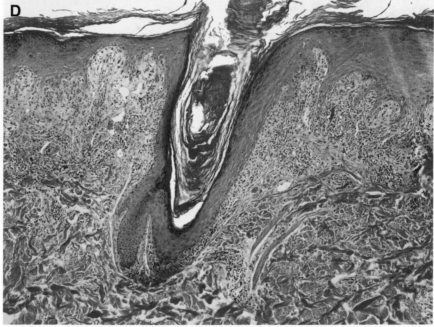

from it.[18] On histology, there is predominantly lobular panniculitis characterized by infiltrates of lymphocytes and plasma cells; germinal center formation may be present (**Fig.** 2A). Vascular changes, including thrombosis, calcification, and (extremely rarely) frank vasculitis may be seen (**Fig.** 2B). Fat necrosis results in hyalinization of the fat, which is highly characteristic of lupus panniculitis (**Fig.** 2C). Over time, there is less inflammation and more hyalinization (**Fig.** 2D).

## THROMBOTIC VASCULOPATHY

Fibrin thrombi within dermal vessels may be encountered in patients with antiphospholipid syndrome, which may occur in patients with

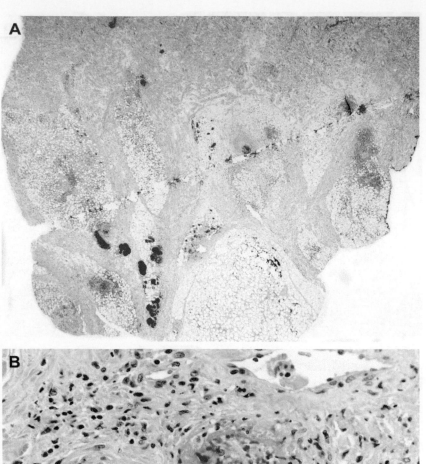

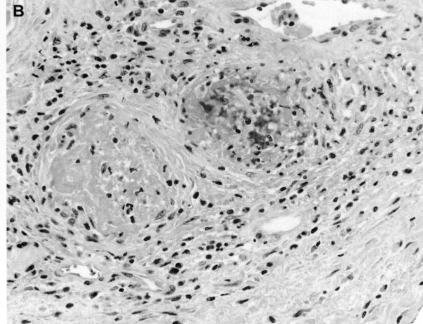

*Fig. 2.* Lupus panniculitis. (*A*) At scanning magnification, a lobular panniculitis with apparent follicular lymphoid aggregates is evident (H&E, original magnification ×20). (*B*) Thrombosis of subcutaneous vessels may be seen (H&E, original magnification ×600).

SLE and other autoimmune conditions (**Fig.** 3A). These patients develop antibodies (anticardiolipin, beta-2 glycoprotein, and lupus anticoagulant) that prolong phospholipid-dependent coagulation assays in vitro and are associated with increased risk of venous and arterial thromboses. Of these, antibodies against bota-2 glycoprotein are the most common. The so-called lupus anticoagulant affects 10% of patients with SLE and incurs an increased risk for deep vein thrombosis and pulmonary embolism. Cutaneous necrosis is often the first manifestation of antiphospholipid antibody syndrome (**Fig.** 3B). Recurrent miscarriages, renal vein thrombosis, and thrombotic vasculopathy involving dermal vessels can also occur.[19]

*Fig. 2. (continued).* (*C*) Hyaline necrosis of the subcutaneous fat is characteristic of lupus panniculitis; note the prominent plasma cells, frequently present in the inflammatory phase (H&E, original magnification ×200). (*D*) Later lesions show hyalinization of the subcutaneous fat and less inflammation (H&E, original magnification ×400).

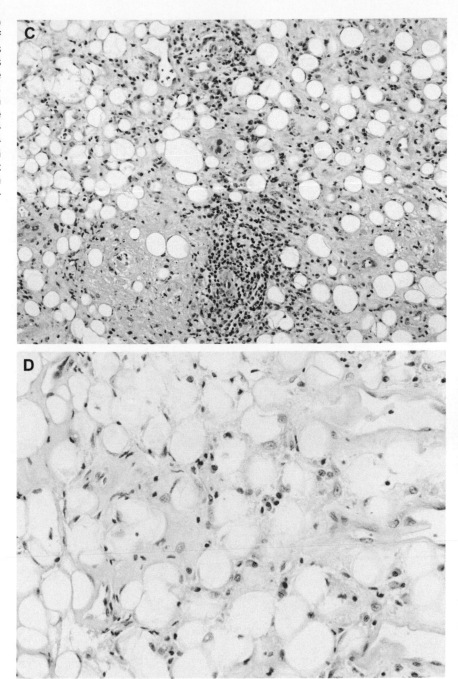

## VASCULITIS

Vasculitis has been reported in up to a third of patients with SLE.[13] The most common pattern is cutaneous small vessel vasculitis manifesting as leukocytoclastic vasculitis (**Fig.** 4A, B). There is neutrophilic infiltration and fibrinoid necrosis of the vascular wall in small vessels of the superficial plexus. Medium and large vessel involvement has also been documented and may involve retinal, pulmonary, gastrointestinal, or central nervous system vasculature (**Fig.** 4C, D).

Lymphocytic vasculitis, characterized by prominent cuffed lymphocytic infiltrates with involvement of the vascular wall of superficial and deep dermal vessels in the fingers and toes, is characteristic of chilblain lupus erythematosus (lupus perniosis), which is regarded as a

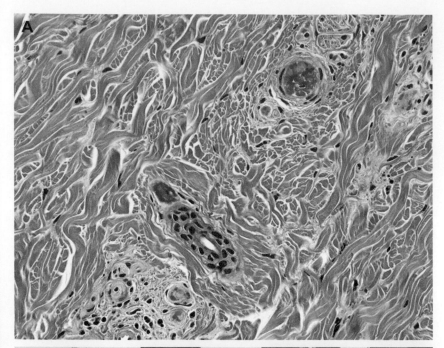

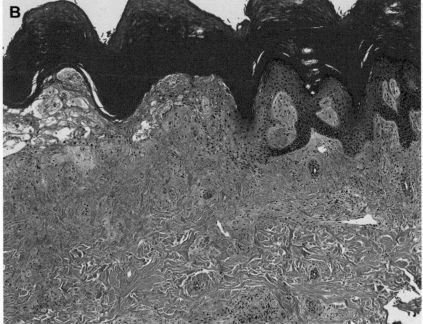

*Fig. 3.* Thrombotic vasculopathy (H&E, original magnification ×200). (*A*) Fibrin thrombi within dermal vessels. This patient with lupus erythematosus developed anti–β2-microglobulin antibodies. (*B*) Cutaneous necrosis may be the initial manifestation of antiphospholipid antibody syndrome (H&E, original magnification ×100).

form of chronic cutaneous lupus erythematosus. Perieccrine lymphocytic infiltrates and papillary dermal edema are also frequently encountered (**Fig. 5**).

## NEUTROPHILIC DERMATOSIS

The presence of neutrophilic infiltrates in biopsies from patients with bullous lupus erythematosus and SLE-associated leukocytoclastic vasculitis is well established. Bullous lupus erythematosus is characterized by subepidermal blister formation with variable numbers of neutrophils (**Fig. 6A**). Sometimes, papillary dermal microabscesses form, simulating dermatitis herpetiformis or linear immunoglobulin (Ig) A bullous dermatosis.[2,14] However, neutrophilic dermatosis (as such) has not been traditionally associated with CTD, but

**Fig. 4.** Small vessel vasculitis (leukocytoclastic vasculitis). (*A*) There is neutrophilic infiltration of the superficial dermal vessels with abundant karyorrhectic debris and extravasated red blood cells in leukocytoclastic vasculitis (H&E, original magnification ×200). (*B*) Fibrinoid necrosis of the vascular wall of a small dermal vessel, which is a defining histopathologic feature of vasculitis, but may prove difficult to find (H&E, original magnification ×600).

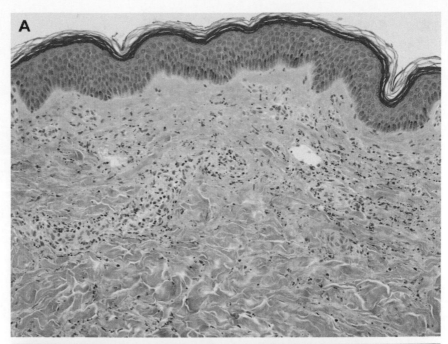

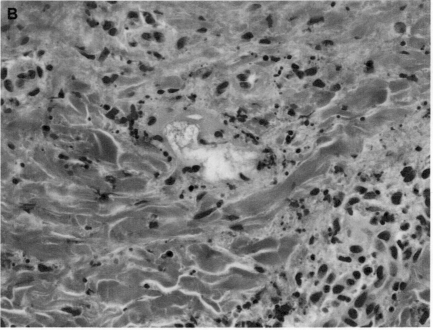

there is a recent body of literature describing neutrophilic tissue reactions in patients with SLE and this has been designated systemic lupus–associated neutrophilic dermatosis.[4–7] In patients with neutrophilic dermatosis and lupus, neutrophilic dermatosis was the initial manifestation of SLE in one-third of the cases in a recent study.[5,6] Approximately half of the reported cases of SLE-associated neutrophilic dermatosis show cellular neutrophilic infiltrates virtually indistinguishable from Sweet syndrome (**Fig. 6**B). These cases are characterized by mid-dermal neutrophilic infiltrates with abundant karyorrhectic debris and papillary dermal edema. An estimated one-third of patients have paucicellular neutrophilic infiltrates, which are subtle and have been described as urticarialike in some reports (**Fig. 6**C). These infiltrates consist of sparse neutrophils, frequently in

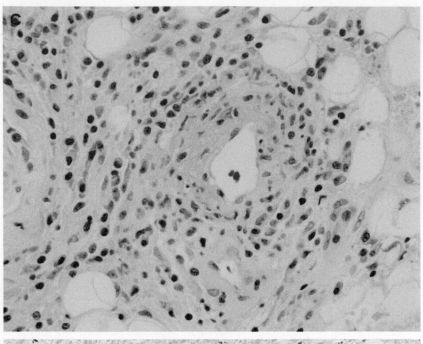

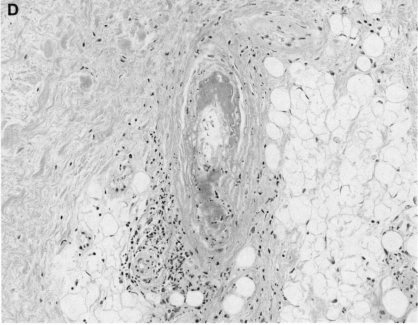

Fig. 4. (continued). (C) Mononuclear infiltration of a medium-sized vessel in a patient with SLE; note the abundance of plasma cells commonly seen in CTDs (H&E, original magnification ×600). (D) Fibrinoid necrosis of a medium-sized vessel wall in a patient initially diagnosed with mixed connective tissue disease, and later classified as SLE (H&E, original magnification ×400).

the papillary dermis. The remaining described cases (~20%) showed infiltrates somewhere in between with moderate numbers of neutrophils (Fig. 6D).[5,6] Of note, classic histologic changes of lupus, such as interface alteration, mucin deposition, and thickening of the basement membrane, were present in less than half of the patients in a recent study and these features tended to exist in patients with an established diagnosis of SLE.[6] The frequent lack of classic histologic features in patients whose initial presentation of SLE is a neutrophilic dermatosis emphasizes the importance of considering CTD in all patients with neutrophilic dermatosis.

*Fig. 5.* Lupus perniosis. A cuffed perivascular and perieccrine lymphocytic infiltrate, sometimes with involvement of the vascular wall (so-called lymphocytic vasculitis) is characteristic of lupus perniosis.

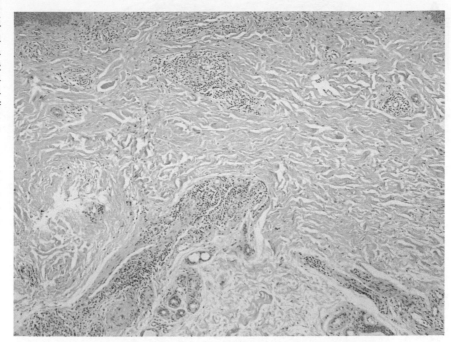

## DIFFERENTIAL DIAGNOSIS

### INTERFACE DERMATITIS

Vacuolar interface dermatitis can be seen in patients with drug reactions. The presence of frequent eosinophils or mixed inflammatory patterns (eg, interface alteration and psoriasiform hyperplasia) strongly favors a hypersensitivity reaction and should help in the distinction. Erythema multiforme (EM) is also characterized by an interface dermatitis. Prominent dyskeratosis in a pauci-inflammatory background and history of characteristic targetoid lesions in EM should help differentiation (Fig. 7A). Note that cutaneous eruptions with clinical and histologic features of EM have been described in patients with lupus (Rowell syndrome; Fig. 7B). Acute graft-versus-host disease typically shows subtle vacuolar interface dermatitis, which in early lesions may show preferential involvement of the bulge region of hair follicles. Discrete apoptotic keratinocytes surrounded by lymphocytes (so-called satellitosis) are characteristic but not always present (Fig. 7C). History of allogeneic stem cell transplant, and time of the biopsy with respect to the transplant, as well as clinical information such as presence of gastrointestinal symptoms, are most important in allowing correct classification. Florid interface alteration in scalp biopsies requires careful clinical correlation to distinguish DLE from lichen planopilaris, because histologic findings can be very similar (Fig. 7D).[20] Note that vacuolar interface dermatitis is a frequent manifestation of other CTD (eg, dermatomyositis, mixed connective tissue disease) and careful clinical and serologic correlations are necessary to arrive at the correct diagnosis. Hypertrophic lupus erythematosus can mimic lichen planus histologically. The presence of deep perivascular and periadnexal infiltrates and mucin deposition can be of help in distinguishing these possibilities. Hypertrophic lupus may also mimic well-differentiated squamous cell carcinoma and distinction may be extremely difficult. To complicate matters, some reports have described well-differentiated squamous cell carcinomas occurring in patients with hypertrophic lupus.[21] Although such association is controversial for obvious reasons, caution should be taken when making a diagnosis of squamous cell carcinoma in a patient with hypertrophic lupus.

In addition, blurring of the dermal-epidermal junction mimicking interface alteration may occur in processes such as melanocytic neoplasia, secondary syphilis, and cutaneous T-cell lymphoma and pathologists should be aware of these potential pitfalls (Box 2, Fig. 8).

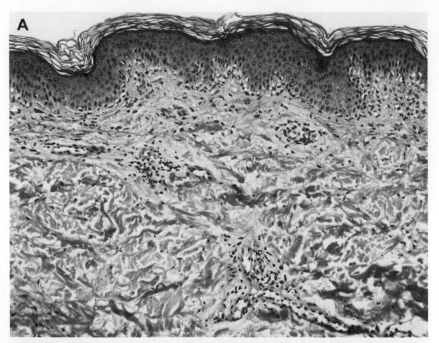

*Fig. 6.* Neutrophilic infiltrates in lupus erythematosus. (*A*) A sparse neutrophilic infiltrate along the dermal-epidermal junction is characteristic of bullous lupus (H&E, original magnification ×200). (*B*) Systemic lupus–associated neutrophilic dermatosis. A cellular neutrophilic infiltrate with prominent karyorrhectic debris indistinguishable from Sweet syndrome can be seen (H&E, original magnification ×200).

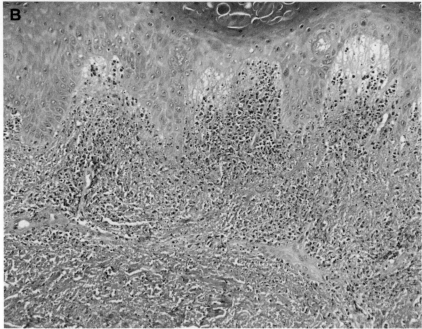

## PANNICULITIS

The most important entity in the differential diagnosis of lupus panniculitis is subcutaneous panniculitislike T-cell lymphoma (SPTCL). Subcutaneous, predominantly lobular infiltrates of lymphocytes and plasma cells are present in both lupus panniculitis and SPTCL. It has been reported that typical changes of discoid lupus, such as interface alteration, thickening of the basement membrane, dermal mucin deposition, and superficial and deep dermal perivascular lymphoid infiltrates, can be identified in approximately 50% of cases of lupus panniculitis, and thus may help in this distinction when present.[15–17] Lymphoid follicles with germinal center

*Fig. 6.* (*continued*). (*C*) Some cases of systemic lupus–associated neutrophilic dermatosis show only subtle superficial dermal neutrophilic infiltrates (H&E, original magnification ×200), (*D*) or moderately cellular infiltrates (H&E, original magnification ×100).

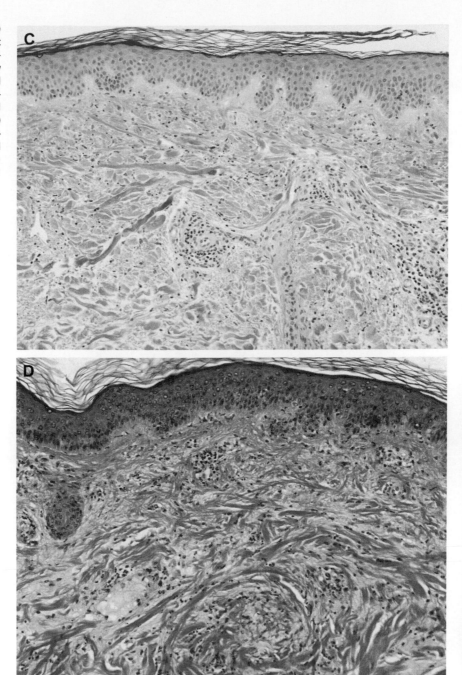

formation have also been described in 50% of cases and are characteristic of lupus panniculitis.[22,23] In SPTCL, there is infiltration of the subcutaneous fat by lymphocytes with variable atypia, consisting of irregular hyperchromatic nuclei. Karyorrhectic debris is frequently encountered. The presence of so-called rimming, atypical lymphoid cells surrounding individual adipocytes, should alert pathologists to the possibility of SPTCL

(**Fig. 9A**). Immunohistochemistry is most helpful in recognizing this entity and it shows a cytotoxic T-cell phenotype consisting of CD3-positive, CD8-positive, CD4-negative lymphoid cells, coexpressing TIA-1, perforin, and granzyme B. Expression of TCRβF1 and a negative CD56 confirms an αβ phenotype, distinguishing it from cutaneous γδ T-cell lymphoma, which has a poor prognosis (**Fig. 9B–D**).[24]

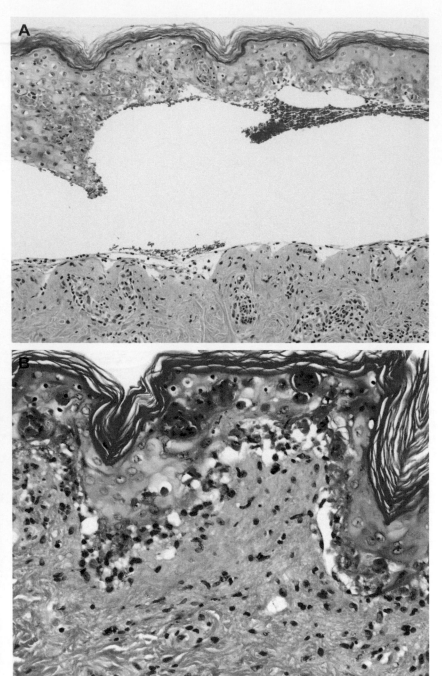

*Fig. 7.* Differential diagnoses of interface dermatitis. (*A*) EM shows florid dyskeratosis in a pauci-inflammatory background (H&E, original magnification ×200). (*B*) Patients with lupus erythematosus may develop EM-like eruptions, Rowell syndrome (H&E, original magnification ×200).

Morphea profunda can mimic lupus panniculitis clinically and histologically. As mentioned earlier, the presence of epidermal changes such as interface alteration, atrophy, and thickening of the basement membrane favor lupus panniculitis. In contrast, prominent sclerosis of the dermis and subcutis favors morphea profunda. However, note that in some cases the distinction cannot be made by histopathology alone.[25]

## THROMBOTIC VASCULOPATHY

Fibrin thrombi within dermal vessels may be seen in patients with SLE and antiphospholipid syndrome. Consumptive coagulopathy (eg,

*Fig. 7. (continued).* (*C*) Acute graft-versus-host disease shows subtle interface alteration and rare apoptotic keratinocytes surrounded by lymphocytes (H&E, original magnification ×200). (*D*) Lichen planopilaris may show florid interface folliculitis with prominent lymphoid inflammation, which may be confused with DLE (H&E, original magnification ×400).

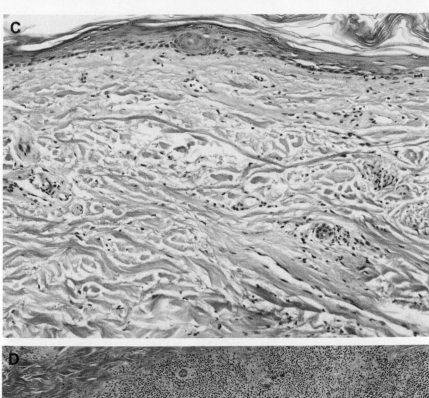

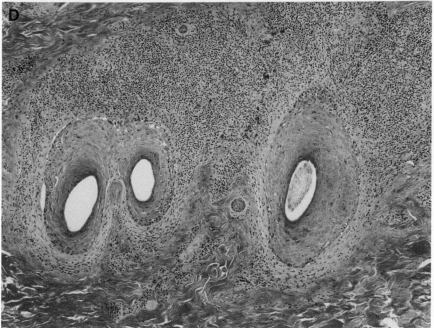

---

**Box 2**
**Pitfalls: interface dermatitis**

! Interface alteration with subepidermal effacement and clefting separation, chronic inflammation, and pigmentary incontinence may be seen in melanocytic neoplasms (ie, melanoma in situ, melanoma regression).

! The presence of a lichenoid interface pattern, in particular if there are foci of neutrophils and/or eosinophils or granulomas, should raise consideration of secondary syphilis.

! Interface alteration with prominent dyskeratotic cells may be a manifestation of cutaneous T-cell lymphoma. Papillary dermal fibrosis and lymphoid atypia may suggest the correct diagnosis, but are not always present.

! Subtle interface alteration should raise consideration of acute graft-versus-host disease or complex allograft rejection (eg, face transplant, limb transplant).

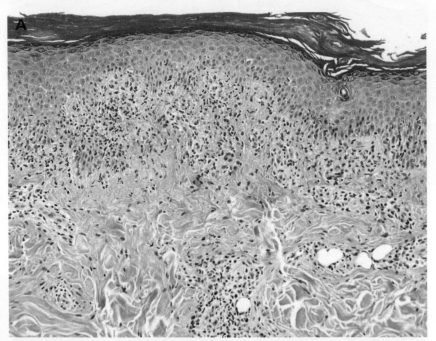

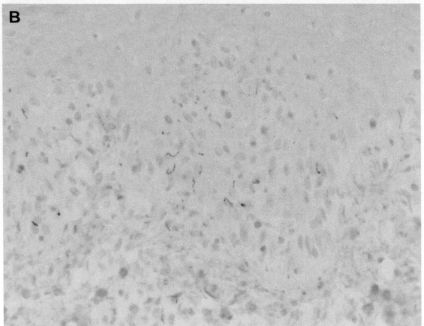

*Fig. 8.* Secondary syphilis. (*A*) Lichenoid interface alteration may be a manifestation of secondary syphilis. Neutrophils and perivascular plasma cells are helpful clues to the diagnosis, but are not always present (H&E, original magnification ×200). (*B*) Scattered treponemes are present in the epidermis and highlighted by a spirochetal immunostain (anti–*Treponema pallidum*, original magnification ×600).

Disseminated intravascular coagulation [DIC]) and other thrombotic disorders, such as purpura fulminans and cryoglobulinemia, may present with thrombotic vasculopathy. In such cases, the clinical course and laboratory findings are usually distinct and necessary to arrive at a diagnosis. The main role of the pathologist in this scenario is in excluding other possibilities (such as vasculitis) that can have a similar clinical presentation.

## VASCULITIS

Leukocytoclastic vasculitis (LCV) is a histologic pattern and not an entity. LCV may be associated with numerous diseases, but the clinical and histologic manifestations are the same regardless of cause and thus are nonspecific. LCV may be seen in the setting of autoimmune diseases, infections, immune

*Fig.* **9.** Subcutaneous panniculitis–like T-cell lymphoma. (*A*) Rimming of individual adipocytes by atypical lymphoid cells is characteristic (H&E, original magnification ×400). (*B–D*) A CD4-positive, CD8-negative, TCRβF1-positive immunophenotype confirms the diagnosis (anti-CD4, anti-CD8, and anti- TCRβF1, original magnification ×400).

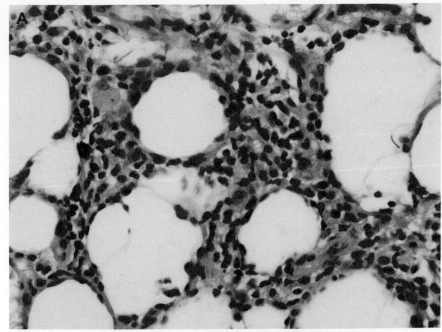

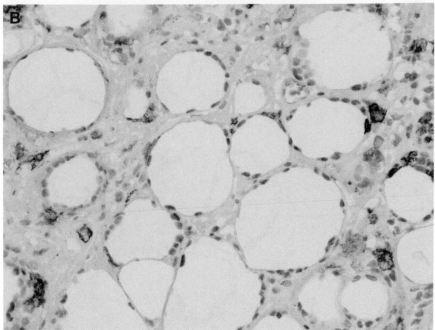

complex diseases such as cryoglobulinemia, new medications, and so forth.[26] Excluding an infectious cause is important for treatment reasons.[14] Identification of microorganisms may prove difficult in tissue sections, and thus obtaining concurrent cultures may be desirable if an infectious cause is suspected.

## NEUTROPHILIC DERMATOSIS

Cell-rich neutrophilic infiltrates resembling Sweet syndrome must be worked up with histochemical stains to rule out infection. Concurrent microbiological cultures are highly desirable in this situation. Once infection is ruled out, neutrophilic dermatoses should be considered. Sweet syndrome is most frequently associated with acute myeloid leukemia,

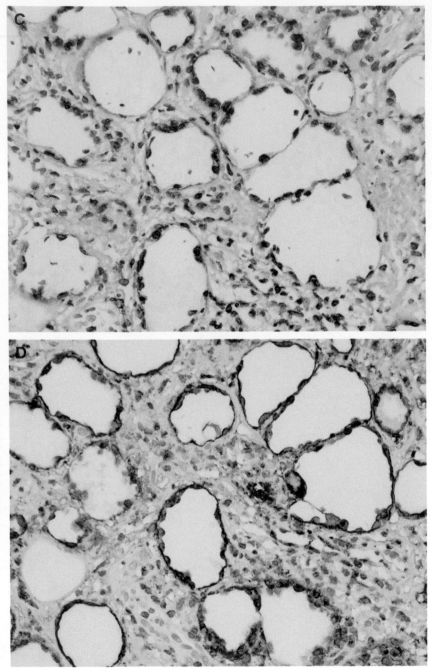

Fig. 9. (continued).

but it has been reported in patients with solid tumors (breast or colon adenocarcinomas), and in patients taking granulocyte colony–stimulating factor. Similar lesions have been reported after jejunoileal bypass and inflammatory bowel disease surgery, known as bowel-associated dermatosis-arthritis syndrome.[27] Paucicellular (and moderately cellular) neutrophilic infiltrates may also be seen in early lesions of LCV, the evanescent eruption of Still disease (**Fig. 10**), and rheumatic fever.[5–7] Careful clinical correlation and laboratory findings should help in making the distinction.

Lymphocytic (small vessel) vasculitis, as seen in chilblain lupus erythematosus, may be seen in

*Fig. 10.* A sparse dermal neutrophilic infiltrate is seen on a biopsy from a patient with the evanescent eruption of Still disease (H&E, original magnification ×200). Some cases show nonspecific perivascular lymphoid infiltrates.

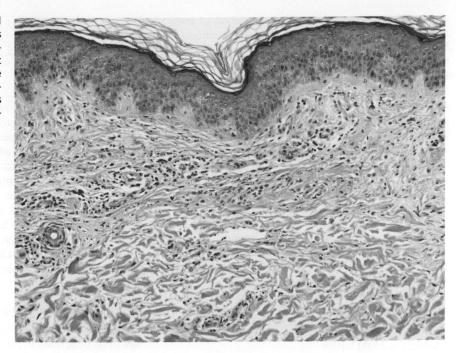

arthropod bite reactions, scabies, drug-induced and other hypersensitivity reactions, polymorphous light eruption, and treated LCV.[14]

## DIAGNOSIS

The diagnosis of SLE is based on clinical and serologic findings (anti–double-stranded DNA and anti-Smith antibodies being highly correlative). There are no diagnostic criteria, but the SLE classification criteria designed for research purposes (American College of Rheumatologists [ACR] 1997 or Systemic Lupus International Collaborating Clinics [SLICC] 2012) are frequently used to determine salient clinical features of the disease, with the understanding that the sensitivity and specificity of both are suboptimal. Accordingly, some authorities have proposed the following diagnostic categories and respective parameters. Definite SLE is diagnosed in patients fulfilling ACR 1997 (4 of 11 parameters) or 2012 SLICC criteria (4 of 17 criteria including 1 of the ACR 11, or nephritis compatible with SLE on biopsy and antinuclear antibodies or anti–double-stranded DNA antibodies). Probable SLE is assigned to patients who do not fulfill ACR or SLICC criteria, but in whom SLE is still the most likely diagnosis (eg, 2 or 3 ACR or SLICC criteria) or have other manifestations not included in either classification (eg, pneumonitis, optic neuritis, Reynaud phenomenon, verrucous endocarditis). Possible SLE is considered when patients have only 1 criterion of the ACR/SLICC schemas and at least 1 or 2 of the features listed earlier. Biopsy of an involved organ (eg, skin) may be necessary in some cases, with the main utility being excluding alternative diagnoses.[28]

## PROGNOSIS

Cutaneous lupus erythematosus not associated with systemic disease (SLE) has a better prognosis. Cutaneous lupus erythematosus, as detailed earlier, is highly variable and therapy is based on severity. Topical treatment is frequently a useful starting point and may prove beneficial even in patients receiving systemic therapy. Systemic therapy for treatment of cutaneous lupus is generally reserved for patients with generalized skin involvement, scarring, or refractory disease. Vitamin D deficiency should be monitored and supplemented when necessary, because sun protection practices are necessary given the inherent photosensitive nature of lupus erythematosus. Smoking cessation is also recommended, given that smoking is known to reduce therapeutic effectiveness and increase the risk of peripheral vascular and lung disease.[12]

SLE may follow a fairly benign clinical course, or have rapid progression with multiorgan involvement and death. The 5-year survival has improved from 40% in the 1950s to more than 90% since the 1980s. Major contributing factors in prognosis are earlier disease recognition and institution of therapy and timely treatment of complications.[28] Nonetheless, mortalities for patients with SLE are up to 5 times higher than the general population. Predictors of decreased survival in SLE include male gender, black race, presence of antiphospholipid antibodies, younger age at diagnosis, hypertension, and presence of proliferative glomerulonephritis. Causes of death in patients with SLE include stroke, renal disease, cardiovascular disease, infection, and other complications from immunosupression.[29–33]

A significant increase in risk of death from diffuse large B-cell lymphoma has been documented for patients with SLE who develop this malignancy compared with the general population.[34–36] There also seems to be increased incidence of vulvar, pulmonary, liver, and thyroid cancers in patients with SLE.[37,38]

## DERMATOMYOSITIS

### CLINICAL FEATURES

Dermatomyositis is a chronic autoimmune disorder affecting primarily skeletal muscle and skin. As with other CTDs, the cause is unknown, but potential association with malignancy should be investigated. Dermatomyositis typically presents in women between the ages of 40 and 50 years. Photosensitivity is an important clinical feature, and a higher incidence has been documented in regions with higher surface ultraviolet light exposure.[39] The onset may be abrupt or insidious over several months. Skin findings may present before or after characteristic symmetric weakness of proximal muscle groups. Some patients experience cutaneous disease exclusively (amyopathic dermatomyositis). Involvement of the pharyngeal musculature presents with dysphagia or voice changes and portends severe disease, frequently associated with interstitial lung disease.

Characteristic cutaneous findings in dermatomyositis include periorbital swelling and erythema, called a heliotrope rash, erythematous papules over the metacarpophalangeal joints (known as Gottron papules), and nail changes including dilated nail-fold capillaries, ragged cuticles, and cuticular hemorrhage. Poikiloderma, characterized by erythema, telangiectasia, and hyperpigmentation and hypopigmentation in a V distribution over the chest (V sign), neck and shoulders (shawl sign), and lateral thighs (holster sign) are characteristic. Uncommon skin findings include flagellate erythema, panniculitis, scleromyxedematous lesions and pityriasiform eruptions.[40]

## MICROSCOPIC FEATURES

### HISTOLOGIC PATTERNS SEEN IN DERMATOMYOSITIS

#### Interface Dermatitis

Dermatomyositis may show nonspecific inflammation or can manifest histologically with interface alteration. So-called classic cases are characterized by subtle interface alteration with epidermal atrophy and typically show capillary ectasia and sparse perivascular lymphocytic inflammation (Fig. 11). However, these findings are not unique to dermatomyositis and are similar to those of other CTDs, particularly SLE. Therefore, correlation with clinical findings, serologies, and other laboratory values (muscle enzyme levels) are necessary for an accurate clinical-pathologic diagnosis.

#### Neutrophilic Dermatosis

Hypercellular (Sweet-like) neutrophilic dermatosis has been described in patients with dermatomyositis, but it seems to be a much less common association than with SLE. In the rare cases described, no interface dermatitis or other common manifestations of CTD were identified.[41]

### DIFFERENTIAL DIAGNOSIS

#### Interface Dermatitis

Biopsies of cutaneous lesions of dermatomyositis may show changes that are virtually identical to those seen in SCLE or ACLE and thus it may not be possible to distinguish them histologically. It has been proposed that the most useful test in such cases may be the so-called lupus band test by direct immunofluorescence, which is negative in dermatomyositis, and positive (deposition of IgA, IgM, IgG, C3, and fibrin at the dermal-epidermal junction in a linear or granular pattern) in most lupus erythematosus lesions.[14]

#### Neutrophilic Dermatosis

As mentioned earlier, Sweet-like neutrophilic dermatosis has been described anecdotally in dermatomyositis but should be investigated for infection with special stains and microbiological cultures. It is important to know of this potential, albeit rare, association.

#### Diagnosis

The diagnosis of dermatomyositis is based on clinical and laboratory findings. In patients with characteristic clinical presentation and laboratory findings (proximal symmetric weakness, heliotrope rash, Gottron papules, marked increase of muscle

*Fig. 11.* Dermatomyositis. Subtle interface alteration in a patient with dermatomyositis (H&E, original magnification ×200).

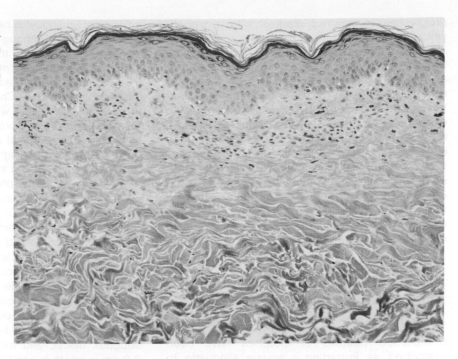

enzyme levels), and no alternative explanation, the diagnosis can be made without a biopsy. Electromyogram and MRI studies may provide further information about the characteristic inflammatory myopathy. In patients with typical clinical findings and skin changes, a skin biopsy showing vacuolar interface alteration may help confirm a diagnosis of DM. For patients with symmetric proximal weakness and increased enzyme levels but no skin findings, a muscle biopsy may prove helpful in making the diagnosis. Antibodies associated with DM include PM-1, Jo-1 (associated with interstitial lung disease), Ku, and Mi2.

### Prognosis

Overall, most patients with DM have a favorable course after treatment with corticosteroids. As with SLE, sun protection is essential. Once a diagnosis of DM is established, additional studies are warranted to investigate significant associated diseases. A detailed clinical history and thorough physical examination with pelvic, breast, and rectal examinations should be pursued to investigate the possibility of malignancy. Cancer screening, including a computed tomography scan of the chest, abdomen, and pelvis, as well as transvaginal ultrasonography and mammography are frequently performed. If there is suspicion of cardiac muscle involvement, an echocardiogram and electrocardiogram should be obtained. Patients with cough or dyspnea or abnormal chest radiograph should undergo

pulmonary function testing and CT scan of the chest to evaluate for interstitial lung disease. Esophageal motility studies should be performed if there is dysphagia or aspiration pneumonia. The reported mortality for DM is 14%, with metastatic cancer as a frequent cause of death.[41]

## LOCALIZED SCLERODERMA (MORPHEA)

### CLINICAL FEATURES

Localized scleroderma, commonly denominated morphea, is a chronic inflammatory disease presenting with cutaneous induration and, when located over a joint, restricted mobility. Although it bears similarities to systemic sclerosis, the two can be distinguished clinically. Morphea is predominantly restricted to the skin and subcutaneous tissue, whereas systemic sclerosis carries additional risk of internal organ involvement. Morphea occurs equally in adults and children, and is more common in women. It presents with fatigue, myalgias, arthralgias, and induration of the skin that worsens over several months. Morphea is highly associated with lichen sclerosus of the genital skin. Morphea has a fluctuant course with periods of remission followed by relapse, and early intervention in relapses is key to avoid morbidity.[2,12,14,42]

Morphea presents most frequently with erythematous plaques with slight hardening; a lilac border may be seen at the edges of the plaque. This condition is called plaque-type morphea and progresses to scarred plaques with a smooth yellow-white surface. Over time, cutaneous adnexa, such as hair follicles and eccrine units, are obliterated and plaques may increase in size and new ones may develop in other areas. Concurrent involvement of the lower back, the hips, and the inframammary region is common. Rare patients experience a rapid course with widespread involvement of almost the entire skin with the exception of the hands and feet, known as pansclerotic morphea. Children most commonly present with linear plaques that coalesce into a band of scarring that may involve an entire extremity, referred to as linear morphea.[43] The scarring in this subtype frequently involves muscle and bone, and plaques extending over a joint reduce mobility.

## MICROSCOPIC FEATURES

### HISTOLOGIC PATTERNS SEEN IN MORPHEA

#### Dermal Sclerosis

Established plaques of morphea have been described as imparting a square silhouette to punch biopsies, which is thought to derive from loss of elasticity of sclerotic skin (**Fig. 12A**). The epidermis may be atrophic. Dermal sclerosis consists of increased collagen deposition, with diminution of the spaces between normal reticular collagen bundles. Encroachment around hair follicles and eccrine units with loss of periadventitial fat may be encountered and is characteristic. Dermal sclerosis typically extends from the midreticular dermis down into the subcutis. Foci of perivascular lymphoplasmacytic inflammation may be seen (**Fig. 12B**).

### PERIVASCULAR AND PERIECCRINE LYMPHOPLASMACYTIC INFILTRATES

Biopsies from early lesions of morphea typically show superficial dermal edema and inflammatory infiltrates of lymphocytes and plasma cells. These infiltrates are usually more pronounced at the dermal-subcutaneous junction and may involve eccrine glands and extend into subcutaneous septa. Dermal sclerosis may be minimal at this stage, and thus clinical correlation is required to arrive at this diagnosis.

## DIFFERENTIAL DIAGNOSIS

The presence of dermal sclerosis with involvement of the papillary dermis raises consideration of lichen sclerosus. Prototypical cases of lichen sclerosus show sclerosis (hyalinization) of the papillary dermis, vascular ectasia, and a bandlike infiltrate of lymphocytes beneath the zone of sclerosis (**Fig. 13A**). Although in classic cases the sclerosis is confined to the upper dermis, some cases show deep dermal and subcutaneous involvement and are referred to as lichen sclerosus/morphea overlap. Chronic radiation dermatitis also manifests with dermal sclerosis (**Fig. 13B**), but vascular proliferation with endothelial swelling and stromal atypia are frequently a tip-off to making the diagnosis (**Fig. 13C**). Radiation therapy (along with infection and trauma) is a known trigger of morphea, and may therefore complicate distinction in some cases. Eosinophilic fasciitis is another cause of dermal sclerosis, which is typically deep involving subcutaneous septa and extending into the fascia. Septal involvement is characteristic, but not sampled in most instances by cutaneous punch biopsy. Over time, sclerosis extends into the dermis, resulting in a picture virtually identical to that of morphea or scleroderma. It has been proposed that an incisional biopsy including dermis, subcutis, fascia, and muscle of approximately 3.0 cm in length is needed for adequate assessment of eosinophilic fasciitis. The presence of tissue eosinophilia is commonly focal and frequently within the fascia, and thus not identified in many biopsies.[44] Peripheral eosinophilia, although transient, is common and characteristic and should be investigated. Nephrogenic systemic fibrosis (NSF) also causes cutaneous induration and subtle fibrosis of the deep dermis and subcutis. In contrast with morphea, NSF is a more cellular, although often subtle, process (**Fig. 13D**). History of renal failure and imaging studies with gadolinium are paramount in making this diagnosis. Chronic graft-versus-host disease frequently shows sclerodermoid changes. The presence of interface dermatitis along with dermal sclerosis should alert pathologists of this possibility. History of allogeneic stem cell transplant more than 3 months before the biopsy is typical and most helpful in arriving at this diagnosis. Old scars and scarring processes manifest with dermal sclerosis, but clinical correlation should help clarify this possibility. In addition, skin biopsies from patients with progressive systemic sclerosis (scleroderma) show findings identical to those of morphea. Evidence of multisystem involvement and serologic studies are helpful in making this distinction.

## DIAGNOSIS

History and physical examination are frequently sufficient for a diagnosis of morphea. An important consideration initially is distinction from systemic

*Fig. 12.* (*A*) Morphea. Punch biopsy showing a square silhouette (H&E, original magnification ×40). (*B*) Perivascular infiltrates of plasma cells entrapped in sclerotic tissue may be seen (H&E, original magnification ×400).

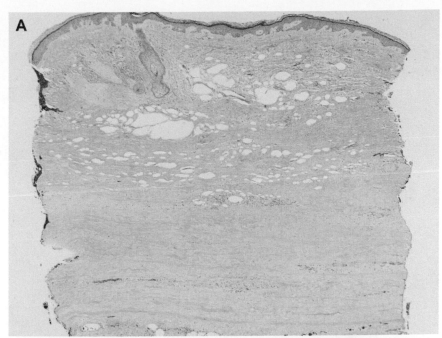

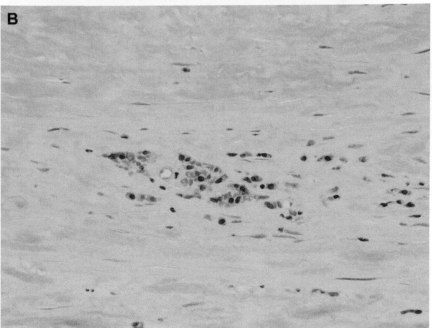

sclerosis. Hand involvement (sclerodactyly, Raynaud phenomenon) strongly suggests systemic sclerosis, because morphea typically does not involve the hands. Skin biopsy is not necessary in typical cases, but is frequently obtained for diagnostic confirmation because there are no specific laboratory tests to confirm the diagnosis of morphea.

## PROGNOSIS

Most patients develop only 1 or 2 plaques of morphea (plaque-type morphea). Despite softening of the skin after institution of treatment, the yellow-white discoloration may persist for years. In these patients, follow-up is important because they may

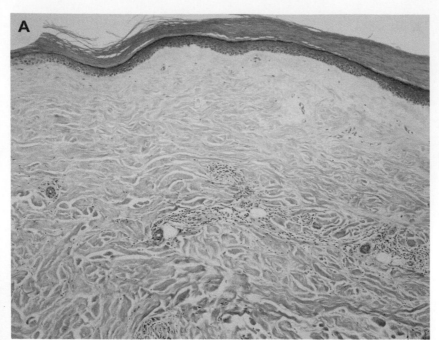

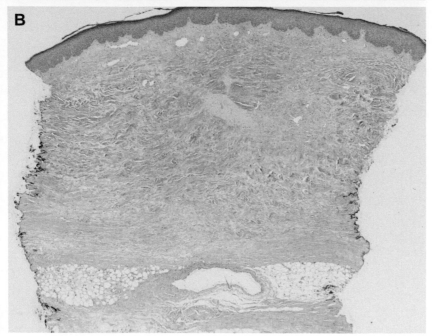

**Fig. 13.** Differential diagnoses of morphea. (*A*) Lichen sclerosus with hyalinization of the papillary dermis and lymphoplasmacytic inflammation beneath (H&E, original magnification ×200). (*B*) Chronic radiation dermatitis. There is diffuse dermal sclerosis and vascular ectasia (H&E, original magnification ×40).

experience recurrence. Generalized morphea is progressive and may involve most of the skin and result in disfigurement. Generalized morphea not only implies a greater number of lesions but also the tendency for them to coalesce. Linear scleroderma has the potential to cause serious complications, such as loss of mobility or growth impairment of an extremity caused by involvement of deeper structures such as muscle and bone. Disease activity in patients with linear scleroderma typically varies from 2 to 5 years, but may recur, particularly in patients with the en coup de sabre variant, which commonly affects the scalp and face in a linear manner.[42]

*Fig. 13.* (*continued*). (*C*) Radiation dermatitis. The presence of stromal atypia is a helpful clue to this diagnosis (H&E, original magnification ×400). (*D*) Nephrogenic systemic fibrosis. Diffuse fibrosis with slight increase in dermal cellularity is seen in contrast with morphea, which manifests as a sclerotic, acellular process (H&E, original magnification ×200).

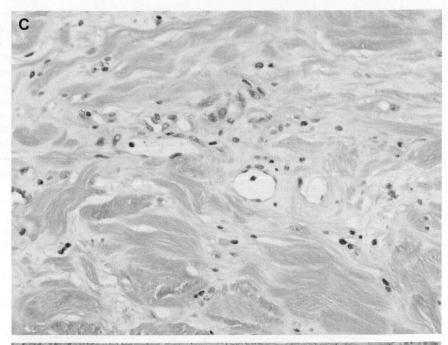

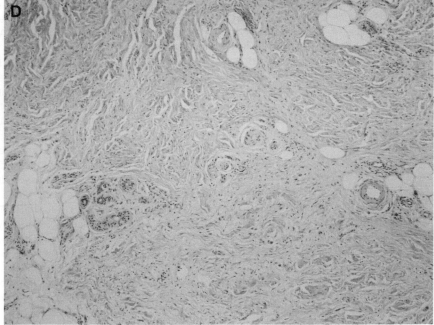

## SUMMARY

CTDs are complex autoimmune disorders with great clinical and histopathologic polymorphism. To arrive at an accurate diagnosis, clinical and serologic correlation is necessary. The main role of histopathology is in suggesting the possibility of CTD as a category and in excluding other disorders with similar clinical manifestations. The spectrum of histologic changes associated with CTD has evolved and neutrophilic dermatosis is an increasingly recognized manifestation. It may be the initial presentation, and therefore CTD should be considered in the differential diagnosis of neutrophilic dermatoses. Lupus erythematosus is perhaps the most common, prototypical, and pleiotropic of these disorders, and pathologists should be acquainted with the histologic changes associated with this disease. Dermatomyositis and localized scleroderma are also encountered frequently in practice. Familiarity with the many manifestations of these diseases allows prompt diagnosis and early treatment.

## REFERENCES

1. Albert LJ, Inman RD. Molecular mimicry and autoimmunity. N Engl J Med 1999;341:2068–74.

2. Luzar B, Calonje E. Idiopathic connective tissue diseases. In: Calonje E, Brenn T, Lazar A, et al, editors. McKee's Pathology of the skin. Elsevier; 2013. p. 711–59.

3. Bertsias GK, Pamfil C, Fanouriakis A, et al. Diagnostic criteria for systemic lupus erythematosus: has the time come? Nat Rev Rheumatol 2013;9: 687–94.

4. Saeb-Lima M, Charli-Joseph Y, Rodriguez-Acosta ED, et al. Autoimmunity-related neutrophilic dermatosis: a newly described entity that is not exclusive of systemic lupus erythematosus. Am J Dermatopathol 2013;35:655–60.

5. Larson AR, Granter SR. Systemic lupus erythematosus-associated neutrophilic dermatosis: a review and update. Adv Anat Pathol 2014;21:248–53.

6. Larson AR, Granter SR. Systemic lupus erythematosus-associated neutrophilic dermatosis-an underrecognized neutrophilic dermatosis in patients with systemic lupus erythematosus. Hum Pathol 2014;45:598–605.

7. Larson AR, Laga AC, Granter SR. The spectrum of histopathologic findings in cutaneous lesions in patients with Still's disease. Am J Clin Pathol 2015; 144:945–51.

8. Tsokos GC. Systemic lupus erythematosus. N Engl J Med 2011;365:2110–21.

9. Lisnevskaia L, Murphy G, Isenberg D. Systemic lupus erythematosus. Lancet 2014;384:1878–88.

10. Walling HW, Sontheimer RD. Cutaneous lupus erythematosus. issues in diagnosis and treatment. Am J Clin Dermatol 2009;10:365–81.

11. Tao J, Zhang X, Guo N, et al. Squamous cell carcinoma complicating discoid lupus erythematosus in Chinese patients: review of the literature, 1964-2010. J Am Acad Dermatol 2012;66:695–6.

12. Kalus A. Rheumatologic skin disease. Med Clin North Am 2015;99:1287–303.

13. Merola JF, Mosoholla SL. Overview of cutaneous lupus erythematosus. In: Pisetsky DS, Callen J, editors. Available at: https://www.uptodate.com. Accessed September 30, 2016.

14. Winfield H, Jaworsky C. Connective tissue diseases. In: Elder D, editor. Lever's histopathology of the skin. Philadelpia (PA): Wolters Kluwer; 2015. p. 329–58.

15. Arps DP, Patel RM. Cutaneous hypertrophic lupus erythematosus. A challenging histopathologic diagnosis in the absence of clinical information. Arch Pathol Lab Med 2013;137:1205–10.

16. Diaz-Jouanen E, DeHoratius RJ, Alarcon-Segovia D, et al. Systemic lupus erythematosus presenting as panniculitis (lupus profundus). Ann Intern Med 1975;82:376–9.

17. Tuffanelli DL. Lupus erythematosus panniculitis (profundus). Arch Dermatol 1971;103:231–42.

18. Requena L, Sanchez YE. Panniculitis: part II: mostly lobular panniculitis. J Am Acad Dermatol 2001;45: 325–61.

19. Erkan D, Zuily S. Clinical manifestations of antiphospholipid syndrome. In: Pisetsky DS, editor. UpToDate. Waltham (MA): UpToDate. Accessed September 16, 2016.

20. Nambudiri VE, Vleugels RA, Laga AC, et al. Clinicopathologic lessons in distinguishing cicatricial alopecia: 7 cases of lichen planopilaris misdiagnosed as discoid lupus. J Am Acad Dermatol 2014;71: e135–8.

21. Perniciaro C, Randle HW, Perry HO. Hypertrophic discoid lupus erythematosus resembling squamous cell carcinoma. Dermatol Surg 1995;21:255–7.

22. Massone C, Kodama K, Salmhofer W, et al. Lupus erythematosus panniculitis (lupus profundus): clinical, histopathological, and molecular analysis of nine cases. J Cutan Pathol 2005;32:396–404.

23. Sanchez NP, Peters MS, Winkelmann RK. The histopathology of lupus erythematosus panniculitis. J Am Acad Dermatol 1981;5:673–80.

24. Jaffe ES, Gaulard P, Ralfkiaer E, et al. Subcutaneous panniculitis-like T-cell lymphoma: definition, classification, and prognostic factors: an EORTC Cutaneous Lymphoma Group Study of 83 cases. Blood 2008;111:838–45.

25. Arps DP, Patel RM. Lupus profundus (panniculitis). a potential mimic of subcutaneous panniculitis-like T-cell lymphoma. Arch Pathol Lab Med 2013;137: 1211–5.

26. Gota C. Overview of cutaneous small vessel vasculitis. In: Matteson EL, Callen J, editors. UpToDate. Waltham (MA): UpToDate. Accessed October 2, 2016.

27. Dicken CH. Bowel-associated dermatosis-arthritis syndrome: bowel bypass syndrome without bowel bypass. Mayo Clin Proc 1984;59:43–6.

28. Wallace DJ. Diagnosis and differential diagnosis of systemic lupus erythematosus in adults. In: Pisetsky DS, editor. UpToDate. Waltham (MA): UpToDate. Accessed September 28, 2016.

29. Rubin LA, Urowitz MB, Gladman DD. Mortality in systemic lupus erythematosus: the bimodal pattern revisited. Q J Med 1985;55:87–98.

30. Abu-Shakra M, Urowitz MB, Gladman DD, et al. Mortality studies in systemic lupus erythematosus. Results from a single center. I. Causes of death. J Rheumatol 1995;22:1259–64.

31. Moss KE, Ioannou Y, Sultan SM, et al. Outcome of a cohort of 300 patients with systemic lupus erythematosus attending a dedicated clinic for over two decades. Ann Rheum Dis 2000;61: 409–13.

32. Bernatsky S, Boivin JF, Joseph L, et al. Mortality in systemic lupus erythematosus. Arthritis Rheum 2006;54:2550–7.

33. Cartella S, Cavazzana I, Ceribelli A, et al. Evaluation of mortality, disease activity, treatment, clinical and immunological features of adult and late onset systemic lupus erythematosus. Autoimmunity 2013;46: 363–8.

34. Zintzaras E, Voulgarelis M, Moutsopoulos HM. The risk of lymphoma development in autoimmune diseases: a meta-analysis. Arch Intern Med 2005;165: 2337–44.

35. Bernatsky S, Ramsey-Gold man R, Rajan R, et al. Non-Hodgkin's lymphoma in systemic lupus erythematosus. Ann Rheum Dis 2005;64:1507–9.

36. Lofstrom B, Backlin C, Sundstrom C, et al. A closer look at non-Hodgkin's lymphoma in a national Swedish systemic lupus erythematosus cohort: a nested case-control study. Ann Rheum Dis 2007;66: 1627–32.

37. Sweeney DM, Manzi S, Janosky J, et al. Risk of malignancy in women with systemic lupus erythematosus. J Rheumatol 1995;22:1478–82.

38. Mellemkjaer L, Andersen V, Linet MS, et al. Non-Hodgkin's lymphoma and other cancers among a cohort of patients with systemic lupus erythematosus. Arthritis Rheum 1997;40:761–8.

39. Meyer A, Meyer N, Schaeffer M, et al. Incidence and prevalence of inflammatory myopathies: a systematic review. Rheumatology 2015;54:50–63.

40. Miller ML, Vleugels RA. Clinical manifestations of dermatomyositis and polymyositis in adults. In: Targoff IN, Shefner JM, Callen J, editors. UpToDate. Waltham (MA): UpToDate. Accessed September 22, 2016.

41. Owen CE, Malone JC, Callen JP. Sweet-like dermatosis in 2 patients with clinical features of dermatomyositis and underlying autoimmune disease. Arch Dermatol 2008;144:1486–90.

42. Jacobe H. Pathogenesis, clinical manifestations, and diagnosis of morphea (localized scleroderma) in adults. In: Callen J, editor. UpToDate. Waltham (MA): UpToDate. Accessed September 16, 2016.

43. Laxer RM, Zulian F. Localized scleroderma. Curr Opin Rheumatol 2006;18:606–13.

44. Barnes L, Rodnan P, Medsger TA, et al. Eosinophilic fasciitis. A pathologic study of twenty cases. Am J Pathol 1979;96:493–517.

# Immunofluorescence of Autoimmune Bullous Diseases

Gilles F. Diercks, MD, PhD*, Hendri H. Pas, PhD,
Marcel F. Jonkman, MD, PhD

## KEYWORDS

- Pemphigus • Pemphigoid • Immunofluorescence • Autoimmune diseases

---

### Key Points

- Immunofluorescence is mandatory for diagnosing autoimmune bullous diseases.

- Taking a perilesional biopsy from the erythema, 1 to 2 cm adjacent to the blister, yields the highest sensitivity for diagnosing in vivo antibodies.

- Storing a biopsy in normal saline increases the signal-to-noise ratio.

- Pemphigus shows smooth or granular deposition of immunoglobulins on the epithelial cell surface in biopsies of skin or mucosa.

- Bullous pemphigoid and epidermolysis bullosa acquisita are differentiated by serration pattern analysis of the linear deposition of immunoreactants along the epidermal basement membrane.

---

## ABSTRACT

Autoimmune bullous diseases of skin and mucosa are uncommon, disabling, and potentially lethal diseases. For a quick and reliable diagnosis immunofluorescence is essential. This article describes two variants of immunofluorescence. The direct method uses a skin or mucosal biopsy of the patient to detect in vivo bound antibodies. Indirect immunofluorescence uses patient's serum and a substrate to visualize circulating autoantibodies. These two methods supplemented with advanced techniques allow reliable classification of autoimmune bullous diseases; not only the main entities pemphigus and pemphigoid, but also subclasses within these groups. This is important because prognosis and therapy vary among different variants of autoimmune bullous diseases.

## OVERVIEW

This article reviews the role of immunofluorescence in the diagnosis of autoimmune bullous diseases (AIBD) of skin and mucosa. Although the clinical picture, the histologic biopsy, and advanced techniques, such as Western blotting and enzyme-linked immunosorbent assay (ELISA) assays, are also essential in the diagnostic work-up, these are beyond the scope of this review. In this respect, further details are found in a recently published textbook "Autoimmune bullous diseases", edited by Marcel F. Jonkman (Springer International Publishing Switzerland 2016, doi: 10.1007/978-3-319-23754-1).

The first evidence that a blistering disease was caused by autoantibodies was provided by Beutner and Jordon in 1964.[1] They demonstrated in pemphigus vulgaris binding of IgG to the epithelial

---

The authors have nothing to disclose.

Department of Dermatology, Center for Blistering Diseases, University Medical Center Groningen, University of Groningen, Groningen, The Netherlands

* Corresponding author. Department of Dermatology, Center for Blistering Diseases, University Medical Center Groningen, Hanzeplein 1, 9700 RB, The Netherlands.

E-mail address: g.f.h.diercks@umcg.nl

Surgical Pathology 10 (2017) 505–512
http://dx.doi.org/10.1016/j.path.2017.01.011

surgpath.theclinics.com

cell surface (ECS) in the epidermis. A few years later binding of IgG to the basement membrane zone could be shown in bullous pemphigoid.[2] With new discoveries and advanced techniques AIBD could be further subclassified with major implications because certain AIBD are more refractory to therapy (eg, epidermolysis bullosa acquisita [EBA]),[3] whereas others are associated with neoplasmata (eg, paraneoplastic pemphigus [PNP][4] and antilaminin 332-pemphigoid).[5]

## DIRECT VERSUS INDIRECT IMMUNOFLUORESCENCE

For direct immunofluorescence a patient's skin or mucosal biopsy is needed and tests the presence of in vivo deposited antibodies. A 3- to 4-mm punch biopsy is taken of erythematous skin 1 to 2 cm adjacent to the vesicle. In our institution we also take a second biopsy of uninvolved skin from the inner aspect of the upper arm, but this is not per se necessary. It is important not to take a biopsy for immunofluorescence of a bulla in skin or mucosa, because ulceration or destruction of the basement membrane can yield false-negative results.

The biopsy should not be stored in formalin (!), but should be snap-frozen in liquid nitrogen or fixated in Michel solution. However, the best option is to store the biopsy in normal saline at room temperature.[6] The major advantage is a washout of unbound circulating immunoglobulin, resulting in a decreased background staining and increased signal-to-noise ratio (**Fig. 1**).

Indirect immunofluorescence tests the presence of circulating antibodies against antigens involved in pemphigus and pemphigoid. For this adequate substrates are necessary to detect these antibodies. Much used substrates are monkey

esophagus[7] and salt-split human skin.[8] Patient serum is placed on these substrates and with a second step (hence the term "indirect") antihuman immunoglobulin and complement fluorescein isothiocyanate–conjugated antibodies are applied, rendering a positive or negative result.

AIBD are divided into intraepidermal blistering diseases, such as pemphigus, and subepidermal blistering diseases, such as pemphigoid. Immunofluorescence patterns of these groups are discussed next.

## PEMPHIGUS

Clinically, pemphigus vulgaris is characterized by flaccid blisters and erosions in pemphigus vulgaris and by crusted scales and erosions in pemphigus foliaceus.[9] Whereas pemphigus vulgaris is primarily a mucosal disease with or without cutaneous involvement, pemphigus foliaceus only affects the skin. Pemphigus is caused by antibodies directed against desmosomal proteins, in particular desmoglein.[10] This results in acantholysis of keratinocytes and subsequent intraepidermal blister formation. Pemphigus foliaceus shows a subcorneal blister caused by antibodies against desmoglein 1. Pemphigus vulgaris is characterized by suprabasal acantholysis and blister formation caused by antibodies against desmoglein 3 with or without antidesmoglein 1 antibodies.[11]

Direct immunofluorescence of perilesional skin shows a characteristic ECS staining pattern (**Fig. 2**). Although in most textbooks this staining pattern is denoted as a fine line between keratinocytes in most cases a granular immunoglobulin deposition is appreciated. This granular deposition seems to be caused by a clustering of IgG, desmoglein 3, and plakoglobin.[12] It is not possible to discern pemphigus foliaceus from vulgaris on a

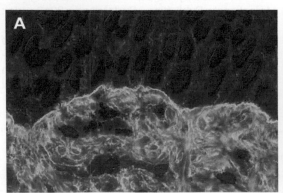 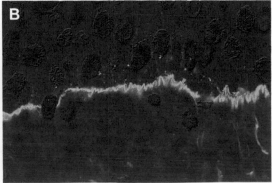

**Fig. 1.** Direct immunofluorescence (IgG) of (*A*) a skin biopsy stored in liquid nitrogen and (*B*) a biopsy stored in normal saline. Note the higher signal-to-noise ratio in (*B*). (*Reprinted from* Jonkman MF, editor. Autoimmune bullous diseases. Switzerland: Springer International Publishing; 2016. http://dx.doi.org/10.1007/978-3-319-23754-1; with permission.)

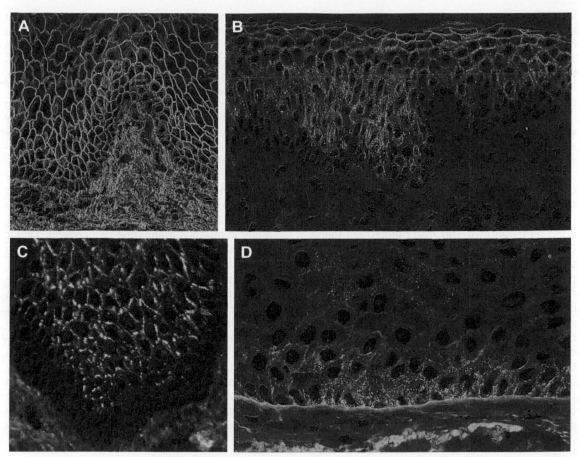

**Fig. 2.** Direct immunofluorescence (IgG) of pemphigus with (*A*) a smooth ECS pattern, (*B*) a fine granular pattern, and (*C*) a coarse granular pattern. (*D*) A case of paraneoplastic pemphigus. IgG deposition intraepidermal and along the epidermal basement membrane. (*Reprinted from* Jonkman MF, editor. Autoimmune bullous diseases. Switzerland: Springer International Publishing; 2016. http://dx.doi.org/10.1007/978-3-319-23754-1; with permission.)

skin or mucosal biopsy, because both show a transepidermal staining pattern. Histopathology, comprising split level or an ELISA assay to the pemphigus antigens desmoglein 1 and 3 is necessary to discriminate between these two entities. Recently, we published a report showing the importance of direct immunofluorescence in pemphigus.[13] Only a minor number of cases showed a negative biopsy, predominantly because these biopsies were taken from healthy skin. This underscores the importance of taking biopsies from perilesional skin.

Monkey esophagus is the substrate of choice to demonstrate circulating antibodies in pemphigus.[7] Although other substrates, such as guinea pig lip or human skin, have been described, monkey esophagus yields a reasonable sensitivity and specificity and is commercially available. In contrast to direct immunofluorescence of skin biopsies, indirect immunofluorescence on monkey esophagus always shows a smooth ECS pattern

(see **Fig. 4**B). One should be aware of false-positive results. A pseudo-ECS pattern could be encountered in patients with anti-A or anti-B antibodies reacting with blood group AB antigens on the monkey epithelial cells.[14] False-negative results are seen in early pemphigus or pemphigus in remission.

In pemphigus erythematosus, a variant of pemphigus with a lupus-like butterfly rash, and nowadays considered as a form of pemphigus foliaceus, in addition to the ECS pattern a granular deposition of IgG along the basement membrane may be observed.[15] These granules are composed of IgG and the shed ectodomain of desmoglein 1.[16]

In many cases of pemphigus ECS depositions consist of IgG but also of IgA. Moreover, variants of pemphigus with only IgA deposition are described called IgA pemphigus.[17] They are divided into two different forms: the subcorneal pustular dermatosis (SPD) type and the intraepidermal neutrophilic IgA dermatosis (IEN) type. In the SPD type the antigen seems to be desmocollin 1, whereas in the IEN type the antigen is still unknown. The direct immunofluorescence of the SPD type shows IgA deposition in the uppermost layers of the epidermis. In the IEN type a transepidermal ECS staining of IgA is found.

PNP is an uncommon, but life-threatening variant of pemphigus and characterized by a severe stomatitis, antibodies against envoplakin, periplakin, and/or $\alpha_2$-macroglobin-like 1 and an underlying neoplasia, mostly a lymphoproliferative disease.[4] In addition to the previously mentioned antigens in PNP, antibodies against desmoplakin, desmogleins, and hemidesmosomal proteins, such as BP230, BP180, and plectin, are found.[18] Direct immunofluorescence shows in most cases an ECS pattern of IgG, equal to other forms of pemphigus. A deposition of IgG along basement membrane is found (see **Fig. 2**D), however this is only seen in a minority of cases.[19] More specific is positive indirect immunofluorescence on rat bladder (see **Fig. 4**E). The transitional epithelium of rat bladder is rich in envoplakin and periplakin, but completely lacks desmogleins, allowing differentiation between PNP and other forms of pemphigus.[20] For a final diagnosis immunoblotting or immunoprecipitation are necessary to demonstrate the specific PNP antibodies. A combination of immunoblotting and rat bladder gives a diagnostic sensitivity and specificity of 100%.[19]

## PEMPHIGOID

Pemphigoid is clinically characterized by tense blisters, erythema, and urticarial plaques, histologically by subepidermal blisters and caused by antibodies against proteins located in the basement membrane zone, in particular the hemidesmosomal proteins BP180 and BP230.[21]

In bullous pemphigoid direct immunofluorescence shows a linear deposition of IgG along the epidermal basement membrane zone (**Fig. 3**A). In addition IgA is seen with IgG, particularly in mucous membrane pemphigoid. Linear deposition of complement is also present in most cases and seems to be related to more severe disease.[22] Pemphigoid gestationis (a pregnancy associated variant of pemphigoid) is in most cases characterized by a strong linear deposition of complement and weak or sometimes absent IgG.[23] In lichen planus pemphigoides (pemphigoid next to lichen planus lesions) shaggy fibrin deposition in addition to IgG is observed.[21] These variants of pemphigoid all have antibodies directed against BP180 or BP 230. However, other proteins might be involved. In anti-p200 pemphigoid, IgG is

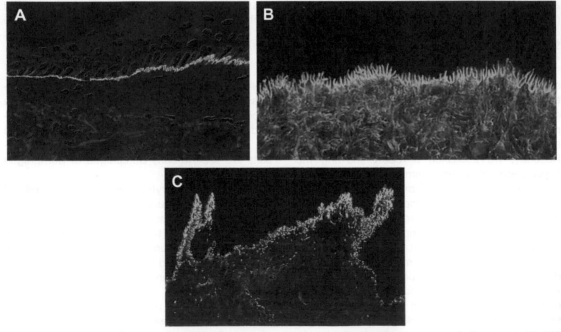

*Fig. 3.* Direct immunofluorescence (IgG) of pemphigoid with (*A*) an n-serrated pattern in bullous pemphigoid, and (*B*) a u-serrated pattern, fitting the diagnosis epidermolysis bullosa acquisita. (*C*) Granular IgA deposition in dermatitis herpetiformis. (*Reprinted from* Jonkman MF, editor. Autoimmune bullous diseases. Switzerland: Springer International Publishing; 2016. http://dx.doi.org/10.1007/978-3-319-23754-1; with permission.)

directed against a yet unidentified 200-kDa protein.[24] Clinically, this disease shows similarities to bullous pemphigoid, with a striking localization of tense blisters on hand and feet.[25] Another antigen is laminin-332, a component of the hemidesmosome. It is important to recognize antilaminin-332 pemphigoid because it is characterized by severe mucosal involvement and 20% to 30% of patients have an underlying malignancy.[26] Both anti-p200 pemphigoid and antilaminin-332 pemphigoid are characterized by linear deposition of IgG with or without IgA and complement.

In EBA the protein involved is type VII collagen, which is part of the anchoring fibrils in the epidermal basement membrane zone.[27] Clinically, EBA is divided into a mechanobullous type, with acral blistering evoked by mechanical trauma, and an inflammatory type, which shows similarities with bullous pemphigoid.[28] Bullous systemic lupus erythematosus also shows autoreactivity to type VII collagen in conjunction with features of systemic lupus erythematosus.[29] Like other forms of pemphigoid, EBA shows linear deposition of IgG along the basement membrane. However, a distinction between EBA and other pemphigoids is made using only a biopsy. In most cases of pemphigoid a serration pattern is discerned. Sublamina densa binding caused by antibodies against type VII collagen show a u-serrated pattern (see Fig. 3B), whereas pemphigoids with binding above the lamina densa (ie, bullous pemphigoid, anti-p200, and antilaminin-332) show an n-serrated pattern (see Fig. 3A).[30]

However, a serration pattern cannot be discerned in all cases, especially in mucosal biopsies. In these cases indirect immunofluorescence of salt-split skin is helpful.[8] Normal human incubated in 1.0-mol sodium chloride produces a reproducible split in the lamina lucida with certain antigens located in the roof of salt-split skin, most importantly BP180 and BP230, whereas laminin-332, p200, and type VII collagen are located in the floor of the split. This implies that bullous pemphigoid

shows an epidermal staining (Fig. 4C) whereas EBA, anti-p200, and antilaminin-332 pemphigoid show a dermal staining (see Fig. 4D). Combining the serration pattern from the biopsy and the results from indirect immunofluorescence on salt-split skin renders a good indication of the antigen involved (Table 1). Advanced techniques, such as immunoblotting and ELISA assays, can give additional information of the exact antigen present. Monkey esophagus can also be used as a substrate to detect antibodies against epidermal basement membrane zone proteins (see Fig. 4A), but we prefer salt-split skin because of its higher sensitivity and the additional information of the epidermal and dermal staining.

When solely linear IgA deposition is found, a diagnosis of linear IgA disease (LAD) is made.[31] The antigen involved is a 120-kDa or 97-kDa shed ectodomain of BP180 or BP180 itself.[32] LAD is divided on its age distribution into a childhood and an adult type. The childhood type seems to be self-limiting in most cases, whereas the adult type is more chronic and refractory to treatment. Direct immunofluorescence shows a linear, n-serrated deposition of IgA along the basement membrane. Indirect immunofluorescence on salt-split skin is characterized by an epidermal staining of IgA. A variant of LAD exists, with a u-serrated linear IgA deposition and a dermal binding of IgA on salt-split skin, in the past called LAD type II, but nowadays better known as IgA-EBA.[33] IgA variants of pemphigoid respond well to dapsone treatment.

Another blistering disease with deposition of IgA is dermatitis herpetiformis.[34] Instead of a linear deposition a granular deposition of IgA along the basement membrane, in particular in the dermal papillae, is observed (see Fig. 3C). Dermatitis herpetiformis is characterized by an itchy polymorphous skin eruption, mainly on knees and elbows. It is associated with celiac disease and the involved antigen is epidermal transglutaminase.[35] Indirect immunofluorescence on monkey esophagus shows a strong binding of IgA to the endomysium of smooth muscle fibers, which are rich in transglutaminase (see Fig. 4F).[36] Dermatitis

Table 1
The combination of serration pattern analysis and salt-split human skin can narrow the possible diagnoses in pemphigoid

| Direct immunofluorescence | n-serrated | | u-serrated | |
|---|---|---|---|---|
| Indirect immunofluorescence | Epidermal | Dermal | Epidermal | Dermal |
| | • Bullous pemphigoid and variants • Linear IgA disease | • Antilaminin-332 • Anti-p200 | | • EBA • Bullous systemic lupus erythematosus |

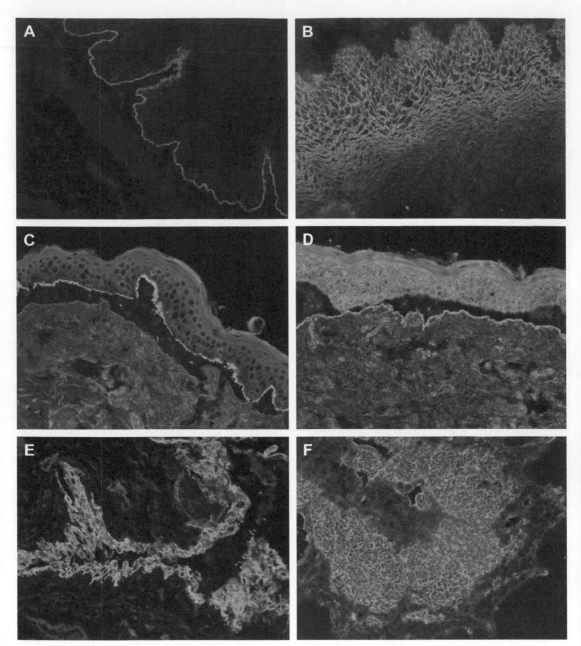

**Fig. 4.** Indirect immunofluorescence. (*A*) Binding of IgG along the basement membrane in pemphigoid on monkey esophagus, and (*B*) in pemphigus IgG binds in a smooth ECS pattern. (*C, D*) Salt-split skin with in (*C*) epidermal binding in bullous pemphigoid and (*D*) dermal binding in epidermolysis bullosa acquisita. (*E*) positive rat bladder in paraneoplastic pemphigus. (*F*) Binding of IgA to the endomysium of smooth muscle fibers in dermatitis herpetiformis.

herpetiformis responds well to dapsone and a gluten-free diet.

## SUMMARY

More than 50 years after the discovery of autoantibodies in AIBD, direct and indirect immunofluorescence still remain the essential armamentarium for the diagnosis. This article underscores that dedicated immunofluorescence microscopy is necessary to subtype the different variants of pemphigus and pemphigoid, which is important for prognosis and treatment.

## REFERENCES

1. Beutner EH, Jordon RE. Demonstration of skin anti-bodies in sera of pemphigus vulgaris patients by in-direct immunofluorescent staining. Proc Soc Exp Biol Med 1964;117:505–10.

2. Jordon RE, Beutner EH, Witebsky E, et al. Basement zone antibodies in bullous pemphigoid. JAMA 1967; 200:751–6.

3. Ishii N, Hamada T, Dainichi T, et al. Epidermolysis bullosa acquisita: what's new? J Dermatol 2010;37: 220–30.

4. Anhalt GJ, Kim SC, Stanley JR, et al. Paraneoplastic pemphigus. An autoimmune mucocutaneous dis-ease associated with neoplasia. N Engl J Med 1990;323:1729–35.

5. Egan CA, Lazarova Z, Darling TN, et al. Anti-epiligrin cicatricial pemphigoid and relative risk for cancer. Lancet 2001;357:1850–1.

6. Vodegel RM, de Jong MC, Meijer HJ, et al. Enhanced diagnostic immunofluorescence using biopsies transported in saline. BMC Dermatol 2004;4:10.

7. Feibelman C, Stolzner G, Provost TT. Pemphigus vul-garis. Superior sensitivity of monkey esophagus in the determination of pemphigus antibody. Arch Der-matol 1981;117:561–2.

8. Gammon W, Briggaman R. Differentiating anti-lamina lucida and anti-sublamina densa anti-BMZ antibodies by indirect immunofluorescence on 1.0 M sodium chloride-separated skin. J Investig Dermatol 1984;82(2):139–44.

9. Jonkman MF. JAMA dermatology patient page. Pemphigus. JAMA Dermatol 2014;150:680.

10. Amagai M, Klaus-Kovtun V, Stanley JR. Autoantibodies against a novel epithelial cadherin in pemphigus vul-garis, a disease of cell adhesion. Cell 1991;67:869–77.

11. Mahoney MG, Wang Z, Rothenberger K, et al. Expla-nations for the clinical and microscopic localization of lesions in pemphigus foliaceus and vulgaris. J Clin Invest 1999;103:461–8.

12. Oktarina DA, van der Wier G, Diercks GFH, et al. IgG-induced clustering of desmogleins 1 and 3 in skin of patients with pemphigus fits with the desmo-glein nonassembly depletion hypothesis. Br J Der-matol 2011;165:552–62.

13. Giurdanella F, Diercks GFH, Jonkman MF, et al. Lab-oratory diagnosis of pemphigus: direct immunofluo-rescence remains the gold standard. Br J Dermatol 2016;175:185–6.

14. Goldblatt F, Gordon TP. Antibodies to blood group antigens mimic pemphigus staining patterns: a use-ful reminder. Autoimmunity 2002;35:93–6.

15. Chorzelski T, Jabłońska S, Blaszczyk M. Immuno-pathological investigations in the Senear-Usher syn-drome (coexistence of pemphigus and lupus erythematosus). Br J Dermatol 1968;80:211–7.

16. Oktarina DA, Poot AM, Kramer D, et al. The IgG 'lupus-band' deposition pattern of pemphigus ery-thematosus: association with the desmoglein 1 ecto-domain as revealed by 3 cases. Arch Dermatol 2012;148:1–6.

17. Hashimoto T. Immunopathology of IgA pemphigus. Clin Dermatol 2001;19:683–9.

18. Zimmermann J, Bahmer F, Rose C, et al. Clinical and immunopathological spectrum of paraneoplastic pemphigus. J Dtsch Dermatol Ges 2010;8:598–606.

19. Poot AM, Diercks GF, Kramer D, et al. Laboratory diagnosis of paraneoplastic pemphigus. Br J Der-matol 2013;169:1016–24.

20. Liu AY, Valenzuela R, Helm TN, et al. Indirect immu-nofluorescence on rat bladder transitional epithe-lium: a test with high specificity for paraneoplastic pemphigus. J Am Acad Dermatol 1993;28:696–9.

21. Schmidt E, Zillikens D. Pemphigoid diseases. Lan-cet 2013;381:320–32.

22. Romeijn TR, Jonkman MF, Knoppers C, et al. Com-plement in bullous pemphigoid: results from a large observational study. Br J Dermatol 2016. http://dx. doi.org/10.1111/bjd.14822.

23. Lipozenčić J, Ljubojevic S, Bukvić-Mokos Z. Pem-phigoid gestationis. Clin Dermatol 2016;30:51–5.

24. Zillikens D, Kawahara Y, Ishiko A, et al. A novel subepidermal blistering disease with autoanti-bodies to a 200-kDa antigen of the basement membrane zone. J Invest Dermatol 1996;106: 1333–8.

25. Meijer JM, Diercks GFH, Schmidt E, et al. Laboratory diagnosis and clinical profile of anti-p200 pemphi-goid. JAMA Dermatol 2016;152(8):897–904.

26. Terra JB, Pas HH, Hertl M, et al. Immunofluores-cence serration pattern analysis as a diagnostic cri-terion in antilaminin-332 mucous membrane pemphigoid: immunopathological findings and clin-ical experience in 10 Dutch patients. Br J Dermatol 2011;165:815–22.

27. Woodley DT, Briggaman RA, O'Keefe EJ, et al. Iden-tification of the skin basement-membrane autoanti-gen in epidermolysis bullosa acquisita. N Engl J Med 1984;310:1007–13.

28. Buijsrogge JJA, Diercks GFH, Pas HH, et al. The many faces of epidermolysis bullosa acquisita after serration pattern analysis by direct immunofluores-cence microscopy. Br J Dermatol 2011;165:92–8.

29. Gammon WR, Briggaman RA. Epidermolysis bullosa acquisita and bullous systemic lupus erythemato-sus. Diseases of autoimmunity to type VII collagen. Dermatol Clin 1993;11:535–47.

30. Vodegel RM, Jonkman MF, Pas HH, et al. U-serrated immunodeposition pattern differentiates type VII collagen targeting bullous diseases from other sub-epidermal bullous autoimmune diseases. Br J Der-matol 2004;151:112–8.

31. Wojnarowska F, Bhogal BS, Black MM. Chronic bullous disease of childhood and linear IgA disease of adults are IgA1-mediated diseases. Br J Dermatol 1994;131:201–4.

32. Pas HH, Kloosterhuis GJ, Heeres K, et al. Bullous pemphigoid and linear IgA dermatosis sera recognize a similar 120-kDa keratinocyte collagenous glycoprotein with antigenic cross-reactivity to BP180. J Invest Dermatol 1997;108:423–9.

33. Vodegel RM, de Jong MC, Pas HH, et al. IgA-mediated epidermolysis bullosa acquisita: two cases and review of the literature. J Am Acad Dermatol 2002; 47:919–25.

34. Kárpáti S. Dermatitis herpetiformis. Clin Dermatol 2012;30:56–9.

35. Sárdy M, Kárpáti S, Merkl B, et al. Epidermal transglutaminase (TGase 3) is the autoantigen of dermatitis herpetiformis. J Exp Med 2002;195:747–57.

36. Chorzelski TP, Beutner EH, Sulej J, et al. IgA anti-endomysium antibody. A new immunological marker of dermatitis herpetiformis and coeliac disease. Br J Dermatol 1984;111:395–402.

# *Moving?*

**Make sure your subscription moves with you!**

To notify us of your new address, find your **Clinics Account Number** (located on your mailing label above your name), and contact customer service at:

**Email: journalscustomerservice-usa@elsevier.com**

**800-654-2452** (subscribers in the U.S. & Canada)
**314-447-8871** (subscribers outside of the U.S. & Canada)

**Fax number: 314-447-8029**

**Elsevier Health Sciences Division**
**Subscription Customer Service**
**3251 Riverport Lane**
**Maryland Heights, MO 63043**

ELSEVIER

# Moving?

**Make sure your subscription moves with you!**

To notify us of your new address, find your Clinics Account Number (located on your mailing label above your name), and contact customer service at:

**Email: journalscustomerservice-usa@elsevier.com**

800-654-2452 (subscribers in the U.S. & Canada)
314-447-8871 (subscribers outside of the U.S. & Canada)

Fax number: 314-447-8029

Elsevier Health Sciences Division
Subscription Customer Service
3251 Riverport Lane
Maryland Heights, MO 63043

 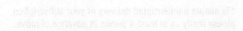

*To ensure uninterrupted delivery of your subscription, please notify us at least 4 weeks in advance of move.

Printed and bound by CPI Group (UK) Ltd, Croydon, CR0 4YY

03/10/2024

01040302-0004